Anatomy

Short Term Book Loan

ONE WEEK

First and second edition authors:

Michael Dykes

Phillip Ameerally

Third edition authors:

Michael Dykes

Will Watson

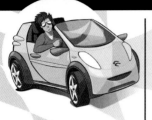

4th Edition
CRASH COURSE

SERIES EDITOR:
Dan Horton-Szar
BSc(Hons) MBBS(Hons) MRCGP
Northgate Medical Practice
Canterbury
Kent, UK

FACULTY ADVISOR:
Susan Whiten
MA PhD
Senior Lecturer in Anatomy and Foundations of Medicine Module Organiser
School of Medicine
University of St Andrews
St Andrews, UK

Anatomy

Louise Stenhouse
BSc(Hons) MBChB(Hons)
Foundation Year 2 Doctor
NHS Fife
Kirkcaldy
Fife, UK

MOSBY

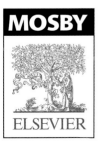

ELSEVIER

Edinburgh London New York Oxford Philadelphia St Louis Sydney Toronto 2012

Commissioning Editor: Jeremy Bowes
Development Editor: Sally Davies
Project Manager: Andrew Riley
Designer: Stewart Larking
Icon Illustrations: Geo Parkin
Illustration Manager: Jennifer Rose

First edition 1998

Second edition 2002

Third edition 2007

Fourth edition 2012

ISBN: 9780723436218

British Library Cataloguing in Publication Data
A catalogue record for this book is available from the British Library

Library of Congress Cataloging in Publication Data
A catalog record for this book is available from the Library of Congress

Notices
Knowledge and best practice in this field are constantly changing. As new research and experience broaden our understanding, changes in research methods, professional practices, or medical treatment may become necessary. Practitioners and researchers must always rely on their own experience and knowledge in evaluating and using any information, methods, compounds, or experiments described herein. In using such information or methods they should be mindful of their own safety and the safety of others, including parties for whom they have a professional responsibility.

With respect to any drug or pharmaceutical products identified, readers are advised to check the most current information provided (i) on procedures featured or (ii) by the manufacturer of each product to be administered, to verify the recommended dose or formula, the method and duration of administration, and contraindications. It is the responsibility of practitioners, relying on their own experience and knowledge of their patients, to make diagnoses, to determine dosages and the best treatment for each individual patient, and to take all appropriate safety precautions.

To the fullest extent of the law, neither the Publisher nor the authors, contributors, or editors, assume any liability for any injury and/or damage to persons or property as a matter of products liability, negligence or otherwise, or from any use or operation of any methods, products, instructions, or ideas contained in the material herein.

Printed in China

Series editor foreword

The *Crash Course* series first published in 1997 and now, 15 years on, we are still going strong. Medicine never stands still, and the work of keeping this series relevant for today's students is an ongoing process. These fourth editions build on the success of the previous titles and incorporate new and revised material, to keep the series up-to-date with current guidelines for best practice, and recent developments in medical research and pharmacology.

We always listen to feedback from our readers, through focus groups and student reviews of the *Crash Course* titles. For the fourth editions we have completely re-written our self-assessment material to keep up with today's 'single-best answer' and 'extended matching question' formats. The artwork and layout of the titles has also been largely re-worked to make it easier on the eye during long sessions of revision.

Despite fully revising the books with each edition, we hold fast to the principles on which we first developed the series. *Crash Course* will always bring you all the information you need to revise in compact, manageable volumes that integrate basic medical science and clinical practice. The books still maintain the balance between clarity and conciseness, and provide sufficient depth for those aiming at distinction. The authors are medical students and junior doctors who have recent experience of the exams you are now facing, and the accuracy of the material is checked by a team of faculty advisors from across the UK.

I wish you all the best for your future careers!

Dr Dan Horton-Szar

Author

Learning anatomy often feels like learning a new language. At the moment you may feel learning is mostly about passing exams. Exams are important, but there is something more important. In the not too distant future you will be a doctor and knowledge of anatomy will be invaluable in almost every interaction you have with patients. A good knowledge of anatomy is, in some ways, like having X-ray vision. The baby you are about to vaccinate – how will you know what lies beneath the area you are about to inject? The man who comes into A&E having cut his hand with a saw – why can't he bend his fingers? The woman with abdominal pain – why does she feel pain where she does? Learning anatomy can seem daunting, especially in the early stages, but it is important to remember that whilst a good knowledge of anatomy will be invaluable to you as a doctor, your knowledge will also be important to your future patients who will put their trust in you to care for them.

The Fourth Edition of this book contains a concise but detailed coverage of the topic. In this new edition, the importance of a good knowledge of anatomy and its relationship to clinical medicine is clear. The hints and tips boxes and clinical boxes provide an understanding of why you are learning what you are learning. New sections on radiology highlight the importance of CT and MRI scanning in medicine, and provide an introduction to interpreting what can often be complex images. The final section of the book contains best-of-five questions and 100 extended matching questions to reinforce your knowledge and allow you to think about anatomy as it relates to medicine. I hope that this book helps you to not only improve your knowledge and understanding, but to appreciate the importance of anatomy in the practice of clinical medicine.

Louise Stenhouse

FY2 Doctor, NHS Fife
2012

Faculty Advisor

The anatomy of the human body is truly awesome and a source of never-ending fascination for many people. Understanding how the structure of the body relates to its functions has been the foundation of medical education and practice for hundreds of years. The fact is that even today all doctors need a good working knowledge of anatomy. Most students would agree that there is a lot of anatomy and that it is not only difficult to know where to start, but also what to focus on!

The purpose of this book is to give you a concise review of 'really useful' anatomy with plenty of diagrams to help you visualise the most important structures and hints about what may be particularly significant from a clinical point of view.

You will need to know your anatomy well to pass your exams, but also, and in the end more importantly, to be able to examine your patients effectively, to recognise abnormality and to perform procedures safely.

Louise Stenhouse (now an FY2 doctor) has brilliantly revised the content of the book both from the point of view of a medical student just starting out and of a junior doctor wanting a concise review. I believe you will find her text accurate, straightforward and logically organised. There is new introductory material in the first chapter to give you some essential background and many new and relevant clinical boxes to highlight the importance of anatomy in clinical practice. With the help of Mark Jones, Consultant Radiologist at the Queen Margaret Hospital, Dunfermline, the radiology has been updated and improved to reflect the ever-increasing importance of medical imaging in modern diagnosis.

I have been involved in teaching anatomy for a while now and I suggest there are three useful approaches to take when you are trying to learn it. Importantly, give yourself plenty of time - you cannot cram it before an exam and expect to have the understanding to apply it to clinical problems. Learn the big picture first, and then tackle the details. And finally, learn anatomy on yourself; aim to visualize the 3D structure of your own body (for example your hand); you will carry those images with you wherever you go and in effect you will be walking around in your very own anatomy atlas. . ...

Good luck, I hope you find the book indispensable both now and as a reference in the future!

Susan Whiten

St Andrews
2012

Acknowledgements

I would like to thank everyone who has helped in the production of this book, especially Susie Whiten for reading my work and for her support, encouragement and patience. I would also like to thank Mark Jones for his enthusiasm and help with the radiological images, and Sally Davies of Elsevier for her guidance.

Louise Stenhouse

The following radiological images were reproduced with permission from Weir J and Abrahams PH, et al Imaging Atlas of Human Anatomy, 2nd edition, Mosby Ltd, 1997:

3.36, 3.40, 5.28, 8.72 and 8.73;

And from Weir J and Abrahams PH, et al Imaging Atlas of Human Anatomy, 4th edition, Mosby Ltd 2011:

3.39, 4.38, 5.29, 5.31, 5.32, 7.43, 7.44 and 7.45.

The radiological and 3D images below have been provided courtesy of Dr Mark Jones, Consultant Radiologist, NHS Fife:

2.09, 3.35, 3.37A, 3.37B, 3.38, 4.35, 4.36, 4.37A, 4.37B, 5.27, 5.30, 5.33, 7.41, 7.42, 8.74, 8.75, 8.76, 8.77, 8.78, 8.79.

Contents

Contents

Basic concepts of anatomy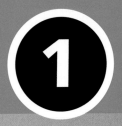

● **Objectives**

In this chapter you will learn to:
- Describe the anatomical position.
- Define the anatomical planes, and anatomical terms used in anatomy and clinical practice.
- Explain the terms of movement.
- Describe the structure and function of skin and bone.
- List the factors which contribute to joint stability.
- Appreciate the classification of muscles according to their actions.
- Understand the organization and function of muscle.
- Appreciate the general organization of the peripheral and central nervous systems.
- Describe the organization of the cardiovascular system.
- Describe the formation of lymph and its drainage into the venous system.
- Explain the structure and function of the gastrointestinal tract.
- Describe the structure and function of the respiratory tract.
- Describe the structure and function of the urinary tract.

DESCRIPTIVE ANATOMICAL TERMS

The anatomical position

This is a standard position used in both anatomy and clinical medicine, to allow an accurate and reproducible description of one body part in relation to another (Fig. 1.1):
- The head is directed forwards with the eyes looking into the distance.
- The body is upright, with the legs together and the feet facing forwards.
- The arms are by the side of the body, with the palms facing forwards and the thumbs laterally.
- The penis is erect.

Anatomical planes

The anatomical planes are as follows (Fig. 1.2):
- The median sagittal plane is a vertical plane passing through the midline of the body from the head to the feet. Any plane parallel to this (i.e. to the left or right of the median sagittal plane) is termed paramedian or sagittal.
- Coronal or frontal planes are vertical planes passing through the body from the head to the feet. They lie perpendicular to sagittal planes.

- Transverse or horizontal planes pass horizontally through the body from the front to the back. They lie at right angles to both the sagittal and coronal planes.

Computerized tomography (CT) and magnetic resonance imaging (MRI) scans commonly produce images of the body in one of more of these planes.

Terms of position

The terms of position commonly used in anatomy and clinical practice are described in Figure 1.3.

Terms of movement

The movements of the body are described as follows (Fig. 1.4):
- Flexion – a movement in the sagittal plane where there is a reduction in the angle between two parts of the body. There are exceptions to this – flexion of the glenohumeral joint increases the angle between the trunk and the upper limb.
- Extension – a backward movement in the sagittal plane where there is an increase in the angle between two parts of the body. Exceptions to this are at the ankle joint, and at the knee joint, as a result of lower limb rotation during embryonic development.
- Abduction – movement away from the median sagittal plane.

1

Fig. 1.1 Anatomical position and regions of the body.

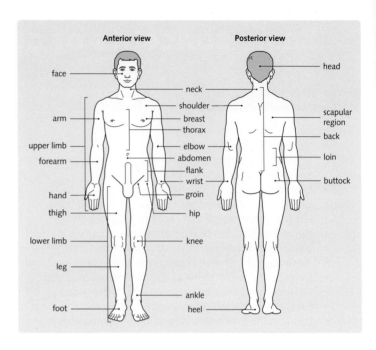

Fig. 1.2 Anatomical planes.

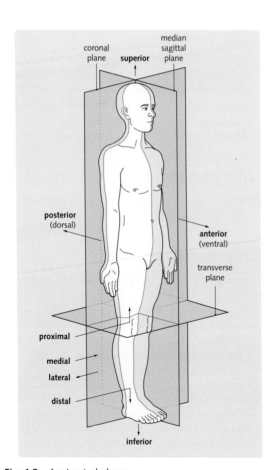

Fig. 1.3 Classification of terms of position commonly used in anatomy and clinical practice.

Position	Description
Anterior	In front of another structure
Posterior	Behind another structure
Superior	Above another structure
Inferior	Below another structure
Deep	Further away from body surface
Superficial	Closer to body surface
Medial	Closer to median sagittal plane
Lateral	Further away from median sagittal plane
Proximal	Closer to the trunk or origin
Distal	Further away from the trunk or origin
Ipsilateral	The same side of the body
Contralateral	The opposite side of the body

- Adduction – movement towards the median sagittal plane.
- Supination – lateral rotation of the forearm causing the palm to face anteriorly.
- Pronation – median rotation of the forearm causing the palm to face posteriorly.
- Eversion – movement of the sole away from the median plane (turning the sole of the foot outwards).

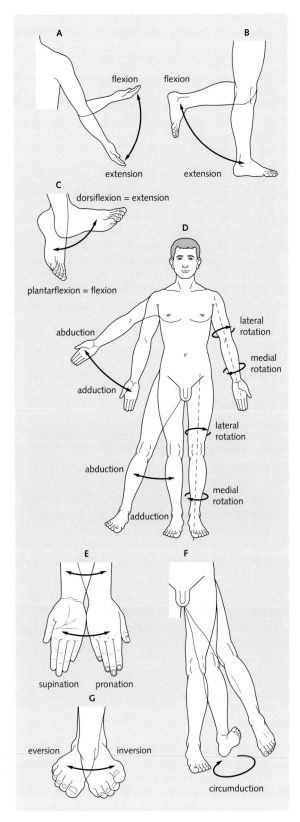

- Inversion – movement of the sole towards the median plane (turning the sole of the foot inwards).
- Rotation – movement of part of the body around its long axis.
- Circumduction – a combination of flexion, extension, abduction and adduction.

The terms used to describe movements of the thumb refer to its being at a right angle to the movements of the fingers (Fig. 1.5).

> **HINTS AND TIPS**
>
> To differentiate supination from pronation, remember that you hold a bowl of **s**oup with a **s**upinated forearm.

OVERVIEW OF ANATOMICAL STRUCTURES AND BODY SYSTEMS

Skin

The skin completely covers the body surface and is the largest organ of the body. The functions of the skin include:

- Protection from ultraviolet light, mechanical, chemical and thermal insults.
- Sensation of pain, temperature, touch and pressure.
- Thermoregulation.
- Metabolic functions, e.g. vitamin D synthesis.

The skin is composed of the following layers (Fig. 1.6):

- The epidermis is the outermost layer of the skin. It is a stratified squamous keratinized epithelium which forms a protective waterproof barrier. The epidermis is avascular, and is continually shed and replaced.
- The dermis lies deep to and supports the epidermis. It is composed largely of interlacing collagen fibres, with some elastic fibres, giving the skin strength and

Fig. 1.4 Terms of movement.
(A) Flexion and extension of forearm at elbow joint.
(B) Flexion and extension of leg at knee joint.
(C) Dorsiflexion and plantarflexion of foot at ankle joint.
(D) Abduction and adduction of right limbs and rotation of left limbs at shoulder and hip joints, respectively.
(E) Pronation and supination of forearm at radioulnar joints.
(F) Circumduction (circular movement) of lower limb at hip joint.
(G) Inversion and eversion of foot at subtalar and transverse tarsal joints.

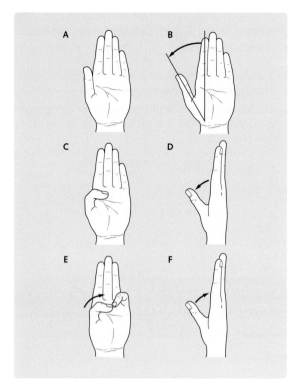

Fig. 1.5 Terms of movement for the thumb.
(A) Neutral hand position
(B) Extension (radial abduction)
(C) Flexion (transpalmar abduction)
(D) Abduction (palmar abduction)
(E) Opposition
(F) Adduction
(Adapted from *Crash Course: Musculoskeletal System* by SV Biswas and R Iqbal. Mosby.)

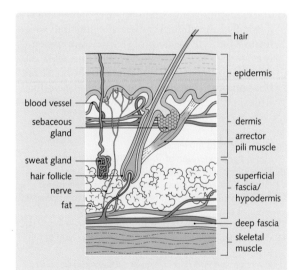

Fig. 1.6 Structure of skin and subcutaneous tissue.

elasticity. It also contains nerve endings (detecting pain, touch, pressure and temperature), blood vessels and glands. It contains mast cells, lymphocytes and macrophages, which play a role in immunity. It is the site of inflammation, growth and repair.

• The hypodermis, or superficial fascia, lies deep to the dermis. It is composed of loose areolar tissue (subcutaneous fatty tissue) which provides thermal insulation and protection for underlying structures.

The skin appendages include:

• Hair follicles (containing hair shafts) – tubular invaginations of the epidermis, into the dermis, lined by stratified squamous epithelium. At the base of each follicle, cell division, growth and maturation results in formation of a column of dead, keratinized cells (the hair shaft) which extrudes from the follicle.

• Sebaceous glands – associated with the hair follicles. They produce sebum, which lubricates the skin and hair and creates a protective bactericidal layer.

• Sweat glands – produce sweat, which plays a role in thermoregulation.

• Nails – located at the distal end of the dorsal surface of each digit. They are composed of a nail plate and a nail bed. The nail plate is composed of tightly packed keratinized cells.

CLINICAL NOTE

Malignant melanoma

Melanocytes are melanin producing cells (melanin determines skin colour), located in the epidermis. A malignant melanoma is a tumour of melanocytes. Women most commonly develop melanoma on the lower limb, men on the trunk. Early signs of melanoma can be summarized as follows: **a**symmetry, **b**order (irregular), **c**olour (variegated), **d**iameter (greater than 6 mm is more likely to be melanoma, although this is by no means absolute), **e**volving/**e**nlarging over time. Diagnosis is made by a full-thickness excision (removal of the melanoma with a small margin of surrounding tissue) or by removal of part of the lesion (biopsy). Melanoma can metastasize to nearby lymph nodes, then to distant organs, commonly the lungs, brain, bone and liver.

Fascia

The fasciae of the body may be divided into superficial and deep layers. Superficial fascia lies deep to the dermis, connecting it to the deep fascia (Fig. 1.6). It supports cutaneous nerves, blood vessels and lymphatics, which supply the dermis and skin. In some places sheets of muscle lie within the fascia, e.g. muscles of facial expression. The thickness of fascia varies at different sites within the body, and superficial fascia is thicker in females than in males.

Deep fascia forms a layer of fibrous tissue around muscles, bones, nerves and deep structures. It also forms intermuscular septa, attaching to bone and dividing the muscles of the limbs into compartments. Deep fascia is very sensitive due to its rich nerve supply. Its thickness varies widely, e.g. it is thickened in the iliotibial tract, but very thin over the rectus abdominis muscle and absent over the face. The arrangement of the fascia determines the pattern of spread of infection as well as the extent to which blood can haemorrhage into tissues.

Bone

Bone is a specialized form of connective tissue with a mineralized extracellular component.
The functions of bone include:

- Locomotion (by serving as a rigid lever)
- Support and protection, e.g. of the brain
- Attachment of muscles
- Calcium homeostasis and storage of other inorganic ions
- Production of blood cells (haematopoiesis).

Classification of bone

Bones are classified according to their position and shape:

- The axial skeleton consists of the skull, vertebral column, sacrum, ribs and sternum.
- The appendicular skeleton, consists of the pelvic girdle, pectoral girdle, and the bones of the upper and lower limbs.

There are a variety of shapes of bone including:

- Long bones, e.g. femur, humerus
- Short bones, e.g. carpal bones
- Flat bones, e.g. skull vault
- Irregular bones, e.g. vertebrae.

General structure of bone

Bone is surrounded by a vascular connective tissue membrane known as the periosteum (Fig. 1.7), which provides nutrition to the underlying bone. Periosteum is osteogenic, containing osteoproginator cells which can differentiate into osteoblasts if required, e.g. after a fracture.

Bone is formed from several components:

- Compact bone – an outer layer, providing strength and rigidity
- Cancellous (trabecular) bone – this lies deep to compact bone, and is also found at the epiphyses of long bones. It consists of a network of trabeculae, laid down in the direction of stresses placed upon the bone.
- Bone marrow – found in the medullary cavity of long bones and the interstices of cancellous bone. At birth

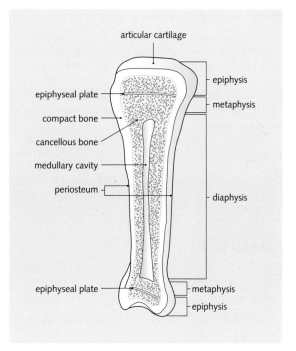

Fig. 1.7 Internal structure of a long bone.

all bone marrow is red (haematopoietic). With age, this is replaced by yellow (fatty) marrow, which is inactive. In adults only the ribs, sternum, vertebrae, clavicle, pelvis and skull bones contain red marrow.
- Endosteum – lining the bone marrow cavity and the canals. It is composed of a single layer of osteogenic cells.

CLINICAL NOTE

Osteoporosis

Bone undergoes constant remodelling. Osteoclasts resorb bone, whilst osteoblasts lay down new bone. In osteoporosis, osteoclasts outperform osteoblasts. Osteoporosis may occur due to ageing, lack of exercise, prolonged use of steroids, low intake of calcium and vitamin D and a lack of oestrogen.

The consequence is a reduction in bone density (BMD) and deterioration in the micro-architecture of bone, leading to a loss of bone strength and an increased risk of fracture. Osteoporotic fractures may occur with minimal or no trauma. The vertebrae, the distal radius (Colles' fracture) and the femoral neck are most commonly affected. At these sites, there is a high ratio of cancellous (trabecular) to cortical bone. Cancellous bone undergoes a faster rate of turnover than cortical bone and so any mismatch in the rate of bone remodelling is more likely to affect this type of bone.

Blood supply of bones

Bones receive a dual blood supply. Major nutrient arteries supply the bone marrow and the majority of the cortex, whilst vessels from the periosteum contribute to the supply of cortical bone. The latter assumes greater importance in the elderly. Stripping of the periosteum, e.g. during surgery or following trauma, may result in bone necrosis.

Joints

These are unions between bones. There are three major types of joints – fibrous, cartilagenous and synovial (Fig. 1.8).

Synovial joints

These are moveable joints, reinforced by ligaments. They have the following features:

- The bone ends are covered by hyaline articular cartilage.
- The joint is surrounded by a fibrous capsule.

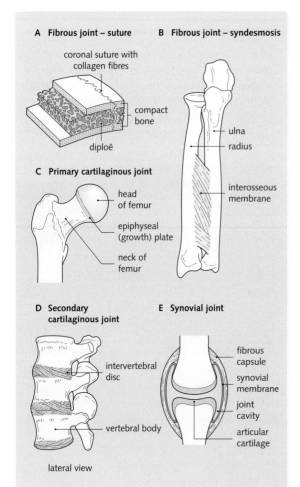

Fig. 1.8 Types of joints.

- The joint and its capsule are lined by a synovial membrane which secretes synovial fluid to lubricate the joint and transport nutrients.
- Some synovial joints, e.g. the temporomandibular joints, are divided into two cavities by an articular disc.

Blood and nerve supply of joints

Joints receive a blood supply from surrounding arteries, the branches of which anastomose to form vascular networks. A nerve which innervates a joint also tends to supply the muscles which move the joint, and the skin over the attachments of the muscles (Hilton's law). Sensory innervation of the joint capsule and ligaments allows sensation of pain and stretch. This contributes to proprioception, and is necessary for motor control and posture.

Stability of joints

Several factors contribute to joint stability:

- Bone – e.g. in a ball-and-socket joint such as the hip joint, bony contours contribute to stability.
- Ligaments – these are important in most joints, acting to prevent excessive movement.
- Muscles – these are an important stabilizing factor in most joints.

Muscles and tendons

Muscle action

Muscles can be classified according to their action:

- Agonist (prime mover) – the major muscle responsible for a particular movement, e.g. biceps brachii is the prime mover in flexing the elbow.
- Antagonist – any muscle that opposes the action of the prime mover: as the prime mover contracts the antagonist relaxes, e.g. triceps brachii relaxes during elbow flexion.

> **HINTS AND TIPS**
>
> If a joint is very stable (e.g. the hip) it has a reduced range of movement compared with a less stable joint (e.g. the shoulder).

- Fixator – a muscle which stabilizes one part of the body, during movement of another part of the body, e.g. muscles which hold the scapula steady when deltoid moves the humerus.
- Synergist – a muscle which performs, or assists in performing, the same set of movements as agonist muscles.

Muscle organization and function

Muscle fibres lie either parallel or oblique to the long axis of the muscle. Parallel muscle fibres allow maximal range of movement e.g. sartorius and sternocleidomastoid muscles. Oblique fibres allow increased power/force, at the expense of a reduced range of movement e.g. deltoid muscles. Muscles with oblique fibres are referred to as pennate muscles, which can be unipennate, bipennate or multipennate.

Motor nerves control the contraction of skeletal muscle. Each motor neuron, together with the muscle fibres it supplies, constitutes a motor unit. The size of motor units varies considerably; where fine precise movements are required (e.g. eye muscles), a single neuron may supply only a few muscle fibres. Where powerful contraction is required, a single neuron may supply several hundred muscle fibres (e.g. gluteus maximus muscle).

CLINICAL NOTE

Clinical examination

During a neurological and musculoskeletal examination, muscle power is assessed by asking the patient to perform movements against resistance (e.g. asking the patient to flex the elbow while the examiner tries to oppose this movement). Power is graded (0 to 5) using the UK Medical Research Council (MRC) scale:

Grade 0: no movement
Grade 1: Flicker of muscle contraction
Grade 2: Movement with gravity eliminated
Grade 3: Movement against gravity
Grade 4: Movement against gravity and some resistance
Grade 5: Normal power.

Muscle attachments

Skeletal muscles are aggregations of contractile fibres which move the joints. Muscles are usually connected to bone via tendons, at sites known as origins and insertions. Some flat muscles are attached by a flattened tendon, known as an aponeurosis. Where the symmetrical halves of a muscle fuse the intersection is known as a raphe. Where tendons cross joints they are often enclosed by a synovial sheath, a layer of connective tissue lined by a synovial membrane and lubricated by synovial fluid. Sacs of connective tissue filled with synovial fluid, known as bursae lie between tendons and bony areas, acting as cushioning devices.

Nervous system

The nervous system is composed of the central nervous system (CNS) and the peripheral nervous system (PNS). The PNS is further divided into the somatic nervous system (comprising the cranial and spinal nerves, supplying the head and trunk/limbs respectively) and the autonomic nervous system (comprising the sympathetic and parasympathetic systems).

The conducting cells of the nervous system are termed neurons. A typical motor neuron consists of a cell body (containing a nucleus), which gives rise to a single axon (nerve fibre) and numerous dendrites (Fig. 1.9). The cell bodies of most neurons are located within the CNS. Aggregations of cell bodies in the CNS and PNS are known as nuclei and ganglia respectively. Axons conduct electrical impulses (action potentials) away from the cell body. They communicate with other neurons at synapses (via neurotransmitter release) or with target organs or glands. They may be myelinated or non-myelinated. Myelinated fibres conduct impulses faster than unmyelinated fibres. Dendrites extend outward from the cell body. They receive signals from other neurons and transmit them to the cell body.

The somatic nervous system is composed of motor (efferent) and sensory (afferent) neurons. The former carries impulses from the CNS to skeletal muscles. The latter carries sensory information to the CNS.

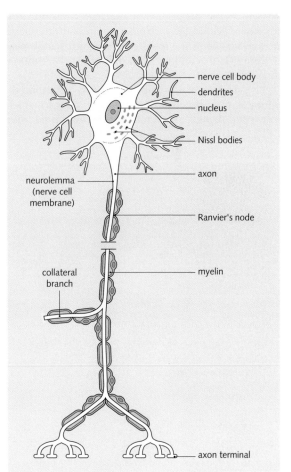

Fig. 1.9   Structure of a typical motor neuron.

Labels: nerve cell body; dendrites; nucleus; Nissl bodies; axon; Ranvier's node; myelin; axon terminal; neurolemma (nerve cell membrane); collateral branch

Central nervous system

The CNS is composed of the brain and spinal cord, both of which are covered by the meninges (composed of three layers – the dura, arachnoid and pia mater).

The brain lies within the cranial cavity, surrounded by cerebrospinal fluid (CSF). The brain is divided into two cerebral hemispheres, known collectively as the cerebrum, which are connected by the corpus callosum. Each cerebral hemisphere consists of four lobes – frontal, temporal, parietal and occipital lobes. Ridges on the surface of the cerebrum are known as gyri. Grooves between the gyri are known as sulci. The frontal and parietal lobes are separated by the central sulcus.

Deeper grooves are known as fissures, which divide the regions of the brain. The longitudinal fissure separates the two cerebral hemispheres. The transverse fissure separates the cerebrum from the cerebellum. The Sylvian fissure (lateral fissure/sulcus) separates the temporal lobe from the frontal and parietal lobes (Fig. 1.10).

The outer layer of the cerebrum is known as the cerebral cortex and is composed of grey matter (cell bodies). Deep to this lies white matter (myelinated axons) (Fig. 1.11). The cerebrum and a part of the brain known as the diencephalon together constitute the forebrain. Within the forebrain are areas of deep grey matter, known as the basal ganglia which have a role in a number of neurological conditions (e.g. Parkinson's disease).

The cerebellum is composed of two hemispheres, with a thin outer cortex of grey matter, deep to which lies white matter. The cerebellum is associated with

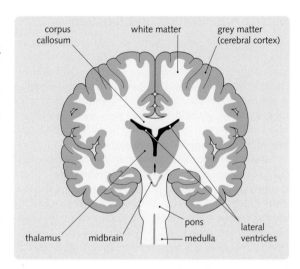

Fig. 1.11 Coronal section of the cerebrum illustrating grey and white matter.

regulation and coordination of movement, posture, and balance.

The brainstem consists of the midbrain, pons and medulla oblongata (Fig. 1.10). Within the brainstem grey matter is arranged into distinct regions known as nuclei. These nuclei give rise to cranial nerves III–XII.

Ventricular system of the brain

The brain contains several cavities known as ventricles, which are continuous with each other. Ventricles are lined with ependyma which secretes CSF. The ventricular system is composed of two lateral ventricles, connected to the third ventricle via the interventricular foramina. The cerebral aqueduct connects the third ventricle to the fourth ventricle, contained within the brainstem. CSF within the ventricles reaches the subarachnoid space around the brain and spinal cord, via apertures in the fourth ventricle (Fig 1.12). CSF eventually returns to the venous system via arachnoid villi which project into the superior sagittal sinus (Fig. 8.7).

Spinal cord

The spinal cord is cylindrical in shape, and is slightly flattened anteriorly and posteriorly. The cord extends from the foramen magnum of the skull (it is a continuation of the medulla oblongata of the brain) to approximately the level of the L2 vertebra in adults (L3 vertebra in infants). The terminal end of the spinal cord is known as the conus medullaris. The pia mater of the meninges extends inferiorly from the conus medullaris, as the filum terminale which attaches to the coccyx. Inferior to the conus medullaris, the lumbosacral spinal nerve

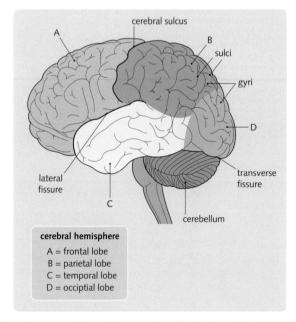

cerebral hemisphere

A = frontal lobe
B = parietal lobe
C = temporal lobe
D = occiptial lobe

Fig. 1.10 Lateral view of the brain illustrating the major features.

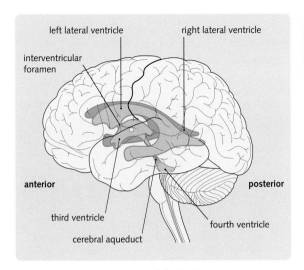

Fig. 1.12   Ventricular system of the brain.

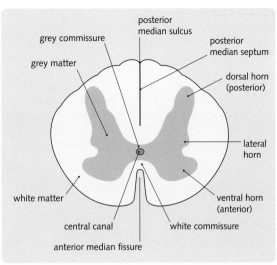

Fig. 1.13   Transverse section of the spinal cord illustrating the major features.

roots together with the filum terminale, comprise the cauda equina.

There are two regions of enlargement within the spinal cord which give rise to the upper and lower limb plexuses. The cervical enlargement (C5–T1 segments of the spinal cord) gives rise to the nerves of the brachial plexus whilst the lumbosacral enlargement (L2–S3) gives rise to the nerves of the lumbosacral plexus (Fig. 2.8).

On the anterior surface of the cord lies the anterior median fissure, whilst on the posterior surface lies the posterior median sulcus, which continues internally as the posterior median septum. A cross section of the spinal cord reveals a central H-shaped structure, composed of grey matter (cell bodies of neurons), surrounded by white matter (axons of neurons). The grey matter is composed of two lateral horns connected by a grey commissure. Within the grey commissure lies the central canal, filled with cerebrospinal fluid. Both the grey and white matter is divided into anterior (ventral), lateral and posterior (dorsal) horns and columns respectively (Fig.1.13).

The cell bodies of motor neurons are located in the ventral (anterior) horn of the spinal cord (Fig. 1.14). The axons of these neurons synapse with the sarcolemma (plasma membrane) of muscle cells at the neuromuscular junction. Depolarization of a motor neuron results in release of neurotransmitter into the synaptic cleft, causing depolarization of the sarcolemma and initiation of muscle contraction.

The receptors of sensory neurons in skin, muscle or viscera respond to specific stimuli, e.g. mechanical, chemical or thermal. The axons of these neurons (known as first order neurons) carry impulses from the receptor to the dorsal (posterior) horn of the spinal cord. First order neurons synapse with second order neurons either at the same level or at a higher level within the spinal cord. The second order neurons carry impulses to higher centres in the brain, where they synapse with third order neurons. Sensory neurons can also synapse directly with motor neurons at the same spinal level or via an interneuron. This is the structural and physiological basis of a reflex arc (Fig. 1.14).

CLINICAL NOTE

Clinical examination/neurology

When testing reflexes the reflex arc is being assessed at a particular spinal cord level. For example, on striking the patellar tendon the quadriceps muscle is stretched. This triggers an action potential within a muscle spindle (receptors within the muscle which monitor muscle length). The action potential travels to the spinal cord via an afferent neuron, where it synapses with an efferent neuron, leading to contraction of the muscle and a knee jerk. The common limb reflexes tested, with their spinal cord levels are:

- Biceps brachii (C5–6)
- Triceps brachii (C7–8)
- Brachioradialis (C6–7)
- Quadriceps femoris (L3–4)
- Gastrocnemius (S1–2)

Although reflexes occur at the level of the spinal cord, they can be influenced by higher centres. For example, after a stroke, loss of inhibitory input from higher centres which would normally dampen reflex activity may be lost and hyper-reflexia (exaggerated limb reflexes) occurs.

Fig. 1.14 Components of a typical spinal nerve.

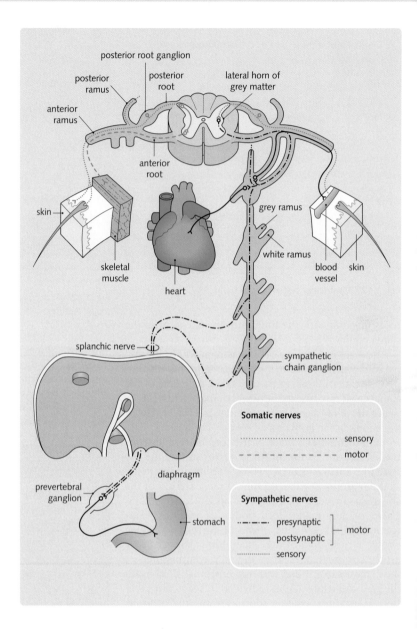

Autonomic nervous system

Autonomic nerves are either sympathetic or parasympathetic. They control involuntary visceral functions. The cell bodies of the preganglionic neurons of the sympathetic nervous system lie within the thoracic and first two lumbar segments of the spinal cord (T1–L2). The preganglionic axons exit via the anterior root of spinal nerves and synapse with post-ganglionic neurons in a ganglion of the sympathetic chain, which runs on either side of the vertebral column. The post-ganglionic axons then re-enter the spinal nerve to supply the body wall and limbs. Some preganglionic axons do not synapse in the sympathetic chain. They can pass through the sympathetic ganglion and travel to autonomic plexuses in the thorax to supply thoracic viscera. Alternatively, they can pass through the ganglion, to form the splanchnic nerves and synapse in a prevertebral ganglion, e.g. coeliac ganglion. Postganglionic axons supply abdominal viscera.

The cell bodies of the parasympathetic preganglionic neurons lie in the nuclei of cranial nerves III, VII, IX, X and in the grey matter of the spinal cord between S2 and S4. Their axons travel in cranial nerves (III, VII, IX, X) and sacral nerves (S2–S4). They synapse in ganglia which lie within, or in close proximity to the viscera they supply.

Spinal nerves

There are 31 pairs of spinal nerves: 8 cervical, 12 thoracic, 5 lumbar, 5 sacral and 1 coccygeal nerve. In the intervertebral foramina, the anterior and posterior roots of each segment of the spinal cord join to form a spinal nerve (Fig. 1.14):

- The anterior root contains motor neurons supplying skeletal muscle. The anterior roots of T1–L2 also contain preganglionic sympathetic fibres, whilst S2–S4 contain preganglionic parasympathetic fibres.
- The posterior root contains sensory neurons whose cell bodies are located in the dorsal root ganglion.

Immediately after formation, the spinal nerve divides into ventral and dorsal rami. The ventral rami supply the limbs and the trunk. The dorsal rami supply the erector spinae muscles of the back along with the overlying skin.

Each spinal nerve provides sensory innervation to an area of skin known as a dermatome (with the exception of the skin of the face, which is supplied by the fifth cranial nerve). There is a degree of overlap in sensory innervation between adjacent dermatomes. Testing for loss of sensation over a dermatome helps to identify the level of a lesion within the spinal cord.

Cardiovascular system

The cardiovascular system functions principally to transport oxygen and nutrients to and remove carbon dioxide and other metabolic waste products from the tissues. The right side of the heart pumps deoxygenated blood to the lungs via the pulmonary circulation. The left side of the heart pumps oxygenated blood into the aorta, and onward to the rest of the body, via the systemic circulation (Fig. 1.15A).

Blood is distributed to the organs via arteries, which branch to become arterioles. Arterioles branch to become capillaries, where gaseous exchange occurs. Deoxygenated blood is returned to the heart via the capillaries which merge to become venules, which in turn become veins (Fig. 1.15B). Superficial veins lie close to the surface of the body, and play a role in thermoregulation. Deep veins, as their name suggests, lie deep within the body, and accompany the arteries supplying a given structure. The deep veins are known as venae comitantes. Valves are present in the low-pressure venous system, acting to prevent back-flow of blood. However, some veins have no true valves, e.g. venae cavae, vertebral, pelvic, head and neck veins.

Not all blood passes through capillaries. Precapillary sphincters, under sympathetic nerve control, regulate flow through the capillary beds. Contraction of these sphincters prevents blood from entering capillaries and blood instead passes directly from arterioles to venules (arteriovenous shunts). The sphincters can also dilate allowing increased blood flow through the capillary beds. This mechanism is important in metabolic regulation, e.g. thermoregulation and oxygen supply to skeletal muscle during exercise.

There may be natural connections between arteries. These are known as anastomoses. New connections can also develop between arteries. If an artery becomes occluded over time, e.g. by atherosclerotic plaques or by thrombi, collaterals (new vessels) may develop, forming an alternative route for blood flow. When such communications are absent (e.g. the central artery of the retina) between arteries, the vessel is known as an end artery. Occlusion of these arteries results in necrosis of the tissue or the structure it supplies.

A typical blood vessel wall is composed of three layers (tunics) (Fig. 1.15C). The proportion of each layer within an individual vessel wall varies, depending upon vessel type and function. Arteries have a well-developed tunica media, composed of smooth muscle. The walls of the largest arteries contain numerous elastic tissue layers; however, veins have relatively little smooth muscle and elastic tissue. Capillary walls are composed of a single layer of endothelium. Larger vessels, e.g. the aorta, are surrounded by an external layer of blood vessels (vasa vasorum) and nerves (vasa nervosa) which supply the vessel wall.

Lymphatic system

The lymphatic system is part of the immune system, and is composed of lymph (lymphatic fluid), lymph nodes, lymph vessels and organs, e.g. the spleen (Fig. 1.16). Lymphatics are found in all tissues except the CNS, eyeball, internal ear, cartilage, bone and the epidermis of the skin.

The lymphatic system has three major functions:

- Removal of excess interstitial fluid from the tissues, helping to maintain fluid balance
- Defending the body against disease
- Absorbing fats from the intestine and transporting them to the circulation.

Lymph originates as plasma. As blood passes through the arterial ends of capillaries, hydrostatic

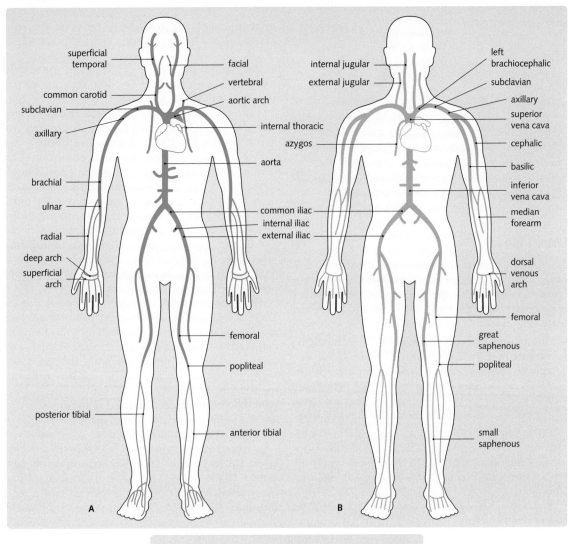

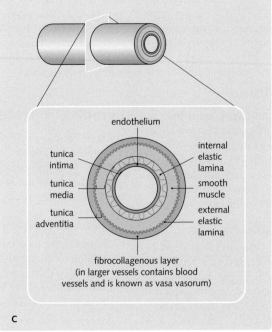

Fig. 1.15 A and B The major arteries and veins of the cardiovascular system. C, Cross section showing the layers (tunics) of a blood vessel wall.

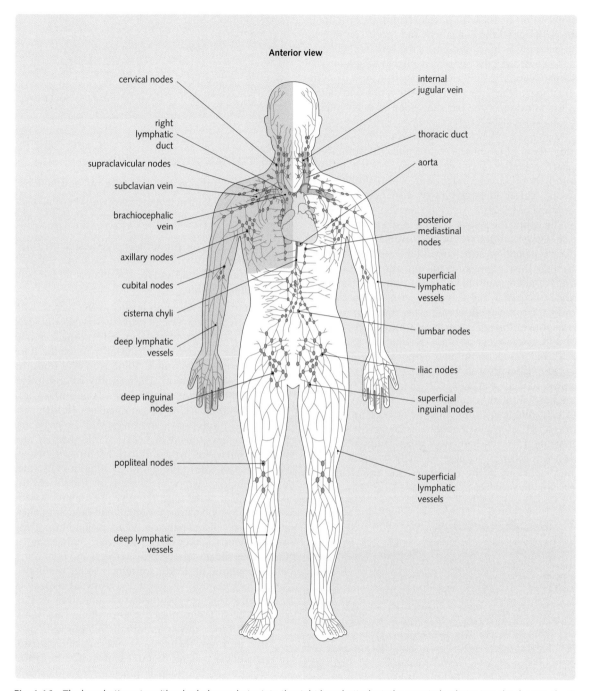

cervical nodes

internal jugular vein

right lymphatic duct

thoracic duct

supraclavicular nodes

aorta

subclavian vein

brachiocephalic vein

posterior mediastinal nodes

axillary nodes

cubital nodes

superficial lymphatic vessels

cisterna chyli

lumbar nodes

deep lymphatic vessels

iliac nodes

deep inguinal nodes

superficial inguinal nodes

popliteal nodes

superficial lymphatic vessels

deep lymphatic vessels

Anterior view

Fig. 1.16 The lymphatic system (the shaded area drains into the right lymphatic duct; the remainder drains into the thoracic duct).

pressure forces plasma through the capillary wall, into the tissues, where it becomes known as interstitial fluid. Interstitial fluid delivers nutrients and oxygen to cells, and removes cellular waste products. Most of the fluid is reabsorbed at the venous ends of capillaries, due to oncotic pressure (created by proteins, e.g. albumin and cations (sodium ions)) within the capillary.

Interstitial fluid which is not reabsorbed enters surrounding lymphatic capillaries, where it becomes known as lymph. Lymphatic capillaries merge to form superficial and deep lymph vessels. Vessels unite to form lymphatic trunks (lumbar, intestinal, bronchomediastinal, subclavian and jugular). The lymphatic trunks drain into the right lymphatic duct and the thoracic duct on the left. The right lymphatic duct drains the right side of the head, neck and thorax, along with the right upper limb, and enters the venous circulation at the junction of the right subclavian and right internal jugular veins. The thoracic duct drains lymph from the remainder of the body and enters the venous circulation at the junction of the left subclavian and left internal jugular veins (Fig. 1.16).

Movement of lymphatic fluid through lymph vessels is the result of (i) muscle contraction, (ii) pulsation of adjacent arteries, (iii) negative intrathoracic pressure within the thorax and (iv) pressure within the lymphatic vessels. Valves in larger vessels also help to prevent backflow of lymph.

The lymphatic system also helps defend against disease. Lymph nodes are located throughout the body, along lymphatic vessels. They filter lymph which passes through them, removing foreign antigens (anything which is not recognized by the immune system as 'self'). Nodes contain T and B lymphocytes and special cells known as antigen-presenting cells. Antigen-presenting cells present foreign antigens to T and B lymphocytes. Lymphocytes recognize these foreign antigens as not 'self', and mount an immune response.

Lymphatics are also involved in the absorption and transport of fats and fat-soluble vitamins. Intestinal villi contain lymphatic capillaries known as lacteals. Fats and fat-soluble vitamins enter the lacteals, mixing with lymph to form chyle (a milky substance with a high fat content). Lacteals drain into larger lymphatic vessels which drain into the cisterna chyli (lying inferior to the diaphragm in the midline). This drains into the thoracic duct.

CLINICAL NOTE

Oncology

Lymph nodes can be a site of tumour spread. Malignant cells may detach from a primary tumour and travel in lymph vessels to reach a lymph node, where they may give rise to a secondary tumour. This process is known as metastasis. In order to be able to predict and examine for likely sites of tumour metastasis, it is important to know the location of major lymph nodes. There are three superficial groups of nodes which are palpable when enlarged:

• Cervical nodes of the neck – lie in a chain on either side of the neck. They drain all structures of the head and neck.
• Axillary nodes – lie in fatty tissue within the axilla. They drain the upper limb and abdominal and thoracic walls, down to the level of the umbilicus.

• Inguinal nodes – lie in the superficial fascia, inferior to the inguinal ligament in the groin. They drain lymph from the lower limb, perineum and external genitalia, the abdominal wall below the umbilicus and the gluteal region.

Gastrointestinal system

The gastrointestinal system has three major functions:

• Digestion of food material starting with chewing (mastication) and continuing in the stomach and duodenum
• Absorption of the products of digestion in the small intestine
• Absorption of fluid and formation of solid faeces in the large intestine.

The process of digestion begins in the mouth with mastication and secretion of salivary enzymes (amylase and lipase). In the stomach, acid and enzyme secretion continue the process. In the second part of the duodenum, pancreatic enzymes, along with bile from the liver, complete digestion. The majority of absorption occurs in the jejunum, which has a large surface area due to the presence of plicae circularis (folds), villi (finger-like projections) and microvilli (microscopic projections on individual cells). Carbohydrates and proteins enter the hepatic portal system (see below) via capillaries within the intestinal villi, and fats enter the lymphatic system via lacteals in the intestinal villi.

The hepatic portal system consists of a number of veins which drain blood from the small and large intestines, stomach, spleen and pancreas. Venous blood from these organs eventually ends in the portal vein. At the entrance to the liver, the portal vein splits into left and right veins, which continue to divide, forming a set of capillaries, known as liver sinusoids. The blood is filtered in the sinusoids and substances absorbed in the intestines are processed. The sinusoids merge to form the hepatic veins. From here, blood travels on into the inferior vena cava, and into the heart. The portal venous circulation anastomoses with the systemic venous circulation at the gastro-oesophageal and recto-anal junctions (portosystemic anastomoses), and with vessels around the umbilicus.

The wall of the gastrointestinal tract is composed of four basic layers with areas of specialization reflecting function:

• Mucosa – is the innermost layer of the gastrointestinal tract.
• Submucosa – connective tissue layer containing blood vessels, autonomic nerves and lymphatics. Within the submucosa lies the enteric nerve plexus, and Mesissner's plexus.

- Muscularis externa – is composed of an inner circular layer and a longitudinal outer layer of muscle. The myenteric (Auerbach's plexus) lies between these two layers.
- Adventitia – the outer layer of the gastrointestinal tract.

The basic structure of the gut wall is illustrated in Figure 1.17. Modifications to this structure reflect the primary function of each area of the intestine, e.g. there are more folds and villi in the jejunum than in the ileum or colon since the jejunum has a more important role in absorption.

Respiratory system

The major function of the respiratory system is gas exchange – oxygen required for metabolic processes is inhaled and carbon dioxide is eliminated in order to maintain the acid–base balance of the body. However, the respiratory system has additional functions:

- Metabolism and activation or inactivation of some proteins, e.g. angiotensin-converting enzyme.
- Phonation (vocal sound production).
- Olfaction.
- Acting as a reservoir for blood.

Anatomically the respiratory system is divided into upper and lower respiratory tracts. The upper respiratory tract consists of the nose, pharynx and larynx. The lower respiratory tract begins at the trachea which divides into two main (primary) bronchi. The main bronchi divide repeatedly into secondary and tertiary bronchi. The tertiary bronchi divide into gradually smaller bronchi, which eventually become terminal bronchioles (bronchi contain cartilage within their walls, bronchioles do not), then respiratory bronchioles and finally alveolar ducts. Clusters of alveolar ducts are

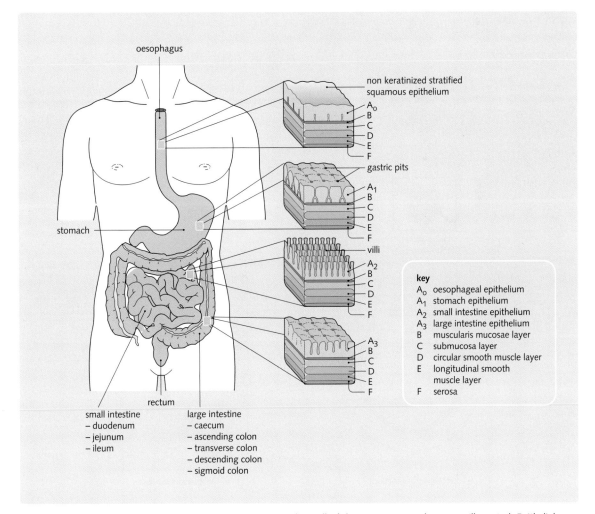

Fig. 1.17   The gastrointestinal system. The layers comprising the wall of the gastrointestinal tract are illustrated. Epithelial adaptions which dictate function are also shown.

referred to as alveolar sacs. The walls of the alveoli are composed of type I and type II pneumocytes (thin epithelial cells) surrounded by a rich capillary network, allowing efficient gas exchange to occur (Fig. 1.18).

Functionally the respiratory tract can be divided into a conducting portion and a respiratory portion. The conducting portion consists of a series of passageways through which air is conducted, and comprises the nasal cavity, pharynx, larynx, trachea, bronchi and terminal bronchioles. The respiratory portion consists of the respiratory bronchioles, alveolar ducts, alveolar sacs and alveoli, and is the site of oxygen and carbon dioxide exchange.

The conducting portion of the respiratory system as far as the bronchi is lined by respiratory epithelium (pseudostratified columnar epithelium). Terminal bronchioles are lined by simple cuboidal epithelium. The respiratory portion is lined by simple squamous epithelium allowing efficient exchange of oxygen and CO_2.

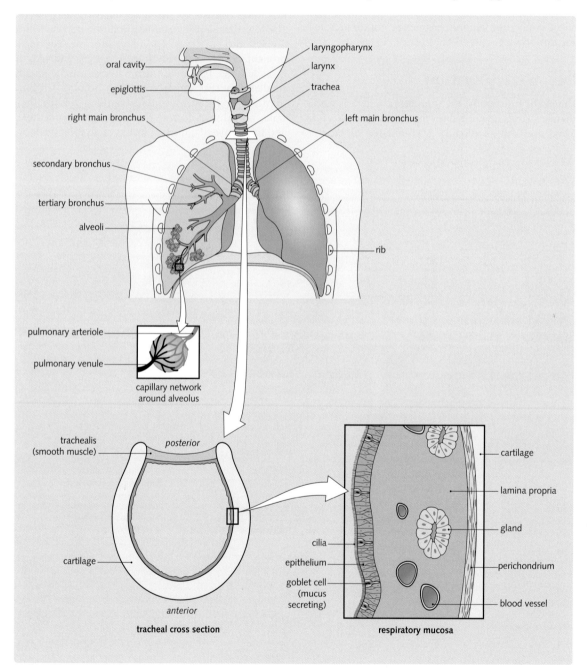

Fig. 1.18 Sagittal section illustrating the conducting and respiratory portions of the respiratory tract.

In addition to serving as a passageway for air, the conducting portion of the respiratory system is adapted to warm, filter and cleanse inhaled air in the following ways:

- Coarse hairs in the nasal vestibule trap large incoming particles.
- There is a rich network of veins underlying the nasal mucosa which warms inhaled air.
- On the lateral walls of the nasal cavity there are bony projections known as conchae. They are covered by epithelium, and act to increase the surface area of the nasal cavity, creating turbulence in the inhaled air. This facilitates the warming and filtration of the air.

- Motile cilia on the luminal surface of the airways beat rhythmically, propelling mucus containing trapped particles upwards towards the pharynx where it is swallowed.
- Goblet cells produce mucus, which humidifies inhaled air and traps foreign particles and bacteria, protecting the deeper portions of the lung. The mucus produced is supplemented by mucous and serous glands, which lie scattered amongst the epithelial cells.

Urinary system

The urinary system comprises the kidneys, ureters, bladder and urethra (Fig. 1.19). The functional unit of the kidney is the nephron.

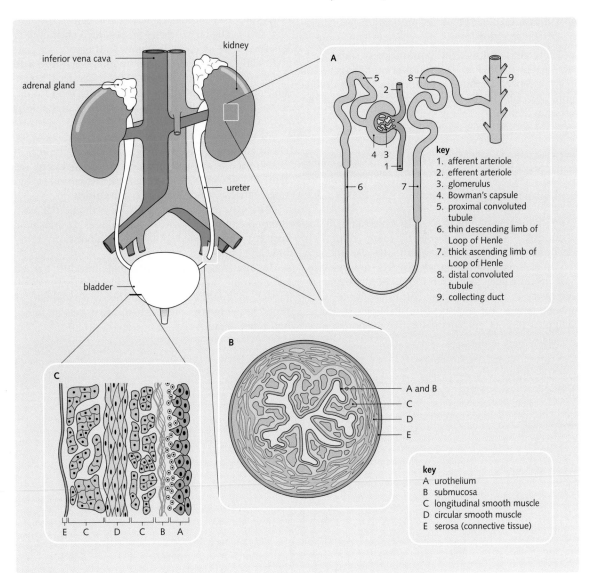

Fig. 1.19 Components of the urinary tract. Inset A shows the structure of a nephron, inset B shows the structure of the ureter and inset C shows the structure of the bladder wall.

17

A nephron is visible using a light microscope. It is composed of a glomerulus and a renal tubule. Blood is filtered at the glomerulus which consists of a knot of capillaries. The filtrate produced travels through the renal tubule, where a variety of substances undergo selective reabsorption and secretion. This results in the formation of urine, which enters the renal pelvis and drains into the bladder via the ureters. The bladder stores urine until it is voided (micturition). In addition to the excretion of waste products, e.g. urea, and reabsorption of filtered substances such as glucose, ions, and proteins, the kidneys also have the following functions:

- Conversion of vitamin D to its active form
- Regulation of blood pressure via renin secretion
- Stimulation of red blood cell production via erythropoietin secretion.

The ureters and bladder have muscular walls. Both are lined by urothelium (transitional epithelium). This is a specialized stratified epithelium allowing distension, especially of the bladder, to accommodate large volumes of urine.

RADIOLOGICAL ANATOMY

Introduction

Plain film radiography (X-ray) is a useful first line investigation in the diagnosis of many conditions e.g. bone/joint injury or disease, and diseases affecting the thoracic and abdominal viscera. The use of a contrast medium such as barium improves the diagnostic effectiveness of plain X-rays. Barium appears radio-opaque (white) on an X-ray film. It allows structures of similar lucency and internal structures not seen on plain X-ray to be distinguished. Contrast studies are commonly used to investigate the gut (e.g. to detect a perforation of the bowel wall or a stricture). A single contrast study uses contrast only. A double contrast study involves introduction of both contrast and air into the intestines.

Angiography involves injection of a contrast medium into an artery or vein via a percutaneous catheter. It is used to assess vascular disease such as atherosclerosis (fatty plaques) in the coronary arteries and aneurysms (a balloon-like swelling) in the abdominal aorta.

Computerized tomography (CT) scanning and magnetic resonance imaging (MRI) produce images in the axial/transverse plane, which can be reconstructed to produce 3D images of the body. In CT scanning, 2D X-rays are taken around a single axis of rotation, producing 'slices'. Digital geometry processing is then used to produce a 3D image of the body. MRI uses a magnetic field and radio waves to produce images. CT and MRI scans are often required to provide further detail on abnormalities highlighted by X-rays and ultrasound scans, or to look for subtle abnormalities which may not be apparent on plain X-rays.

CT scanning is used in evaluation of diseases of the chest, abdomen and pelvis (e.g. in cancer staging). It is also used to evaluate bony structures, including the skull and sinuses. CT scanning is often used to perform interventional procedures such as biopsies.

MRI is the preferred modality for evaluation of brain tumours, multiple sclerosis and injuries to the spinal cord (e.g. in suspected spinal cord compression), vertebrae and joints.

The remainder of the chapters will introduce normal radiographic anatomy and provide a systematic approach to interpreting X-rays. This is a vital skill as foundation doctors are often the first person to see and interpret an X-ray.

In this chapter you will learn to:
- Outline the surface anatomy of the back.
- Describe the major features of a typical vertebra.
- List the distinguishing features of the vertebrae in each region of the vertebral column.
- Describe the joints of the vertebral column.
- Understand the structure of intervertebral discs and describe their functions.
- Discuss the arrangement of the ligaments of the vertebral column.
- Appreciate the potential movements of each region of the vertebral column.
- Describe the major muscle groups supporting the vertebral column.
- Appreciate the general organisation of the spinal cord, and describe the meninges surrounding it.
- Explain the blood supply of the vertebral column and the spinal cord.

REGIONS AND COMPONENTS OF THE BACK

The back consists of the vertebral column, the spinal cord, the roots of the spinal nerves and associated muscles. The vertebral column extends from the skull to the coccyx and supports the weight of the upper body. It is composed of vertebrae, intervertebral discs, and ligaments. The vertebral column houses the spinal cord and meninges, the roots of the spinal nerves and blood vessels.

SURFACE ANATOMY AND SUPERFICIAL STRUCTURES

The surface anatomy of the back is illustrated in Figure 2.1.

Cutaneous innervation of the back

The skin of the back is supplied segmentally (in a dermatomal distribution) by the posterior rami of each of the 31 pairs of spinal nerves (Fig. 1.14). All of the posterior rami of the spinal nerves, with the exception of the first cervical nerve, divide into medial and lateral branches. The posterior ramus of the 1st (suboccipital) cervical nerve supplies the deep muscles in the suboccipital region of the neck but does not supply the skin.

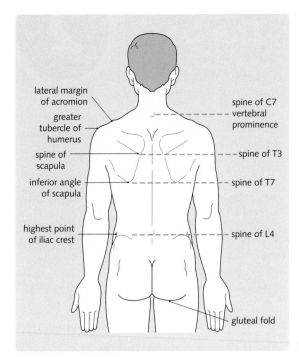

Fig. 2.1 Surface features of the back.

THE VERTEBRAL COLUMN

Osteology of the vertebral column

The vertebral column consists of 33 vertebrae, arranged in five distinct regions. There are seven cervical, twelve thoracic, five lumbar, five sacral and four coccygeal vertebrae. The sacral and coccygeal vertebrae fuse to form the sacrum and coccyx respectively (Fig. 2.2). Vertebrae articulate with each other via intervertebral discs and articular facet (zygapophyseal) joints. There is limited movement between adjacent vertebrae, but movement within the vertebral column as a whole is considerable.

CLINICAL NOTE

Scoliosis, kyphosis and lordosis

Scoliosis is an abnormal lateral curvature of the vertebral column; a true scoliosis also includes some element of vertebral rotation. 80% of cases are idiopathic. The majority of the remainder are neuromuscular in origin (e.g. secondary to cerebral palsy or muscular dystrophy), and a very small number occur secondary to abnormal vertebral development (congenital). Kyphosis describes an abnormal increase in the thoracic curvature, resulting in a 'hunchback'.

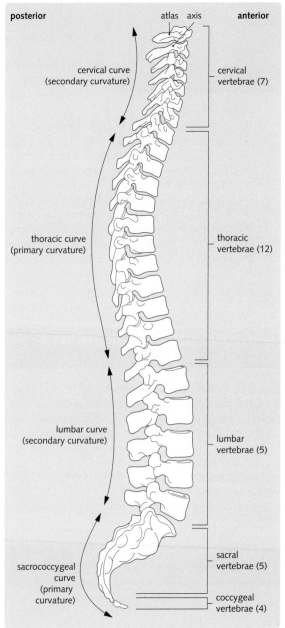

Fig. 2.2 Lateral view of the vertebral column.

It may occur secondary to vertebral wedge fractures as a result of osteoporosis. Lordosis describes an abnormal increase in the lumbar curvature, with anterior rotation of the pelvis. It may occur secondary to pregnancy or obesity, where the centre of gravity shifts anteriorly.

There are four curvatures of the vertebral column in adults (Fig. 2.2). The thoracic and sacral curvatures are kyphoses. They are primary curvatures, developing during the fetal period and are present at birth. The cervical and lumbar curvatures are lordoses. They are secondary curvatures which begin to develop during the fetal period, but become apparent at 3 months (when a baby begins to lift his/her head) and 12–18 months of age (when a child begins to walk) respectively.

Features of a typical vertebra

Figure 2.3A illustrates the features of a typical vertebra:

- A vertebral body – the weight-bearing part of the vertebra. These increase in size from the cervical to the sacrococcygeal region.
- A vertebral foramen – collectively, the foramina form the vertebral canal, through which the spinal cord passes.

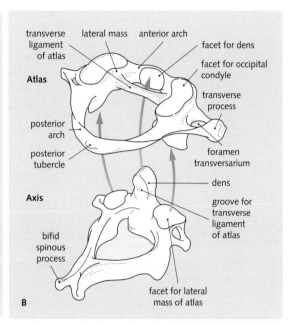

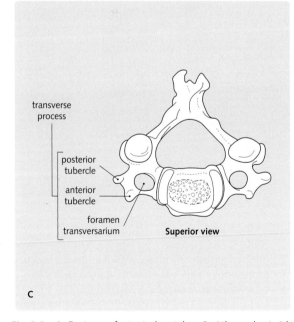

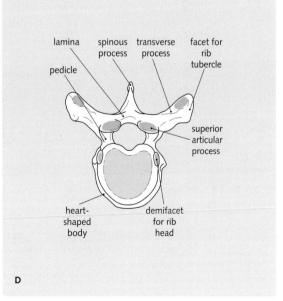

Fig. 2.3   A, Features of a typical vertebra. B, Atlas and axis (showing their articulations). C, Features of a cervical vertebra. D, Features of a thoracic vertebra.

(Continued)

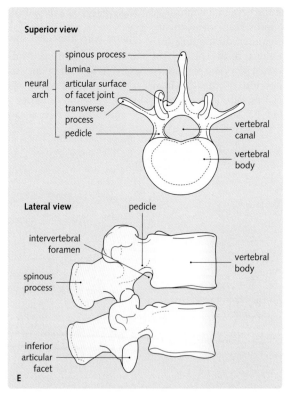

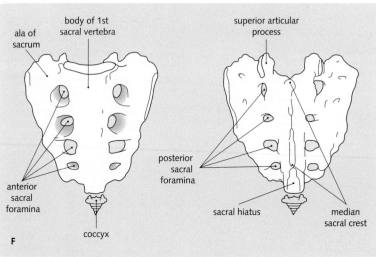

Fig. 2.3–Cont'd E, Features of a lumbar vertebra. F, Anterior and posterior views of the sacrum.

- A vertebral arch – composed of two pedicles and two laminae. The arch forms the lateral and posterior walls of the vertebral canal. A single spinous process projects posteriorly from the junction of the laminae, and transverse processes extend posterolaterally from the junctions of the pedicles and laminae on each side.
- Superior and inferior articular processes – these project superiorly and inferiorly from the junctions of the

pedicles and laminae. The superior articular process of one vertebra articulates with the inferior articular process of an adjacent vertebra to form facet joints.
- Intervertebral foramina – formed by the superior and inferior notches on each of the pedicles. Spinal nerves and vessels pass through the foramina.

In addition, each region of the vertebral column possesses characteristic features (Figs 2.3B–F, 2.4).

Fig. 2.4 Differentiating characteristics of vertebrae by region.

Vertebral region	Differentiating characteristics
Cervical	• Small vertebral bodies – transverse diameter greater than anteroposterior diameter. Concave superior surface, convex inferior surface • Large triangular vertebral foramina • Short and bifid spinous processes (with the exception of C6 and particularly C7) • Foramina transversarii for passage of the vertebral arteries
Thoracic	• Heart-shaped vertebral bodies with costal facets for articulation with the ribs • Small circular vertebral foramina • Long transverse processes (T1–T10 have facets for articulation with the ribs) • Long spinous processes
Lumbar	• Large, kidney-shaped vertebral bodies • Triangular vertebral foramina • Long, thin transverse processes • Bulky, square spinous processes
Sacral	• Fused vertebral bodies • Sacral foramina

Some vertebrae are highly specialized, for example the C1 (atlas), C2 (axis) and the sacrococcygeal vertebrae. The atlas is ring shaped and lacks a vertebral body. The axis features the dens (the odontoid process) projecting superiorly from the vertebral body (Fig. 2.3B).

The sacrococcygeal region forms part of the pelvic girdle. The sacrum consists of five fused vertebrae. There are four anterior and four posterior sacral foramina for passage of the anterior and posterior rami of the sacral spinal nerves. The median sacral crest represents the fused spinous processes of the sacral vertebrae (Fig. 2.3F).

Joints of the vertebral column

Atlanto-occipital joint

The atlanto-occipital joint is formed by the articular surfaces of the lateral masses of C1 vertebra (the atlas) and the occipital condyles. It is a synovial joint surrounded by a loose capsule. Flexion and extension (nodding movements) occur at this joint.

Atlanto-axial joints

The atlanto-axial joints comprise two lateral synovial joints, between the articular surfaces of the lateral masses of the axis and atlas, and a median joint between the dens (odontoid process) of the axis and the anterior arch of the atlas (Fig. 2.3B). The dens is held in place by the transverse ligament of the atlas. These joints allow rotational (shaking) movements of the head where the skull and the atlas rotate as a unit on the axis. Alar ligaments connect the dens to the occipital condyles, preventing excess rotation.

CLINICAL NOTE

Rheumatoid arthritis

Patients with rheumatoid arthritis must undergo careful pre-operative assessment, as they may suffer from atlantoaxial subluxation due to destruction of the transverse ligament and/or erosion of the dens. If the dens is not held firmly against the C1 vertebrae, it can impinge upon the spinal cord and so extension of the neck during anaesthesia can result in spinal cord injury.

Zygapophyseal joints (facet joints)

These are joints between the articular facets present on the superior and inferior articular processes. They are plane synovial joints. Flexion, extension, lateral flexion and rotation can occur within the vertebral column. Which of these movements are possible at any given vertebral level depends upon the shape and orientation of the articular facets (Fig. 2.5).

Fig. 2.5 Movements of the vertebral column.

Vertebral region	Movements
Cervical	The most mobile region of the vertebral column. Flexion, extension, and lateral flexion occur. Rotation occurs mainly at the atlanto-axial joint. Rotation is limited due to the shape and orientation of the articular processes of the facet joints of C3 to C7.
Thoracic	Rotation occurs. Flexion and extension are inhibited by facet joint shape and orientation, long spinous processes, the ribs and sternum.
Lumbar	Flexion, extension, and lateral flexion occur. Rotation is prevented by the shape and orientation of the articular facet joints.

Vertebral fractures and dislocations

Sudden forceful flexion of the vertebral column (e.g. in a car accident) can lead to compression fractures of the vertebrae. It can also result in anterior dislocation of a vertebral body (relative to the vertebrae below), resulting in dislocation or fracture of the articular facets and damage to the spinal cord. Hyperextension of the vertebral column can result in fracture of the vertebral arches, and stretching or tearing of the anterior longitudinal ligament (whiplash).

Intervertebral discs

Intervertebral discs lie between the vertebral bodies of adjacent vertebrae (Fig. 2.6) forming secondary cartilaginous joints. They help to absorb compressive forces. Intervertebral discs are composed of the following:

- Anulus fibrosus – an outer ring composed of concentric layers of fibrocartilage
- Nucleus pulposus – a gelatinous core.

Ligaments of the vertebral column

These are described in Figures 2.6 and 2.7.

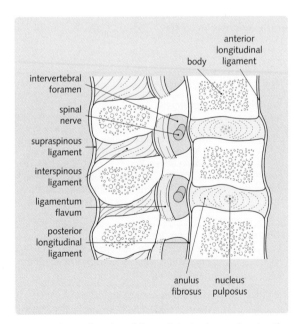

Fig. 2.6 Sagittal section of the vertebral column, showing the intervertebral discs and ligaments.

Fig. 2.7 Ligaments of the vertebral column.

Ligament	Action
Anterior longitudinal	Extends from the anterior tubercle of C1 vertebra (the atlas) to the sacrum. Is attached to the anterior surfaces of the vertebral bodies and intervertebral discs. Prevents hyperextension of the vertebral column and maintains stability of the intervertebral discs.
Posterior longitudinal	Extends from C2 vertebra to the sacrum. Is attached to the posterior aspect of the vertebral bodies and intervertebral discs (therefore lines the anterior surface of the vertebral canal). Prevents hyperflexion of the vertebral column and posterior protrusion of the intervertebral discs.
Supraspinous	Crosses and unites the tips of the spinous processes from C7 to the sacrum (between the skull and C7 this ligament is known as the ligamentum nuchae).
Interspinous	Ligaments uniting adjacent spinous processes.
Ligamentum flavum	Unites adjacent laminae; limits flexion of the vertebral column, assists in extending the spine after flexion, and helps to preserve the curvatures of the vertebral column.

Ligamentum nuchae

The ligamentum nuchae is a strong triangular fibro-elastic ligament that lies in the median sagittal plane. It is essentially a continuation of the supraspinous ligament. It is attached superiorly to the external occipital protuberance and the foramen magnum. It also attaches to the spinous processes of the cervical vertebrae and ends by attaching to the tip of C7 spinous process. It helps to return the head to its normal position following flexion of the neck and provides a site of muscular attachment for trapezius and rhomboid minor.

Herniated intervertebral disc

When the vertebral column is flexed, compression of the anterior part of the intervertebral disc pushes the nucleus pulposus posteriorly, which can cause it to herniate into the vertebral canal. Herniation is more likely if the anulus fibrosus has degenerated/weakened with age (if the intervertebral disc were a jam doughnut, imagine what would happen to the jam if half of the doughnut was squashed), or in an area where the anulus fibrosus is thin, with no ligamentous support (for this reason posterolateral herniations are most common). Herniation is particularly common in the lumbar and lumbosacral regions, where discs are large and the range of movement is greatest. The result is compression of the spinal nerve roots, or of the spinal cord. Compression of any of the nerve roots from L5 to S3 causes sciatica. Most commonly the L5 and/or S1 nerve roots are affected – resulting in back pain which travels down the posterior aspect of the thigh and sometimes into the foot.

Muscles of the vertebral column

An individual's body weight, for the greater part, is anterior to their vertebral column. To support this and move the vertebral column, there are three main groups of muscles which run longitudinally on the posterior aspect of the vertebrae:

- Superficial extrinsic muscles, associated with the upper limb – trapezius, latissimus dorsi, levator scapulae and rhomboids minor and major (Chapter 3).
- Intermediate extrinsic muscles – serratus posterior superior and inferior, and levatores costarum. These connect the vertebrae and the ribs and bring about accessory respiratory movements.
- Deep intrinsic muscles of the back – this is a complex group of muscles, the most important of which are the erector spinae muscles, forming the ridges of muscle on either side of the vertebral column. The more superficial long muscles support the curves of the spine and bring about extension, and the shorter deeper muscles are involved with smaller rotatory movements.

Back of the neck

At the back of the neck is a complex arrangement of muscles connecting the skull to the spine and pectoral girdle.

CLINICAL NOTE

Metastasis via vertebral veins

Blood may return from the pelvis and abdomen to the heart via the vertebral venous plexuses and via the azygos veins to the superior vena cava. Abdominal and pelvic tumours, along with tumours of the breast, may metastasize to the vertebrae in this way.

THE SPINAL CORD AND MENINGES

The spinal cord lies in the vertebral canal. It commences immediately below the foramen magnum and ends as the conus medullaris, approximately opposite the L2 vertebra in adults and the L3 vertebra in children (Fig. 2.8). There are 31 pairs of spinal nerves, each composed of a dorsal and a ventral root (Fig. 1.14). Each spinal nerve exits through an intervertebral foramen. During fetal development the vertebral column grows at a faster rate than the spinal cord, meaning that postnatally the spinal cord does not occupy the entire length of the vertebral canal. Therefore, the level at which any given spinal nerve originates from the cord does not correspond with the vertebral level at which that spinal nerve exits. In other words, from superior to inferior, there is an increasing distance between the origin of a spinal nerve and its exit from the vertebral canal. Spinal nerve roots, therefore, become longer and increasingly oblique at lower levels of the spinal cord. The lumbar and sacral nerve roots are the longest of all, forming the cauda equina, inferior to the conus medullaris.

There are two areas of enlargement in the spinal cord:

- A cervical enlargement from the C5 to T1 spinal cord segments. Anterior rami from these segments form the brachial plexus, innervating the upper limbs.
- A lumbosacral enlargement from the L2 to S3 spinal cord segments. Anterior rami from these segments form the lumbar and sacral plexuses, innervating the lower limbs.

Spinal meninges and cerebrospinal fluid

The meninges and the cerebrospinal fluid (CSF) surround and protect the spinal cord.

HINTS AND TIPS

The first cervical nerve (C1) exits the vertebral canal between the skull and the first cervical vertebrae (i.e. superior to the first cervical vertebrae). C2–C7 nerves also exit **above** their respective vertebrae. However, there are only seven cervical vertebrae, but eight cervical nerves, and so the C8 nerve exits between the C7 and T1 vertebrae. All subsequent spinal nerves, therefore, exit **below** their respective vertebrae.

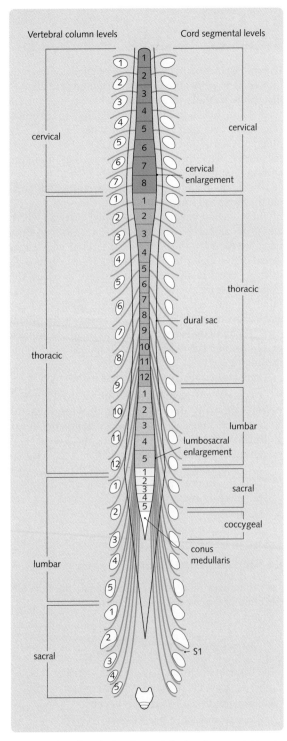

Fig. 2.8 Spinal cord, showing vertebral and segmental levels.

Dura mater

The dura mater is the outermost covering of the spinal cord. It is attached superiorly to the foramen magnum (where it is continuous with the dura of the brain), and inferiorly to the coccyx by the filum terminale. It is a tough fibrous membrane separated from the vertebral periosteum by the epidural space, which contains fat, connective tissue and the internal vertebral venous plexus. The dura mater extends along the spinal nerve roots and blends with the epineurium of the spinal nerves.

Arachnoid mater

The arachnoid mater is a delicate membrane lying deep to, but apposed to, the dura. It covers the spinal cord and spinal nerve roots. Between the two layers lies a potential space – the subdural space. The subarachnoid space lies between the arachnoid and the pia mater and it contains CSF.

Pia mater

The pia mater is a fine vascular membrane which closely adheres to the spinal cord. It covers the roots of the spinal nerves and the spinal blood vessels. Inferior to the conus medullaris, the pia continues as the filum terminale. It pierces the dural sac at the S2 vertebral level to attach to the coccyx. The pia mater extends laterally forming the denticulate ligaments, which pierce the arachnoid space and attach to the internal surface of the dura.

CLINICAL NOTE

Lumbar puncture

Lumbar puncture is most commonly performed to obtain a sample of cerebrospinal fluid (CSF) for analysis (e.g. if meningitis is suspected). It is also undertaken in order to inject chemotherapeutic or anaesthetic drugs. The patient is positioned on their left side, curled up, thus flexing the back and opening up the intervertebral spaces. An imaginary line between the iliac crests indicates the level of the L4 vertebra. A hollow needle is inserted into the L3/4 or L4/5 intervertebral space. The needle passes through the skin, supraspinous ligament, infraspinous ligament, ligamentum flavum, dura (the latter two demonstrate a perceptible 'give' as the needle passes through them) and arachnoid mater to enter the subarachnoid space. If raised intracranial pressure is suspected (headache, vomiting, reduced GCS, papilloedema) lumbar puncture should not be attempted, as it may result in herniation (coning) of the cerebellum and brainstem through the foramen magnum. Compression of the brainstem may lead to respiratory depression, which may prove fatal.

Anaesthesia

In epidural anaesthesia, an anaesthetic agent is injected into the extra(epi)dural space, affecting lumbar and sacral nerve roots: the procedure is as above except that the dura is not penetrated and the patient must not lie on their side (this would result in unilateral anaesthesia).

In spinal anaesthesia, the anaesthetic agent is passed into the subarachnoid space for a more profound and longer-lasting anaesthesia.

Blood supply of the spinal cord and vertebrae

Arterial supply to the spinal cord consists of the following:

- An anterior spinal artery, arising from the vertebral arteries. It travels in the anterior median fissure of the spinal cord and supplies the anterior aspect of the cord.
- Two posterior spinal arteries arising from the vertebral arteries. Each artery supplies the posterior cord on the ipsilateral side.
- Segmental arteries (branches of the vertebral, ascending cervical, deep cervical, posterior intercostal and lumbar arteries) which give rise to radicular arteries. Particularly in the lower regions of the spinal cord, radicular arteries supplement the

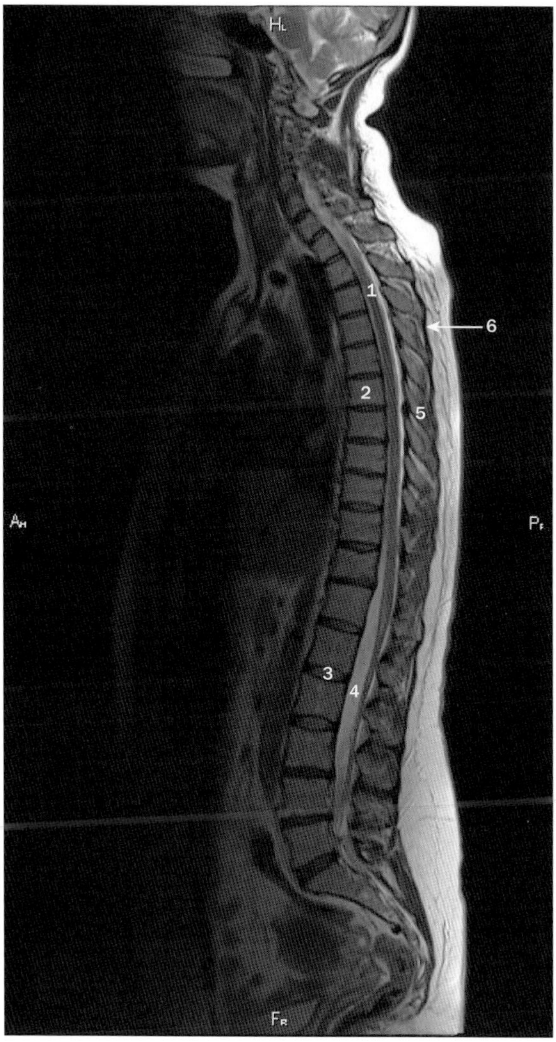

Fig. 2.9 MRI (sagittal section) showing the spinal cord, vertebrae and intervertebral discs.

1. Spinal cord
2. Vertebrae
3. Intervertebral discs
4. Cerebrospinal fluid in subarachnoid space
5. Spinous processes
6. Supraspinous ligament

blood supply provided by the anterior and posterior spinal arteries. Segmental arteries also supply the vertebrae.

The veins of the vertebrae and spinal cord drain into three anterior and three posterior longitudinal veins, which drain to internal vertebral venous plexuses (in the epidural space). The internal venous plexuses pass superiorly, through the foramen magnum of the skull and communicate with veins within the skull. They also communicate with the external vertebral venous plexus (on the outer surface of the vertebrae) via intervertebral veins located in the intervertebral foramina. The external plexus drains into the systemic segmental veins, then into vertebral and ascending lumbar veins ending in the azygos vein on the right and the hemiazygos vein on the left. The spinal cord has no lymphatic vessels.

RADIOLOGICAL ANATOMY

Plain radiography is a useful tool in detecting degenerative changes of the vertebral column such as osteoarthritis, and osteoporosis. MRI scanning in particular is valuable in diagnosis of disease of the spine and spinal cord, e.g. disease of the intervertebral discs, spinal cord compression and spinal tumours, etc. (Fig. 2.9).

The upper limb 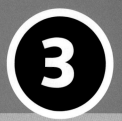 3

● Objectives

In this chapter you will learn to:
- Give an overview of the regions of the upper limb and appreciate its blood supply, nerve supply and lymphatic drainage.
- Describe the joints of the pectoral girdle, particularly the glenohumeral (shoulder) joint.
- Explain the movements of the glenohumeral joint and the muscles responsible for each movement.
- State the origins, insertions, actions and nerve supply of the muscles which form the rotator cuff.
- Describe the boundaries of the axilla and describe its contents.
- Understand the formation of the brachial plexus between the neck and axilla.
- Discuss the arterial supply and venous drainage of the the arm.
- Describe the elbow joint.
- List the muscles involved in elbow flexion and extension, and state their nerve supply.
- Describe the boundaries of the cubital fossa and its contents.
- Name the muscles, vessels and nerves in each compartment of the forearm, and appreciate their involvement in the movement of the wrist and the digits.
- State the boundaries and contents of the anatomical snuffbox.
- List the boundaries of the carpal tunnel and the structures passing through it.
- Appreciate the arrangement of a dorsal digital expansion.
- List the intrinsic muscles of the hand and state their nerve supply.
- Explain the arrangement of the long flexor tendons and synovial sheaths within the hand.
- Describe the cutaneous nerve supply of the hand.
- Be able to examine an X-ray of the upper in limb in a systematic manner, recognizing the major features.

REGIONS AND COMPONENTS OF THE UPPER LIMB

The upper limb is joined to the trunk by the pectoral girdle. The pectoral girdle and the glenohumeral joint together comprise the shoulder region. The arm lies between the shoulder and the elbow. The forearm lies between the elbow and the radiocarpal (wrist) joint. The hand is distal to the radiocarpal joint.

The pectoral girdle is composed of the scapula and the clavicle. The acromion of the scapula articulates with the lateral end of the clavicle to form the acromioclavicular joint. The medial end of the clavicle articulates with the manubrium of the sternum to form the sternoclavicular joint. The humerus lies in the arm. It articulates proximally with the glenoid fossa of the scapula to form the glenohumeral joint, and distally with the radius and ulna to form the elbow joint. The radius articulates with the carpal bones at the radiocarpal joint.

The arterial supply to the upper limb is via the subclavian artery. The right subclavian artery arises from the brachiocephalic trunk (the first branch of the arch of the aorta). The left subclavian artery arises directly from the arch of the aorta. At the lateral border of the first rib the subclavian artery becomes the axillary artery. At the lower border of teres major the axillary becomes the brachial artery. In the cubital fossa (which lies anterior to the elbow joint) the brachial artery divides into the radial and ulnar arteries which supply the forearm and hand.

Venous drainage of the upper limb begins in the hand. The dorsal venous network on the dorsum of the hand is a superficial network of veins, which drains into the cephalic and basilic veins. From here, blood is returned to the axillary vein, which eventually becomes the subclavian vein.

The nerve supply to the upper limb is derived from the brachial plexus: the median, musculocutaneous and ulnar nerves supply the flexor (anterior) compartment; the radial nerve supplies the extensor (posterior) compartment.

SURFACE ANATOMY AND SUPERFICIAL STRUCTURES

Surface anatomy

The surface anatomy of the shoulder region is shown in Figure 3.1.

Clavicle

The clavicle is shaped like an italic letter *f*, and is palpable along its length. The medial two-thirds of the clavicle are convex anteriorly. The lateral third is concave anteriorly. Its sternal end articulates with the manubrium of the sternum, forming the sternoclavicular joint. The acromial end articulates with the acromion of the scapula to form the acromioclavicular joint.

Scapula

The tip of the coracoid process can be palpated in the deltopectoral triangle. The deltopectoral triangle is bounded medially by pectoralis major, laterally by the deltoid muscle (which forms the smooth round curve of the shoulder) and superiorly by the clavicle. The acromion process forms the point of the shoulder and is easily palpable due to its subcutaneous position. The spine of the scapula is palpable along its length, and the medial border of the scapula can also be palpated along its length as far as the inferior angle (opposite the T7 vertebra).

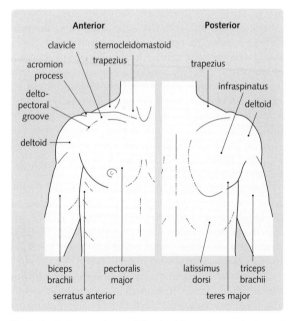

Fig. 3.1 Surface anatomy of the shoulder region – anterior and posterior views.

Elbow region

The medial and lateral epicondyles of the humerus and the olecranon process of the ulna can be palpated. The head of the radius is also palpable, in a depression on the posterior aspect of the extended elbow, distal to the lateral epicondyle. The pulse of the brachial artery can be palpated along the medial aspect of the arm, and within the cubital fossa, where it lies medial to the tendon of biceps brachii. The tendon of biceps brachii is palpable as it enters the fossa.

Wrist and hand

The styloid processes of the radius and ulna may be palpated at the wrist. On the anterior surface of the wrist, the scaphoid tuberosity and the pisiform bone can be seen and palpated on the radial and ulnar sides respectively. The long flexor tendons of the forearm muscles cross the anterior aspect of the wrist and are covered by the flexor retinaculum. The radial artery is palpable on the anterolateral surface of the wrist. The anatomical snuffbox (a depression between the extensor muscle tendons of the thumb) is visible on the posterior aspect of the wrist, on the lateral side, when the thumb is fully extended. On the posterior aspect of the hand, the metacarpal bones can be palpated and the extensor tendons which cover them are visible. The metacarpal heads form the knuckles of a clenched fist. On the palmar surface of the hand, the metacarpal heads are covered by the palmar aponeurosis, the intrinsic muscles of the hand and the long flexor tendons.

Musculature

The only bony attachment of the upper limb to the trunk is through the sternoclavicular joint. The limb is mainly suspended by a series of muscles, which adds greatly to the mobility of the shoulder region. The muscles form the anterior, posterior and medial walls of the axilla, which can be palpated as the anterior and posterior axillary folds (see below).

During flexion of the arm, the biceps brachii muscle becomes visible on the anterior surface of the arm. The tendon of the long head of biceps brachii is palpable in the intertubercular groove (between the greater and lesser tubercles of the humerus). Triceps brachii muscle is palpable along the posterior aspect of the arm.

Proximally in the forearm, individual muscles cannot be distinguished. However, when the wrist is flexed the muscle bellies of the flexors can be palpated anterolaterally and when the wrist is extended the extensor muscles can be palpated posterolaterally. Anteriorly at the wrist, the long flexor tendons can be identified from medial to lateral; flexor carpi ulnaris, flexor digitorum superficialis, palmaris longus and flexor carpi radialis.

Over the lateral aspect of the radiocarpal joint, the tendons of abductor pollicis longus, extensor pollicis brevis and longus form the borders of the anatomical snuffbox.

The intrinsic muscles of the hand control the fine movments of the digits. The muscles of the thenar eminence lie at the base of the thumb and those of the hypothenar eminence lie on the medial border of the hand. On the dorsal surface, the dorsal interossei, are palpable between the metacarpal bones. Other intrinsic muscles lie deeper and are not palpable.

Superficial venous drainage

The dorsal and palmar veins of the hand drain into the dorsal venous network which is often visible on the dorsum of the hand (Fig. 3.2). The basilic and cephalic veins arise from the medial and lateral sides of the venous network respectively. The basilic vein travels proximally along the medial aspect of the forearm. In the inferior half of the arm it pierces the deep fascia, becoming the the axillary vein at the lower border of teres major. The cephalic vein travels proximally along the anterolateral aspect of the forearm. Anterior to the cubital fossa it communicates with the basilic vein

via the median cubital vein, which is usually easy to identify. The cephalic vein then continues superiorly in the arm, passing along the deltopectoral groove between pectoralis major and deltoid muscles, and into the deltopectoral triangle. Finally, it pierces the clavipectoral fascia and drains into the axillary vein.

Lymphatic drainage

Lymphatic vessels in the hand coalesce to form trunks, which travel proximally in the forearm and the arm alongside the cephalic, basilic and deep veins. Lymph vessels accompanying the cephalic vein drain into the infraclavicular nodes or the axillary nodes. Some vessels along the basilic vein are interrupted at the elbow by a supratrochlear node, but ultimately they all drain into the axillary nodes. Lymph from the axillary nodes drains to the apical nodes, then to the supraclavicular nodes, and finally into the subclavian trunk. The subclavian trunk is joined by the jugular trunk (containing lymph from the head and neck), forming the right lymphatic trunk, and the thoracic duct on the left. These drain into the right and left subclavian veins respectively.

Cutaneous innervation of the upper limb

Figure 3.3 illustrates the dermatomes of the upper limb. Knowledge of the dermatomes is helpful in ascertaining the level at which a spinal injury has occurred.

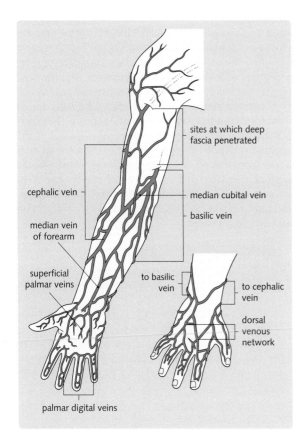

Fig. 3.2 Superficial venous drainage of the upper limb.

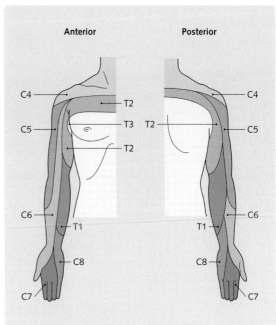

Fig. 3.3 Dermatomes of the upper limb.

THE SHOULDER REGION AND AXILLA

Pectoral girdle

The pectoral girdle (clavicle and scapula) connects the upper limb to the axial skeleton (Fig. 3.4). The clavicle acts as a strut, holding the upper limb away from the trunk and improving the range of movement at the glenohumeral joint. At both the sternoclavicular and acromioclavicular joints there are very strong ligaments to prevent dislocation (see below).

Clavicle

The clavicle lies in a subcutaneous position. It articulates with the sternum medially and the acromion process of the scapula laterally (Fig. 3.5). Medially, supporting the sternoclavicular joint, the costoclavicular ligament attaches the sternal end of the clavicle to the first rib and laterally, supporting the acromioclavicular joint, the coracoclavicular ligament attaches the infero-lateral surface of the clavicle to the coracoid process. These strong ligaments prevent joint dislocation. The subclavius is a small muscle which inserts into a longitudinal groove on the inferior surface of the clavicle.

Scapula

The scapula is a flat, triangular bone which lies on the posterior thoracic wall. It features superior, medial and lateral borders, and superior, inferior and lateral angles (Fig. 3.6). The glenoid cavity on the lateral edge of the scapula,

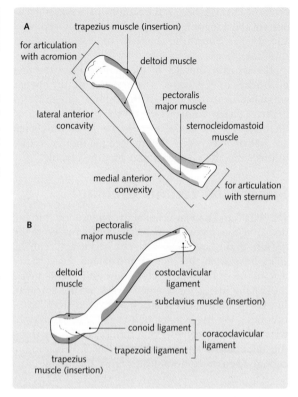

Fig. 3.5 Superior (A) and inferior (B) aspects of the right clavicle and its muscular attachments.

articulates with the head of the humerus. The coracoid process lies anterior to the glenoid cavity and provides attachment for muscles and ligaments. The subscapular fossa forms the anterior surface of the scapula. The posterior surface is divided by the spine of the scapula, into the supraspinous and infraspinous fossae. The spine features a lateral expansion – the acromion process. Medially, the scapula is attached to the vertebral column via trapezius, levator scapulae and rhomboid major and minor muscles. Laterally it is attached to the humerus via the rotator cuff and deltoid muscles.

CLINICAL NOTE

Fractures of the clavicle

Fractures of the clavicle occur most commonly at the narrowest point – the junction of the outer and middle thirds. Fractures can occur as a result of direct trauma, or by falling onto an outstretched arm, when the force of a fall is transmitted to the sternoclavicular joint through the clavicle. The weight of the upper limb depresses the lateral fragment, whilst the medial fragment causes 'tenting' (which describes the appearance) of the skin.

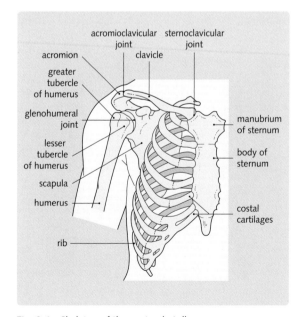

Fig. 3.4 Skeleton of the pectoral girdle.

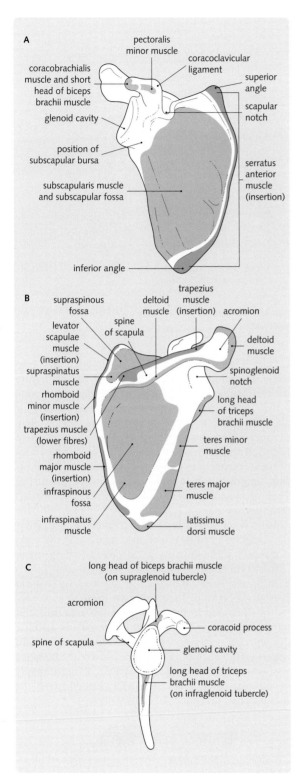

Fig. 3.6 Anterior (A), posterior (B), and lateral (C) aspects of the right scapula and its muscular attachments.

Joints of the pectoral girdle

Sternoclavicular joint

The sternoclavicular joint is an atypical synovial joint – its articular sufaces are covered by fibrocartilage rather than hyaline cartilage. The presence of an articular disc separates the joint into two cavities, which prevents the clavicle from overriding the sternum. The joint is surrounded by a capsule and is reinforced by anterior and posterior sternoclavicular ligaments, and the costo-clavicular ligament. As the lateral end of the clavicle moves, its medial end moves in the opposite direction, moving around the axis of the coracoclavicular ligaments. The joint is supplied by the medial supra-clavicular nerve (C3–C4).

Acromioclavicular joint

The acromoclavicular joint is also an atypical synovial joint, between the lateral end of the clavicle and the medial surface of the acromion. The joint is surrounded by a capsule and is reinforced by several ligaments. Superiorly, the capsule is thickened to form the acromio-clavicular ligament. However, the major support for the joint is the coracoclavicular ligament. This ligament is composed of two parts – the trapezoid and conoid ligaments, which connect the inferior aspect of the clavicle to the coracoid process of the scapula. The joint is supplied by the lateral supraclavicular nerve (C3–C4).

Glenohumeral joint

Humerus

The proximal humerus is shown in Figure 3.7. The head articulates with the glenoid cavity of the scapula. The greater tubercle of the humerus lies lateral to the intertubercular sulcus and the lesser tubercle lies on the medial side. The anatomical neck lies between the tubercles and the humeral head. The surgical neck lies more distally, between the tuberosities and the shaft, and is related to the axillary nerve and circumflex arter-ies. The spiral groove lies on the posterior surface of the shaft and is related to the radial nerve.

> **CLINICAL NOTE**
>
> **Orthopaedics**
>
> The surgical neck of the humerus is commonly fractured. The importance of this fracture is its relationship to the axillary nerve and the anterior and posterior circumflex arteries. The axillary nerve supplies the deltoid muscle. It also provides a cutaneous supply to the skin. Humeral

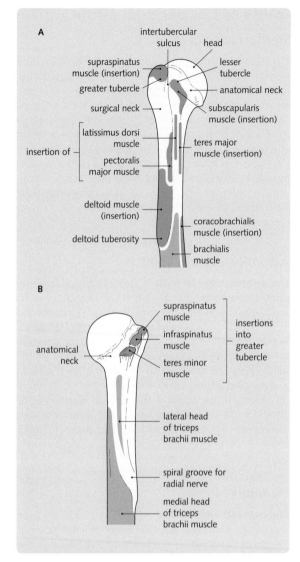

Fig. 3.7 Anterior (A) and posterior (B) views of the distal end of the humerus and its muscle attachments.

fractures or glenohumeral joint dislocation can result in damage to the axillary nerve, leading to weakness of shoulder abduction and loss of cutaneous sensation (anaesthesia) over the deltoid muscle. Injury to the circumflex arteries may result in haematoma.

The glenohumeral joint is a multiaxial, ball-and-socket synovial joint (Fig. 3.8). There is a wide range of movement at the joint, which comes at the expense of joint stability. The head of the humerus is large compared with the shallow glenoid cavity, and the joint

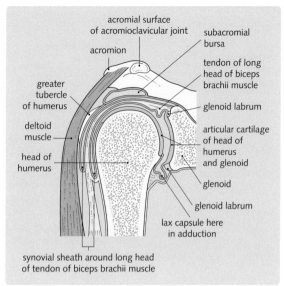

Fig. 3.8 Coronal section of the glenohumeral joint and related structures.

capsule is relatively lax, both of which result in a relatively unstable joint. However, several factors help to increase the stability of the joint. The glenoid labrum, a rim of fibrocartilage, attaches to the margins of the glenoid cavity. This serves to deepen the shallow glenoid fossa. The joint capsule is attached to the margins of the glenoid labrum and around the anatomical neck of the humerus. It is reinforced anteriorly by the superior, middle and inferior glenohumeral ligaments. These are referred to as intrinsic ligaments due to the fact that they are part of the joint capsule. Superiorly, the capsule is reinforced by a further intrinsic ligament – the coracohumeral ligament. Also reinforcing the superior aspect of the joint is the coracoacromial ligament, which forms part of the coraco-acromial arch (along with the acromion and coracoid process). Its position prevents superior dislocation of the joint.

The tendons of the rotator cuff muscles – supraspinatus, infraspinatus, teres minor and subscapularis stabilize the superior, posterior and anterior aspects of the joint respectively, by helping to keep the head of the humerus applied to the shallow glenoid cavity. The nerve supply to the joint comes from the lateral pectoral nerve, the suprascapular nerve and the axillary nerve.

HINTS AND TIPS

The names of the muscles which form the rotator cuff – subscapularis, infraspinatus, teres minor and subscapularis – can be more easily remembered by the acronym SITS.

Fig. 3.9 Movements of the glenohumeral joint and the muscles involved.

Movement	Muscles
Flexion	Pectoralis major, anterior fibres of deltoid
Extension	Posterior fibres of deltoid, latissimus dorsi, teres major
Abduction	Deltoid, supraspinatus
Adduction	Pectoralis major, latissimus dorsi
Lateral rotation	Infraspinatus, teres minor, posterior fibres of deltoid
Medial rotation	Pectoralis major, anterior fibres of deltoid, latissimus dorsi, teres major, subscapularis
Circumduction	Varying combinations of flexion, extension, abduction, and adduction muscles

The movements at the glenohumeral joint and the muscles involved in each movement are described in Figure 3.9. The movement of abduction deserves special mention: a maximum of 120° of abduction is possible at the glenohumeral joint. Further abduction is achieved by serratus anterior and trapezius, resulting in lateral rotation of the inferior angle of the scapula. The glenoid fossa then comes to point superiorly.

Muscles of the shoulder region

Figure 3.10 outlines the major muscles of the shoulder region.

Axilla

This pyramidal shaped space lies between the upper part of the humerus and the thoracic wall. Vessels and nerves pass from the neck, through the axilla, travelling distally to supply the upper limb. The axilla is composed of an apex, four walls and a base. Its boundaries are as follows:

- The apex communicates with the root of the neck. Its boundaries are the lateral border of the first rib medially, the clavicle anteriorly and the superior border of the scapula posteriorly
- Anterior wall: pectoralis major and minor muscles, subclavius, and the clavipectoral fascia
- Posterior wall: the lateral border of the scapula, subscapularis, latissimus dorsi and teres major muscles
- Medial wall: ribs 1–4, with their associated intercostal muscles, and the overlying serratus anterior muscle

- Lateral wall: intertubercular sulcus of the humerus
- Base: composed of skin, and superficial and deep fascia.

The clavipectoral fascia is a strong sheet of connective tissue which is attached to the clavicle. It splits to enclose the subclavius muscle. Inferior to subclavius muscle the fascia forms a single layer and upon reaching pectoralis minor muscle, it splits once more to enclose the muscle. Inferior to pectoralis minor it continues as the suspensory ligament of the axilla, and is attached to the floor of the axilla. The sheet of fascia which lies between subclavius and pectoralis minor has several structures passing through it:

- Cephalic vein
- Thoracoacromial artery
- Lymphatic vessels from the infraclavicular nodes
- Lateral pectoral nerve.

The contents of the axilla are shown in Figure 3.11 and include:

- Axillary artery
- Axillary vein
- Brachial plexus
- Axillary lymph nodes.

Axillary artery

The axillary artery is a continuation of the third part of the subclavian artery. It commences at the lateral border of the first rib, becoming the brachial artery at the lower border of teres major. The axillary artery (along with the brachial plexus) is enclosed in the axillary sheath – a fascial sheath derived from the prevertebral fascia of the neck. It is divided into three parts by pectoralis minor (Fig. 3.12):

- The first part lies proximal to pectoralis minor and has one branch — the superior thoracic artery. This supplies both pectoral muscles and the thoracic wall.
- The second part lies posterior to pectoralis minor and has two branches — the thoracoacromial artery, which supplies the sternoclavicular joint, pectoral and deltoid muscles, and the lateral thoracic artery, which supplies serratus anterior, the breast and the axillary nodes.
- The third part lies distal to pectoralis major and has three branches—the subscapular artery, which supplies latissimus dorsi and forms part of a scapular anastomosis, and the anterior and posterior circumflex humeral arteries, which supply the shoulder joint.

Axillary vein

The axillary vein commences at the lower border of the teres major muscle and is the continuation of the basilic vein. It travels proximally through the axilla,

Fig. 3.10 Major muscles of the shoulder region.

Name of muscle (nerve supply)	Origin	Insertion	Action
Latissimus dorsi (thoracodorsal nerve)	Iliac crest, lumbar fascia, spinous processes of lower six thoracic vertebrae, lower ribs, scapula	Floor of intertubercular sulcus of humerus	Extends, adducts, and medially rotates arm
Levator scapulae (C3 and C4 and dorsal scapular nerve)	Transverse processes of C1–C4	Medial border of scapula	Elevates scapula
Rhomboid minor (dorsal scapular nerve)	Ligamentum nuchae, spines of C7 and T1	Medial border of scapula	Elevates and retracts medial border of scapula
Rhomboid major (dorsal scapular nerve)	Spines of T2–T5	Medial border of scapula	Elevates and retracts medial border of scapula
Trapezius (spinal part of XI nerve and C2 and C3)	Occipital bone, ligamentum nuchae, spinous processes of thoracic vertebrae	Lateral third of clavicle, acromion, spine of scapula	Elevates scapula, retracts scapula and pulls medial border of scapula downwards
Subclavius (nerve to subclavius)	First costal cartilage	Clavicle	Depresses and stabilizes the clavicle
Pectoralis major (medial and lateral pectoral nerves)	Clavicle, sternum, upper six costal cartilages	Lateral lip of intertubercular sulcus of humerus	Adducts arm, rotates it medially, and flexes humerus
Pectoralis minor (medial pectoral nerve)	Third, fourth, and fifth ribs	Coracoid process of scapula	Depresses point of shoulder protracts shoulder
Serratus anterior (long thoracic nerve)	Upper eight ribs	Medial border and inferior angle of scapula	Protracts the scapula
Deltoid (axillary nerve)	Clavicle, acromion, spine of scapula	Lateral surface of humerus (deltoid tubercle)	Abducts, flexes and medially rotates, extends and laterally rotates arm
Supraspinatus (suprascapular nerve)	Supraspinous fossa of scapula	Greater tubercle of humerus, capsule of shoulder joint	Rotator cuff muscle Initiates abduction of the arm (first 15°)
Subscapularis (upper and lower subscapular nerves)	Subscapular fossa	Lesser tubercle of humerus	Rotator cuff muscle Medially rotates arm
Teres major (lower subscapular nerve)	Lateral border of scapula	Medial lip of intertubercular sulcus of humerus	Medially rotates and adducts arm
Teres minor (axillary nerve)	Lateral border of scapula	Greater tubercle of humerus, capsule of shoulder joint	Rotator cuff muscle Laterally rotates arm
Infraspinatus (suprascapular nerve)	Infraspinous fossa of scapula	Greater tubercle of humerus, capsule of shoulder joint	Rotator cuff muscle Laterally rotates arm

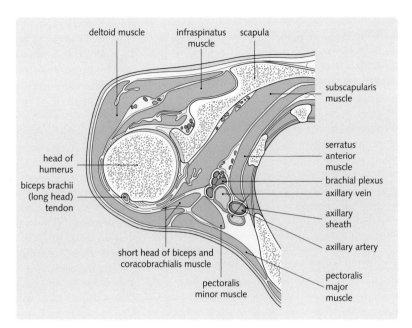

Fig. 3.11 A transverse section demonstrating the contents and muscular boundaries of the axilla.

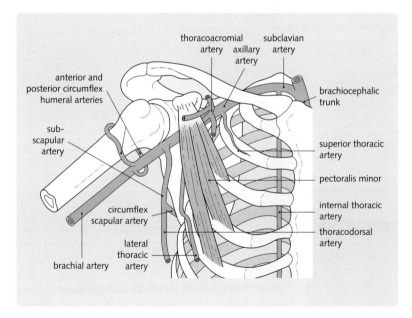

Fig. 3.12 Axillary artery and its branches.

lying medial to the axillary artery, becoming the subclavian vein at the lateral border of the first rib. The axillary vein lies outside the axillary sheath containing the axillary artery and the cords of the brachial plexus. This allows venous expansion and increased venous return during exercise.

Brachial plexus

The brachial plexus is formed from the anterior rami of spinal nerves C5–C8 and T1. Figure 3.13 illustrates the division of the plexus into roots (deep to the scalene muscles), trunks (found in the posterior triangle of the neck), divisions (behind the clavicle) and cords (named according to their position relative to the

Fig. 3.13 Brachial plexus showing the roots, trunks, divisions, cords and branches.

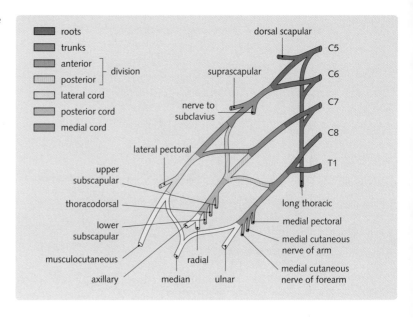

axillary artery). Figure 3.14 lists the branches of the brachial plexus along with their distribution.

CLINICAL NOTE

Surgery

During breast surgery, removal of axillary lymph nodes is common. This carries a risk of injury to the long thoracic nerve which originates from the C5–C7 roots of the brachial plexus, crosses the thoracic wall and supplies serratus anterior muscle. Serratus anterior acts to hold the scapula against the posterior wall of the thorax, and to assist in lateral rotation of the scapula – allowing the arm to be raised above the head. Damage to the long thoracic nerve and paralysis of serratus anterior muscle, leads to 'winging' of the scapula (this can be demonstrated by asking the patient to push against a wall with an outstretched arm) and difficulty in raising the arm above the head.

Axillary lymph nodes

These comprise (Fig. 3.15):

- Lateral group
- Pectoral group
- Subscapular group
- Central group
- Infraclavicular group (receives lymph from upper limb)
- Apical group.

These lymph nodes drain the lateral part of the thoracic wall including the breast, as well as the upper limb. The lateral, pectoral and subscapular groups drain into the central group of nodes. The central and infraclavicular groups of nodes drain into the apical nodes, then into the supraclavicular nodes, which eventually drain into the right lymphatic trunk and the thoracic duct on the left.

Quadrangular and triangular spaces

A number of spaces are formed by the arrangement of the muscles and bones in the axillary region which form 'gateways' between the axilla, the scapular region and the arm (Fig. 3.16). The triangular space links the axilla with the posterior scapular region. It contains the circumflex scapular artery and vein. The artery is a branch of the subscapular artery and, together with the dorsal scapular and suprascapular arteries, it forms part of an anastomosis around the scapula. If the axillary artery becomes occluded, a collateral circulation

Fig. 3.14 Branches of the brachial plexus and their distribution.

Branches	Distribution
Roots	
Dorsal scapular nerve (C5)	Rhomboid major, rhomboid minor, and levator scapulae muscles
Long thoracic nerve (C5–C7)	Serratus anterior muscle
Upper trunk	
Suprascapular nerve (C5, C6)	Supraspinatus and infraspinatus muscles
Nerve to subclavius (C5, C6)	Subclavius muscle
Lateral cord	
Lateral pectoral nerve (C5–C7)	Pectoralis major muscle
Musculocutaneous nerve (C5–C7)	Coracobrachialis, biceps brachii, brachialis muscles, and the skin along the lateral border of the forearm (lateral cutaneous nerve of the forearm)
Lateral root of median nerve (C5–C7)	Joins the medial root (C8, T1) to form the median nerve (see below)
Posterior cord	
Upper subscapular nerve (C5–C6)	Subscapularis muscle
Thoracodorsal nerve (C6–C8)	Latissimus dorsi muscle
Lower subscapular nerve (C5–C6)	Subscapularis and teres major muscles
Axillary nerve (C5–C6)	Deltoid and teres minor muscles. Skin over the lower half of the deltoid muscle (upper lateral cutaneous nerve of arm)
Radial nerve (C5–C8, T1)	Triceps, brachialis, anconeus, and posterior muscles of forearm. Skin of the posterior aspects of arm, forearm, the lateral half of the dorsum of the hand, and dorsal surface of the lateral three-and-a-half digits.
Medial cord	
Medial pectoral nerve (C8, T1)	Pectoralis major and minor muscles
Medial cutaneous nerve of the arm (C8, T1)	Skin of the medial side of the arm
Medial cutaneous nerve of the forearm (C8, T1)	Skin of the medial side of the forearm
Ulnar nerve (C8, T1)	In the forearm, flexor carpi ulnaris and medial half of flexor digitorum profundus. In the hand, hypothenar muscles, adductor pollicis, third and fourth lumbricals, palmar and dorsal interossei, palmaris brevis muscles. Skin of the medial half of the dorsum and palm of hand, skin of the palmar, and dorsal surfaces of the medial one-and-a-half digits (palmar and dorsal digital cutaneous branches).
Median nerve (C5–C8, T1)	In the forearm, pronator teres, flexor carpi radialis, flexor digitorum superficialis (median nerve). Flexor pollicis longus, lateral half of flexor digitorum profundus and pronator quadratus (anterior interosseous branch). In the hand, thenar muscles, first two lumbricals (median nerve). Skin of lateral half of palm and palmar surface of lateral three-and-a-half digits (palmar and digital cutaneous branches).

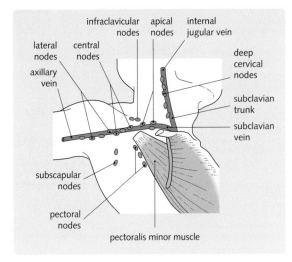

Fig. 3.15 Arrangement of the right axillary lymph nodes.

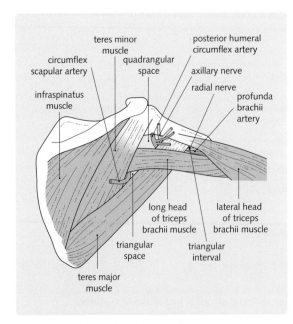

Fig. 3.16 Quadrangular and triangular spaces.

may develop, allowing blood to flow from the first part of the subclavian artery to the third part of the axillary artery. The quadrangular space allows passage of the axillary nerve and posterior circumflex humeral artery and vein from the axilla to the posterior scapular and deltoid regions. The triangular interval (lower triangular space) contains the radial nerve and the profunda brachii artery as they pass into the posterior compartment of the arm, within the radial groove of humerus.

THE ARM

The arm lies between the shoulder and elbow joint. It is divided into flexor (anterior) and extensor (posterior) compartments which are separated by lateral and medial intermuscular septa, arising from the deep fascia of the arm.

Flexor and extensor compartments of the arm

The bony skeleton of the arm and the sites of muscle attachment within the flexor and extensor compartments are shown in Figure 3.17. The muscles of the arm are described in Figure 3.18.

> **HINTS AND TIPS**
>
> Biceps brachii, brachialis and coracobrachialis muscles comprise the muscular components of the flexor compartment of the arm. This can be remembered by the mnemonic BBC All are innervated by the musculocutaneous nerve.

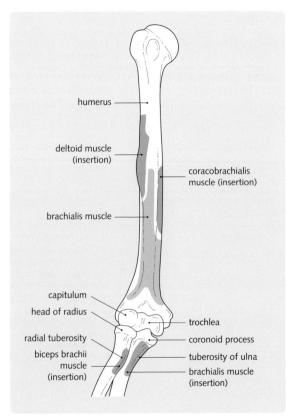

Fig. 3.17 Skeleton of the arm, showing sites of muscle attachment.

Fig. 3.18 Muscles of the arm.

Name of muscle (nerve supply)	Origin	Insertion	Action
Flexor compartment			
Biceps brachii–long head (musculocutaneous nerve)	Supraglenoid tubercle of scapula	Tuberosity of radius and bicipital aponeurosis into deep fascia of forearm	Supinator of flexed forearm, flexor of elbow joint, weak flexor of shoulder joint
Biceps brachii–short head (musculocutaneous nerve)	Coracoid process of scapula		
Coracobrachialis (musculocutaneous nerve)	Coracoid process of scapula	Shaft of humerus	Flexes and adducts shoulder joint
Brachialis (musculocutaneous nerve and radial nerve)	Anterior surface of humerus	Ulnar tuberosity and coronoid process	Flexes elbow joint
Extensor compartment			
Triceps–long head (radial nerve)	Infraglenoid tubercle of scapula	Olecranon process of ulna	Extends elbow joint
Triceps–lateral head (radial nerve)	Posterior surface of humerus (upper part)		
Triceps–medial head (radial nerve)	Posterior surface of humerus (lower part)		

Adapted from *Clinical Anatomy, An Illustrated Review with Questions and Explanations,* 2nd edn, by RS Snell, Little Brown & Co

Vessels of the arm

Arterial supply

The brachial artery is a continuation of the axillary artery. It commences at the lower border of teres major muscle (Fig. 3.19) and terminates in the cubital fossa (at the neck of the radius), where it divides into radial and ulnar arteries. It supplies the flexor compartment of the arm. The artery is superficial and palpable throughout its course, being covered by skin and fascia only. Within the cubital fossa, it lies medial to the tendon of biceps brachii.

The profunda brachii artery arises from the lateral side of the brachial artery. It passes into the extensor compartment of the arm via the triangular interval (Page 40), and travels in the radial groove of the humerus along with with the radial nerve. It supplies the extensor compartment of the arm, and ends by dividing into two collateral branches, which anastomose with recurrent radial and ulnar branches to form a collateral circulation around the elbow.

Venous drainage

Usually a pair of veins accompany the brachial artery (venae comitantes of the brachial artery). The venae comitantes receive tributaries which correspond to branches of the brachial arteries. The basilic vein travels superficially along the medial aspect of the arm, penetrates the deep fascia in the middle of the arm and joins with the venae comitantes to form the brachial vein. It becomes the axillary vein at the inferior border of the teres major muscle. The cephalic vein travels along the lateral aspect of the arm. It penetrates the clavipectoral fascia and drains into the axillary vein.

Nerves of the arm

Musculocutaneous nerve

The musculocutaneous nerve is the terminal branch of the lateral cord of the brachial plexus. It pierces coracobrachialis muscle in the arm, then travels distally between biceps brachii and brachialis muscles,

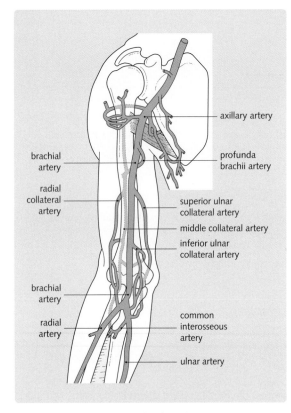

brachial artery

profunda brachii artery

axillary artery

radial collateral artery

superior ulnar collateral artery

middle collateral artery

inferior ulnar collateral artery

brachial artery

radial artery

common interosseous artery

ulnar artery

Fig. 3.19 Brachial artery and its branches.

ulnar collateral artery. It continues distally, travelling between the medial intermuscular septum and the medial head of triceps to reach the posterior aspect of the medial epicondyle of the humerus. It then passes between the two heads of flexor carpi ulnaris muscle to enter the forearm. The ulnar nerve has no branches in the arm.

> **HINTS AND TIPS**
>
> Pressure on the ulnar nerve as it crosses behind the medial epicondyle of the humerus results in a tingling sensation in the medial one and a half digits of the hand. This is the same sensation which is felt when you hit your 'funny bone'.

Radial nerve

The radial nerve is a continuation of the posterior cord of the brachial plexus. It exits the axilla via the triangular interval and enters the posterior compartment of the arm, along with the profunda brachii artery (Fig. 3.16). Both travel distally, from medial to lateral, in direct contact with the spiral groove of the humerus. On the lateral side of the humerus, the radial nerve pierces the lateral intermuscular septum to enter the flexor compartment of the arm. It passes anterior to the lateral epicondyle of the humerus, deep to the brachioradialis muscle, and enters the forearm. Branches of the radial nerve which originate in the axilla and arm provide a motor supply to the three heads of triceps brachii and anconeus, and a sensory supply to the skin of the arm as the posterior cutaneous nerve of the arm, the lower lateral cutaneous nerve of the arm, and the posterior cutaneous nerve of the forearm. Branches at the level of the elbow joint provide a motor supply to the lateral fibres of brachioradialis and extensor carpi radialis longus.

providing a nerve supply to all three of these muscles in the flexor compartment. It terminates by piercing the deep fascia at the elbow to become the lateral cutaneous nerve of the forearm.

Median nerve

The median nerve is formed by the lateral and medial roots of the brachial plexus. It enters the flexor compartment of the arm and intially lies lateral to the brachial artery. In the middle of the arm, the nerve crosses anterior to the brachial artery, coming to lie on its medial side. It enters the cubital fossa between the brachial artery and the tendon of biceps where it lies deep to the bicipital aponeurosis. The median nerve has no branches in the arm, however a branch to pronator teres (one of the muscles of the forearm) may arise proximal to the elbow joint.

Ulnar nerve

The ulnar nerve exits the axilla medial to the axillary artery and travels distally through the anterior compartment of the arm. Approximately halfway down the arm it pierces the medial intermuscular septum to enter the extensor compartment, accompanied by the superior

> **HINTS AND TIPS**
>
> The radial nerve runs in the spiral groove, making it vulnerable to damage in the event of a midshaft fracture of the humerus. Damage results in paralysis of the extensor muscles of the forearm, resulting in wrist drop. Triceps brachii muscle is unaffected by this type of injury since the branches of the radial nerve which supply it originate proximal to the radial groove.

The medial cutaneous nerve of the arm is a direct branch of the brachial plexus which supplies the skin over the medial aspect of the arm.

THE ELBOW JOINT AND CUBITAL FOSSA

Elbow joint

The elbow joint is a synovial hinge joint between the distal end of the humerus and the proximal end of the radius and the ulna (Fig. 3.20). The articular surfaces comprise:

- The capitulum of the humerus which articulates with the head of the radius
- The trochlea of the humerus which articulates with the trochlear notch of the ulna.

Movements of the elbow joint are limited to flexion and extension. Independent rotation of the radius occurs at the proximal radioulnar joint in the movements of pronation and supination of the forearm. The joint capsule is lax anteroposteriorly, but it is thickened medially to form collateral ligaments:

- The ulnar collateral ligament lies on the medial side of the joint capsule, and passes from the the medial epicondyle of the humerus to the ulna.
- The radial collateral ligament lies on the lateral side of the joint capsule and attaches the lateral epicondyle of the humerus to the anular ligament of the radius.
- The anular ligament of the radius is attached to the margins of the radial notch of the ulna. It holds the head of the radius in the radial notch of the ulna. This articulation between the radius and ulna forms the proximal radioulnar joint.

The nerve supply of the elbow joint arises from the musculocutaneous, median, ulnar and radial nerves.

Cubital fossa

The cubital fossa is a triangular region lying anterior to the elbow joint. Its boundaries are:

- Laterally: brachioradialis
- Medial: pronator teres
- Base: an imaginary line drawn between the medial and lateral epicondyles of the humerus
- Floor: proximally, brachialis muscle and distally, supinator
- Roof: skin, superficial fascia, and the bicipital aponeurosis.

Figure 3.21 shows the contents of the cubital fossa. The contents of the cubital fossa from medial to lateral

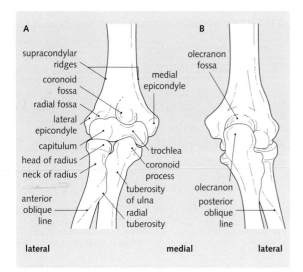

Fig. 3.20 Anterior (A) and posterior (B) aspects of the humerus and the upper end of the ulna and radius.

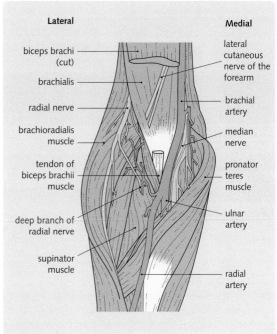

Fig. 3.21 Contents of the cubital fossa.

are: the median nerve, the brachial artery and the tendon of biceps brachii.

Note:

- The brachial artery lies deep to the bicipital aponeurosis. It usually divides into the radial and ulnar arteries within the cubital fossa (although this can vary between individuals).
- The median nerve exits the cubital fossa between the ulnar and humeral heads of pronator teres.
- The medial cutaneous nerve of the forearm (a direct branch of the medial cord of the brachial plexus) lies superficial to pronator teres.
- The radial nerve enters the anterior compartment of the arm between brachialis and brachioradialis. It commonly divides into a deep motor and superficial cutaneous branch in the cubital fossa.
- The lateral cutaneous nerve of the forearm emerges between biceps and brachialis.
- Superficially, the median cubital vein lies between the basilic and cephalic veins.

CLINICAL NOTE

Measurement of blood pressure

During measurement of blood pressure, the cuff of the sphygmomanometer is wrapped around the arm, and the stethoscope is placed over the brachial artery, in the cubital fossa. As the cuff is slowly deflated Korotkov sounds (K1–K5) are heard upon auscultation. The first sound heard after cuff pressure is released is known as K1 – the pressure reading on the sphygmomanometer at which this is heard, represents the systolic blood pressure. The sounds heard upon auscultation are due to turbulent arterial blood flow as a result of narrowing of the arterial lumen by the cuff. K5 denotes the point at which sounds heard upon auscultation disappear. This equates to diastolic blood pressure.

CLINICAL NOTE

Venepuncture

Venepuncture is a procedure which allows blood samples to be taken for a variety of biochemical, microbiological or immunological investigations. The median cubital vein in the median cubital fossa, is a commonly used site for venepuncture. A tourniquet is applied to the arm above the cubital fossa, to hinder venous return from the forearm, making the medial cubital vein more prominent.

THE FOREARM

The forearm lies between the elbow and wrist joints. It contains the radius and the ulna, united by the interosseous membrane; a strong thin membrane attached to each bone at its interosseous border. The interosseous membrane provides attachments for muscles. Superiorly it is incomplete, allowing the passage of the posterior interosseous vessels. Inferiorly it is pierced by the anterior interosseous vessels.

Radioulnar joints

Pronation and supination occur at the proximal and distal radioulnar joints. At the proximal radioulnar joint, the head of the radius is held within the anular ligament, which is attached to the anterior and posterior edges of the radial notch of the ulna. The head of the radius rotates within the anular ligament during pronation and supination.

At the distal radioulnar joint the head of the ulna articulates with the ulnar notch of the radius. The distal ends of the radius and ulna are held together by an articular disc (known as the triangular ligament). The disc also separates the distal radioulnar joint from the radiocarpal joint. The distal radius rotates medially and laterally over the ulna during pronation and supination respectively.

Supinator, biceps brachii and brachioradialis supinate the hand. Pronator teres and pronator quadratus pronate the hand.

HINTS AND TIPS

Remember that flexion and extension occur at the elbow joint; rotation occurs at the proximal and distal radioulnar joints.

CLINICAL NOTE

Colles' fracture

A Colles' fracture may occur in postmenopausal women, in whom osteoporosis is common. The fracture often occurs as a result of a fall onto an outstretched hand. The distal end of the radius (approximately 2.5 cm from the distal end) is fractured, dorsally (posteriorly) displaced and in some cases comminuted (broken into small pieces). The injury produces a 'dinner fork' deformity of the wrist.

As in the arm, the forearm is divided into flexor (anterior) and extensor (posterior) compartments (Fig. 3.22).

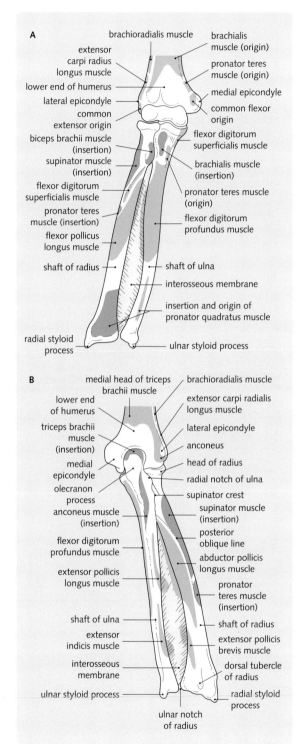

A
brachioradialis muscle
extensor carpi radius longus muscle
lower end of humerus
lateral epicondyle
common extensor origin
biceps brachii muscle (insertion)
supinator muscle (insertion)
flexor digitorum superficialis muscle
pronator teres muscle (insertion)
flexor pollicus longus muscle
shaft of radius
radial styloid process

brachialis muscle (origin)
pronator teres muscle (origin)
medial epicondyle
common flexor origin
flexor digitorum superficialis muscle
brachialis muscle (insertion)
pronator teres muscle (origin)
flexor digitorum profundus muscle
shaft of ulna
interosseous membrane
insertion and origin of pronator quadratus muscle
ulnar styloid process

B
medial head of triceps brachii muscle
lower end of humerus
triceps brachii muscle (insertion)
medial epicondyle
olecranon process
anconeus muscle (insertion)
flexor digitorum profundus muscle
extensor pollicis longus muscle
shaft of ulna
extensor indicis muscle
interosseous membrane
ulnar styloid process

brachioradialis muscle
extensor carpi radialis longus muscle
lateral epicondyle
anconeus
head of radius
radial notch of ulna
supinator crest
supinator muscle (insertion)
posterior oblique line
abductor pollicis longus muscle
pronator teres muscle (insertion)
shaft of radius
extensor pollicis brevis muscle
dorsal tubercle of radius
radial styloid process
ulnar notch of radius

Fig. 3.22 Anterior (A) and posterior (B) aspects of the right radius and ulna, showing sites of muscular attachments.

Flexor compartment of the forearm

Muscles of the flexor compartment

The muscles of the flexor compartment can be divided into superficial and deep groups. There are six superficial muscles, all of which originate from the medial epicondyle of the humerus. This is known as the common flexor origin (Fig. 3.22A). There are three deep muscles which originate from the forearm bones and the interosseous membrane (Fig. 3.23).

Arteries of the flexor compartment

The brachial artery enters the forearm through the cubital fossa, where it divides into the radial and ulnar arteries (Fig. 3.24). The ulnar artery passes deep to pronator teres and accompanies the ulnar nerve, both structures becoming superficial at the wrist. The radial artery accompanies the superficial branch of the radial nerve to the wrist. The radial pulse is palpable over the distal radius.

Nerves of the flexor compartment

Median nerve

The median nerve enters the forearm between the two heads of pronator teres. It crosses the ulnar artery and runs deep to flexor digitorum superficialis until just proximal to the wrist, where it becomes superficial between the tendon of this muscle, and the tendon of flexor carpi radialis.

Branches of the median nerve in the forearm comprise:

- Muscular branches to all of the muscles in the flexor compartment of the arm, with the exception of flexor carpi ulnaris and the medial half of flexor digitorum profundus (which are supplied by the ulnar nerve). Superficial muscles are supplied directly by the median nerve, whilst the deep muscles are supplied by the anterior interosseous nerve.
- The anterior interosseous nerve: this arises from the median nerve as it passes between the two heads of pronator teres. It travels distally with the anterior interosseous artery (a branch of the ulnar artery) through the forearm, on the anterior surface of the interosseous membrane, between flexor pollicis longus and flexor digitorum profundus. It supplies the deep muscles of the flexor compartment – flexor pollicis longus, the lateral part of flexor digitorum profundus and pronator quadratus. It also provides articular branches to the distal radioulnar, wrist and carpal joints.
- The palmar cutaneous nerve: this arises proximal to the wrist joint and provides a sensory supply to the skin over the thenar eminence and the central part of the palm of the hand.
- Unnamed articular branches to the elbow and proximal radioulnar joints.

Fig. 3.23 Muscles of the flexor compartment of the forearm.

Name of muscle (nerve supply)	Origin	Insertion	Action
Superficial			
Pronator teres – humeral head (median nerve)	Common flexor origin and medial supracondylar ridge	Lateral aspect of shaft of radius	Pronation of forearm and flexion of elbow
Pronator teres – ulnar head (median nerve)	Coronoid process of ulna		
Flexor carpi radialis (median nerve)	Common flexor origin	Second and third metacarpal bones	Flexion and abduction of wrist joint
Flexor carpi ulnaris – humeral head (ulnar nerve)	Common flexor origin	Pisiform and through pisometacarpal ligament to fifth metacarpal bone	Flexion and abduction of wrist joint
Flexor carpi ulnaris – ulnar head (ulnar nerve)	Olecranon process and posterior border of ulna		
Palmaris longus (median nerve)	Common flexor origin	Palmar aponeurosis	Flexion of wrist joint
Flexor digitorum superficialis – humeroulnar head (median nerve)	Common flexor origin and coronoid process of ulna	Middle phalanges of medial four digits	Flexion of PIP and MCP joints of the medial four digits and wrist joint
Flexor digitorum superficialis – radial head (median nerve)	Anterior oblique line of radius		
Deep			
Pronator quadratus (anterior interosseous nerve)	Anterior surface of ulna	Anterior surface of radius	Pronation of forearm
Flexor pollicis longus (anterior interosseous nerve)	Anterior surface of radius and interosseous membrane	Distal phalanx of thumb	Flexion of interphalangeal and MCP joints
Flexor digitorum profundus (medial half by ulnar nerve and lateral half by anterior interosseous nerve)	Anterior surface of ulna and interosseous membrane	Distal phalanges of medial four digits	Flexion of DIP, PIP, MCP, and wrist joint

DIP, distal interphalangeal; PIP, proximal interphalangeal; MCP, metacarpophalangeal.

CLINICAL NOTE

Allen's test

Allen's test is commonly performed to assess the patency of the arterial supply to the hand, before cannulating the radial artery or, less commonly, before taking an arterial blood gas sample. These procedures can result in radial artery spasm or occlusion of the artery by a clot, therefore an adequate collateral circulation to the hand is required to prevent ischaemia. The patient is asked to elevate their hand and make a fist for 20–30 seconds. The radial and ulnar arteries are occluded at the wrist by applying pressure. If sufficient pressure is applied, the hand will blanch (become pale). Pressure on the ulnar artery is released and the colour of the hand is observed. If the hand refills with blood within 5–7 seconds, turning pink, the ulnar artery is patent. This means that there is an adequate collateral circulation and it is safe to take an arterial blood sample or cannulate the radial artery.

- A dorsal branch, which passes deep to the tendon of flexor carpi ulnaris to reach the dorsal aspect of the hand. It provides sensory innervation to the dorsal surface of the medial one-and-a-half digits.

Radial nerve

The radial nerve enters the forearm deep to the brachioradialis muscle. It immediately divides into a superficial and a deep branch. The deep branch passes laterally around the radius between the two heads of the supinator muscle, into the extensor compartment of the forearm, where it becomes the posterior interosseous nerve. The deep branch and the posterior interosseous nerve provide a motor supply to muscles of the extensor compartment of the forearm. The superficial branch continues distally in the forearm deep to brachioradialis, accompanied by the radial artery. The nerve and artery then pass onto the dorsum of the hand. The superficial branch of the radial nerve provides a sensory supply to the skin over the dorsal surface of the lateral three and a half digits, as far as the distal interphalangeal joints. Cutaneous sensation beyond the distal interphalangeal joints is supplied by the median nerve.

Extensor compartment of the forearm

Muscles of the extensor compartment

The muscles of the extensor compartment of the forearm can be divided into superficial and deep groups (Fig. 3.25). The superficial group of muscles consists of seven muscles, all of which arise from the lateral epicondyle and the supracondylar ridge of the humerus. This is known as the common extensor origin. The deep group consists of five muscles (Figs 3.22A and B).

Vessels of the extensor compartment

The arterial supply to the extensor compartment of the forearm is provided by the anterior and posterior interosseous arteries along with branches of the radial artery. The common interosseous artery is a branch of the ulnar artery, which arises near its origin. It divides into the anterior and posterior interosseous arteries. The anterior interosseous artery travels distally on the anterior surface of the interosseous membrane. As it does so, it gives off branches which pass through the membrane, to supply the deep muscles of the extensor compartment of the forearm. The artery eventually passes through an opening in the distal end of the interosseous membrane to anastomose with the posterior interosseous artery. The anterior interosseous artery contributes to the palmar and dorsal carpal arches of the hand. The posterior interosseous artery passes posteriorly proximal to the upper border of the interosseous membrane.

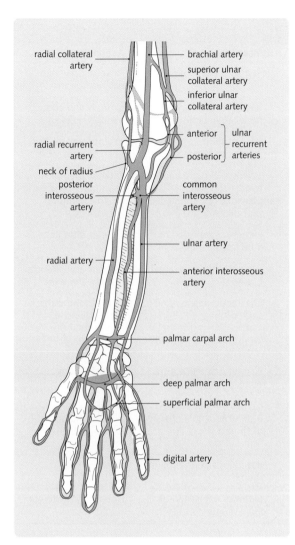

Fig. 3.24   Arterial supply of the right forearm.

Ulnar nerve

The ulnar nerve passes posterior to the medial epicondyle of the humerus and enters the anterior compartment of the forearm, passing between the two heads of flexor carpi ulnaris. It then travels distally between flexor carpi ulnaris and flexor digitorum profundus, accompanied by the ulnar artery. In the distal half of the forearm, both the artery and nerve become superficial, lying lateral to the tendon of flexor carpi ulnaris. In the forearm, branches of the ulnar nerve comprise:

- Muscular branches to flexor carpi ulnaris and the medial half of flexor digitorum profundus
- A palmar cutaneous branch, which supplies the skin over the medial part of the palm

Fig. 3.25 Muscles of the extensor compartment of the forearm.

Name of muscle (nerve supply)	Origin	Insertion	Action
Brachioradialis (radial nerve)	Lateral supracondylar ridge of humerus	Styloid process of radius	Flexes elbow and rotates forearm
Extensor carpi radialis longus (radial nerve)		Base of second metacarpal bone	Extends and abducts hand at wrist joint
Extensor carpi radialis brevis (posterior interosseous nerve)		Base of third metacarpal bone	Extends and abducts hand at wrist joint
Extensor digitorum (posterior interosseous nerve)	Common extensor origin	Extensor expansion of middle and distal phalanges of the medial four digits	Extends the medial four fingers and hand at wrist joint
Extensor digiti minimi (posterior interosseous nerve)		Extensor expansion of little finger	Extends little finger
Extensor carpi ulnaris (posterior interosseous nerve)		Base of fifth metacarpal bone	Extends and adducts hand at the wrist
Anconeus (radial nerve)		Olecranon process and shaft of ulna	Extends and stabilizes the elbow joint
Supinator (posterior interosseous nerve)	Common extensor origin and supinator crest of ulna	Neck and shaft of radius	Supination of forearm
Abductor pollicis longus (posterior interosseous nerve)	Shafts of radius and ulna and interosseous membrane	Base of first metacarpal bone	Abducts thumb
Extensor pollicis brevis (posterior interosseous nerve)	Shaft of radius and interosseous membrane	Base of proximal phalanx of thumb	Extends metacarpo-phalangeal joint of thumb
Extensor pollicis longus (posterior interosseous nerve)	Shaft of ulna and interosseous membrane	Base of distal phalynx of thumb	Extends thumb
Extensor indicis (posterior interosseous nerve)		Extensor expansion of index finger	Extends index finger

It accompanies the posterior interosseous nerve to supply the deep muscles of the extensor compartment. The posterior interosseous artery also contributes to the palmar and dorsal carpal arches of the hand. The radial artery also provides branches to the muscles of the extensor compartment.

Nerves of the extensor compartment

The radial nerve supplies the extensor compartment of the forearm. It divides into superficial and deep branches in the cubital fossa. The deep motor branch passes between the two heads of supinator, enters the extensor compartment, becoming the posterior interosseous nerve, which travels between the superficial and deep layers of muscles. Brachioradialis and extensor carpi radialis longus are supplied directly by the radial nerve (prior to its division into superficial and deep branches). All of the remaining muscles of the extensor compartment are supplied by the posterior interosseous nerve. The nerve ends at the wrist joint, which it also supplies.

Anatomical snuffbox

When the thumb is fully extended a depression appears proximal to the base of the first metacarpal. This is the anatomical snuffbox. In the anatomical position the anterior border is formed by the tendons of abductor pollicis longus and extensor pollicis brevis. The posterior margin is formed by the tendon of extensor pollicis longus. The cephalic vein and the superficial radial nerve lie superficial to the tendons of the snuffbox. The floor is formed by the radial styloid, scaphoid and trapezium bones. The radial artery crosses the floor en route to the dorsum of the hand.

THE WRIST AND HAND

Figure 3.26 shows the skeleton of the wrist and hand.

Radiocarpal joint

The radiocarpal (wrist) joint is a synovial joint. The joint is composed of the distal end of the radius, the scaphoid, lunate and triquetral bones, and the articular disc which overlies the distal end of the ulna. The disc separates the radiocarpal joint from the distal radio-ulnar joint (Fig. 3.27). The joint capsule is reinforced by radiocarpal, ulnocarpal and collateral ligaments. The nerve supply to the joint is via the anterior and posterior interosseous nerves.

Flexion, extension, abduction, adduction and circumduction are possible at the radiocarpal joint.

The styloid process of the radius extends further distally when compared with the styloid process of the ulna, limiting abduction relative to adduction. Flexion and extension involves the radiocarpal joint, with a contribution from the midcarpal joints (synovial joints between the proximal and distal rows of carpal bones). Adduction occurs mainly at the radiocarpal joint, with the triquetrum articulating with the medial surface of the radius, whereas abduction occurs mainly at the midcarpal joint.

Dorsum of the hand

The skin on the dorsum of the hand is thin and loose, and the dorsal venous network of veins which drains into the cephalic and basilic veins is usually visible. The long extensor tendons of the forearm lie deep to the superficial veins. As the tendons cross the wrist joint they are surrounded by synovial sheaths and bound down by the extensor retinaculum which is attached to the radius, the pisiform and triquetral bones. When the extensor tendons reach the proximal phalanges of the digits, they divide into three slips. A central slip inserts into each middle phalanx and two collateral slips insert into each distal phalanx. The tendons of the interossei and lumbricals insert into the collateral slips of the extensor tendons forming the extensor expansion (Fig. 3.28).

Nerve supply to the dorsum of the hand

Figure 3.29 shows the cutaneous innervation of the hand. Note that the fingertips of the lateral three-and-a-half and the medial one-and-a-half digits are supplied by palmar digital branches of the median and ulnar nerves respectively.

Vessels of the dorsum of the hand

Figure 3.30 shows the blood supply to the dorsum of the hand.

Palm of the hand

Skin

The skin is thick and hairless. Flexure creases and papillary ridges occupy the entire flexor surface, improving the gripping ability of the hand. Fibrous bands bind the skin down to the palmar aponeurosis and divide the subcutaneous fat into loculi, forming a cushion capable of withstanding pressure. A small muscle – palmaris brevis – attaches the dermis of the skin to the underlying palmar aponeurosis and flexor retinaculum on the medial aspect of the hand. Its action of wrinkling the skin over the hypothenar eminence improves the ability to grip objects.

Palmar aponeurosis

The palmar aponeurosis lies deep to the skin and superficial fascia. The central portion is a triangular-shaped thickening of deep fascia, which is continuous with thinner portions of deep fascia, overlying the thenar and hypothenar eminences respectively. Proximally it is attached to the flexor retinaculum and is continuous with the tendon of palmaris longus muscle. Distally it divides into four slips, which cross the metacarpophalangeal joints and attach to the proximal phalanges of the fingers and the fibrous flexor sheaths. The longitudinal slips which enter the digits are linked by transverse fibres. The flexor tendons, nerves and blood vessels of the hand lie deep to the palmar aponeurosis.

Continued

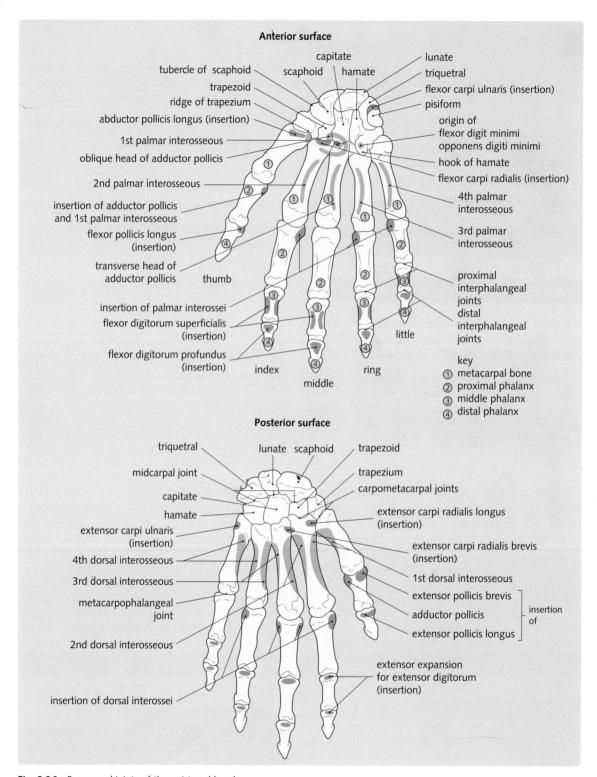

Anterior surface

capitate

tubercle of scaphoid
scaphoid
hamate
lunate
triquetral

trapezoid
flexor carpi ulnaris (insertion)

ridge of trapezium
pisiform

abductor pollicis longus (insertion)
origin of
flexor digit minimi
opponens digiti minimi

1st palmar interosseous

oblique head of adductor pollicis
hook of hamate

flexor carpi radialis (insertion)

2nd palmar interosseous
4th palmar
interosseous

insertion of adductor pollicis
and 1st palmar interosseous

flexor pollicis longus
(insertion)
3rd palmar
interosseous

transverse head of
adductor pollicis   thumb
proximal
interphalangeal
joints

insertion of palmar interossei
distal
interphalangeal
joints

flexor digitorum superficialis
(insertion)
little

flexor digitorum profundus
(insertion)   index   ring

middle

key
① metacarpal bone
② proximal phalanx
③ middle phalanx
④ distal phalanx

Posterior surface

triquetral
lunate scaphoid
trapezoid

midcarpal joint
trapezium

capitate
carpometacarpal joints

hamate
extensor carpi radialis longus
(insertion)

extensor carpi ulnaris
(insertion)

4th dorsal interosseous
extensor carpi radialis brevis
(insertion)

3rd dorsal interosseous
1st dorsal interosseous

metacarpophalangeal
joint
extensor pollicis brevis ⎤
adductor pollicis   ⎬ insertion
                            ⎪ of
extensor pollicis longus ⎦

2nd dorsal interosseous

extensor expansion
for extensor digitorum
(insertion)

insertion of dorsal interossei

Fig. 3.26 Bones and joints of the wrist and hand.

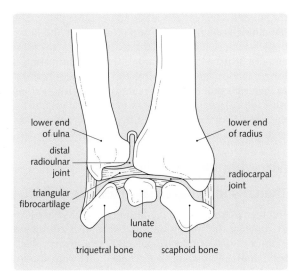

Fig. 3.27 Relationship of the distal radioulnar joint to the radiocarpal joint.

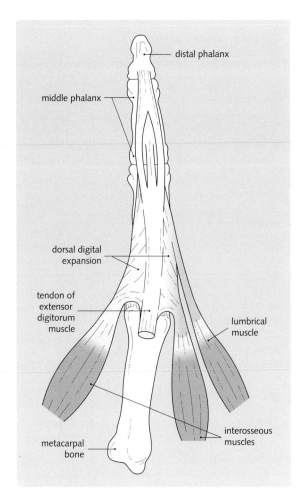

Fig. 3.28 Dorsal digital expansion and extensor tendon.

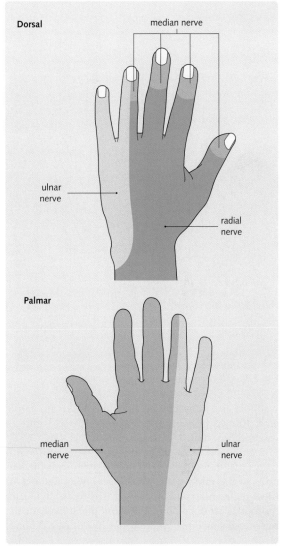

Fig. 3.29 Cutaneous innervation of the dorsal and palmar surfaces of the hand.

distal interphalangeal joints, particularly of the 4th and 5th digits, is observed. Its cause is unclear, however it occurs more frequently after the age of 40, in males, in people with a family history of the condition, and in people with cirrhosis of the liver. It can significantly affect hand function and surgery to release the affected band may be required.

Flexor retinaculum and carpal tunnel

The flexor retinaculum is a strong band of deep fascia which lies anterior to the wrist. It is attached to the pisiform and the hook of the hamate medially, and to the

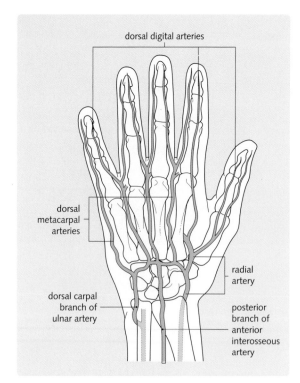

dorsal digital arteries

dorsal metacarpal arteries

dorsal carpal branch of ulnar artery

radial artery

posterior branch of anterior interosseous artery

Fig. 3.30 Vessels of the dorsum of the hand.

scaphoid and trapezium laterally. It converts the carpal arch, formed by the carpal bones (Fig. 3.26) into an osseofibrous tunnel – the carpal tunnel (Fig. 3.31). The tendons of flexor digitorum superficialis muscle initially enter the carpal tunnel in two rows, with the tendons of the middle and ring fingers lying anterior to those of the index and little finger. The flexor digitorum profundus tendons lie in the same plane beneath the superficialis tendons. At the distal row of carpal bones

the superficialis tendons all lie in the same plane. The remaining contents of the carpal tunnel are the flexor pollicis longus tendon and the median nerve (the most anterior structure in the carpal tunnel). The palmaris longus tendon, the ulnar nerve and artery lie superficial to the flexor retinaculum. The flexor retinaculum along with the adjacent carpal bones provide the origins for the muscles of the thenar and hypothenar eminences.

Muscles of the hand

Thenar and hypothenar eminence

The thenar eminence is the prominent region between the base of the thumb and the wrist. It is composed of three muscles: abductor pollicis brevis, flexor pollicis brevis and opponens pollicis. These muscles are responsible for fine movements of the thumb, especially opposition and the pinch grip. The hypothenar eminence lies between the base of the little finger and the wrist. It is composed of the abductor digiti minimi, flexor digiti minimi and opponens digiti minimi (Fig. 3.32).

CLINICAL NOTE

Carpal tunnel syndrome

Carpal tunnel syndrome (CTS) arises from compression of the median nerve due to inflammation of the synovial sheaths surrounding the long tendons of the fingers. Pain and paraesthesia over the lateral three-and-a-half digits (the cutaneous distribution of the median nerve), along with weakness and wasting of the thenar muscles – leading to impaired precision and pinch grip, are common symptoms.

Continued

Fig. 3.31 Cross-section of the right carpal tunnel at the distal row of carpal bones showing its contents. (Adapted from Williams P (ed) (1995) *Gray's Anatomy*, 38th edition, Churchill Livingstone.)

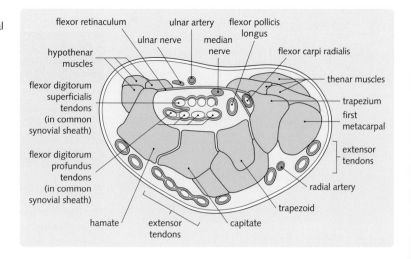

flexor retinaculum

ulnar artery

flexor pollicis longus

ulnar nerve

median nerve

hypothenar muscles

flexor carpi radialis

flexor digitorum superficialis tendons (in common synovial sheath)

thenar muscles

trapezium

first metacarpal

flexor digitorum profundus tendons (in common synovial sheath)

extensor tendons

radial artery

hamate

extensor tendons

trapezoid

capitate

Fig. 3.32   The intrinsic muscles of the hand.

Name of muscle (nerve supply)	Origin	Insertion	Action
Thenar eminence muscles			
Abductor pollicis brevis (recurrent branch of median nerve)	Scaphoid, trapezium and flexor retinaculum	Base of proximal phalanx	Abducts thumb at the MCP joint
Flexor pollicis brevis (recurrent branch of median nerve)	Trapezium and flexor retinaculum	Base of proximal phalanx	Flexes thumb at the MCP joint
Opponens pollicis (recurrent branch of median nerve)	Trapezium and flexor retinaculum	First metacarpal	Rotates metacarpal at carpometacarpal joint to oppose thumb
Hypothenar eminence muscles			
Abductor digiti minimi (deep branch of ulnar nerve)	Pisiform and flexor retinaculum	Base of proximal phalanx	Abducts little finger at the MCP joint
Flexor digiti minimi (deep branch of ulnar nerve)	Hook of hamate and flexor retinaculum	Base of proximal phalanx	Abducts little finger at the MCP joint
Opponens digiti minimi (deep branch of ulnar nerve)	Hook of hamate and flexor retinaculum	Fifth metacarpal	Assists in flexing the carpometacarpal joint, cupping the palm to assist gripping
Other intrinsic hand muscles			
Lumbricals (first and second: median nerve; third and fourth: deep branch of ulnar nerve)	Tendons of flexor digitorum profundus	Extensor expansion of the medial four digits	Extends the DIP and PIP joints of medial four digits. Flexes the MCP joint of the medial four digits
Palmar interossei (deep branch of ulnar nerve)	First, second, fourth and fifth metacarpal bones	Base of proximal phalanx and extensor expansion	Adduct the digits towards the middle finger. Flexes digit at MCP and extends interphalangeal joints
Dorsal interossei (deep branch of ulnar nerve)	Adjacent sides of the five metacarpal bones	Base of proximal phalanx and extensor expansion	Abduct the digits away from the middle finger. Flexes digit at MCP and extends interphalangeal joints
Adductor pollicis (deep branch of ulnar nerve)	Oblique head: capitate, trapezoid and second and third metacarpals. Transverse head: distal part of third metacarpal	Base of proximal phalanx	Adducts thumb
Palmaris brevis (superficial branch of the ulnar nerve)	Palmar aponeurosis and flexor retinaculum	Dermis of the skin on medial border of hand	Wrinkles the skin over the hypothenar eminence and improve the grip of the hand

DIP, distal interphalangeal; PIP, proximal interphalangeal; MCP, metacarpophalangeal.

Cutaneous sensation over the thenar eminence is unaffected – this area is supplied by the palmar branch of the median nerve, which arises proximal to the flexor retinaculum and lies superficial to it. Treatment is by surgical decompression of the carpal tunnel – achieved by dividing the flexor retinaculum.

Other intrinsic muscles of the hand

These include adductor pollicis, four dorsal and four palmar interosseous muscles, and the lumbrical muscles (Fig. 3.32). The dorsal and palmar interossei abduct and adduct the digits respectively, at the metacarpophalangeal joints. They also assist the lumbrical muscles in flexion at the metacarpophalangeal joints with extension of the interphalangeal joints.

HINTS AND TIPS

The mnemonics PAD and DAB are useful in remembering the actions of the palmar and dorsal interossei. Palmar interossei ADduct (PAD) whilst Dorsal interossei ABduct (DAB) the fingers.

Long flexor tendons in the hand

The following flexor tendons enter the hand: flexor carpi ulnaris, flexor carpi radialis, flexor digitorum superficialis and profundus, and flexor pollicis longus (only flexor digitorum superficialis and profundus, and flexor pollicis longus enter directly through the carpal tunnel). The muscle tendons are surrounded by synovial sheaths as they enter the hand through the carpal tunnel and cross the palm to the digits.

Synovial flexor tendon sheaths

Flexor digitorum superficialis and profundus tendons share a common synovial sheath which is incomplete on its radial side. The sheath begins a short distance proximal to the flexor retinaculum and ends distal to it (the flexor sheath surrounding flexor digiti minimi (to the little finger) continues to the distal phalanx). The tendons to the index, middle and ring fingers, are then bare for a short distance in the palm before becoming enclosed again as they pass over the phalanges. The bare area of the tendons of flexor digitorum profundus provides the site of origin for the lumbrical muscles. The separate synovial sheath around the flexor pollicis longus tendon extends from just proximal to the flexor retinaculum to the distal phalanx of the pollux (the thumb) (Fig. 3.33).

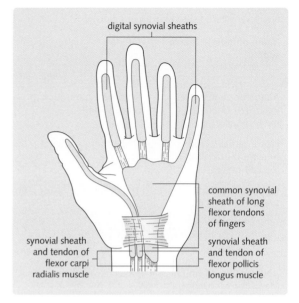

Fig. 3.33 Synovial flexor tendon sheaths in the hand.

digital synovial sheaths

common synovial sheath of long flexor tendons of fingers

synovial sheath and tendon of flexor carpi radialis muscle

synovial sheath and tendon of flexor pollicis longus muscle

HINTS AND TIPS

Penetrating hand injury can cause infection, especially if the thumb or fifth digit synovial sheaths are involved. The infection can track rapidly to the palm leading to tendon necrosis due to loss of blood flow through the vinculae.

Long flexor tendons in the digits

The tendon of flexor digitorum superficialis splits before inserting into each side of the middle phalanx, while the tendon of flexor digitorum profundus runs between the two slips of flexor digitorum superficialis, to insert into the terminal phalanx. The flexor tendons receive their blood supply from small blood vessels known as vinculae (which arise from the periosteum of the phalanges). The tendons and their synovial sheaths are bound down to the phalanges by fibrous flexor sheaths, which form fibrous tunnels extending from the metacarpophalangeal joints to the distal phalanges. The flexor sheaths are strong and thick over the phalanges, but weak and loose over interphalangeal joints to allow movement (Fig. 3.34).

Nerves in the hand

Median nerve

The median nerve emerges from the carpal tunnel to enter the palm. It divides into a recurrent branch, providing motor innervation to the muscles of the thenar eminence and into palmar digital nerves. The latter provide motor innervation to the first and second

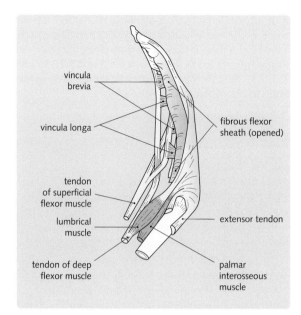

vincula brevia

vincula longa

fibrous flexor sheath (opened)

tendon of superficial flexor muscle

lumbrical muscle

extensor tendon

tendon of deep flexor muscle

palmar interosseous muscle

Fig. 3.34 Long flexor tendons of a finger and its associated vincula.

lumbricals, and sensory innervation to the palmar surface of the lateral three-and-a-half digits of the hand. On the dorsal surface of the hand, they provide sensation to the nail bed and skin of the terminal phalanges of the lateral three-and-a-half digits (Fig. 3.29).

Ulnar nerve

The ulnar nerve and artery pass into the hand together, superficial to the flexor retinaculum. The nerve then divides into deep motor and superficial sensory branches. The motor branch runs with the deep branch of the ulnar artery. It supplies the hypothenar muscles, the two medial lumbricals, the interossei and adductor pollicis. The superficial branch supplies palmaris brevis and provides sensory innervation to the palmar surface of the medial one-and-a-half digits. Sensory innervation to the dorsal surface of the hand and medial one-and-a-half digits is supplied by the dorsal branch of the ulnar nerve – which originates proximal to the flexor retinaculum (Fig. 3.29).

Vessels of the hand

The radial artery crosses the anatomical snuffbox overlying the scaphoid and trapezium, and passes between the two heads of the first dorsal interosseous muscle to enter the palm of the hand. It emerges between the two heads of adductor pollicis, to form the deep palmar arch. The deep palmar arch crosses the palm medially, travelling between the bases of the metacarpal bones and the long flexor tendons. On the medial side of the palm it joins with the deep branch of the ulnar artery. The radial artery

and the deep palmar arch give off several branches supplying the hand and wrist (Fig. 3.24). They include:

- A superficial palmar branch which anastomoses with the superficial palmar arch of the ulnar artery.
- The dorsal carpal artery – a branch of the radial artery arising in the wrist. It travels medially across the wrist giving rise to dorsal metacarpal arteries, which further divide to become dorsal digital arteries, supplying the digits.
- The princeps pollicis artery and the radialis indicis artery supply the thumb and index finger respectively.
- Palmar metacarpal branches arise from the deep palmar arch – these anastomose with the common palmar digital arteries of the superficial palmar arch.

At the wrist the ulnar artery lies between flexor carpi ulnaris and flexor digitorum superficialis. It enters the hand with the ulnar nerve, superficial to the flexor retinaculum. In the hand it forms the superficial palmar arch. The superficial palmar arch travels laterally across the palm, lying deep to the palmar aponeurosis and superficial to the long flexor tendons. On the lateral side of the palm it joins with a palmar branch of the radial artery. The superficial palmar arch gives rise to several branches which include:

- The deep palmar branch which anastomoses with the deep palmar arch of the radial artery
- A single palmar digital artery which supplies the medial side of the little finger
- The common palmar digital arteries which join with the dorsal metacarpal arteries and then divide to form three proper palmar digital arteries, which supply the lateral half of the little finger, the ring and middle fingers, and the medial half of the index finger.

Palmar spaces

The intermediate palmar septum, from the palmar aponeurosis to the third metacarpal, divides the central part of the palm into two fascial spaces: the thenar space lies laterally and the midpalmar space lies medially. The spaces communicate with the subcutaneous tissue of the webs of the fingers. Deep infections of the midpalmar space often spread to these sites.

Nails

These lie on the dorsal surface of the distal phalanges and they are composed of tightly packed keratin.

over the hypothenar and sometimes the thenar eminence may indicate liver disease. Nail changes may be the only clue in a patient with psoriatic arthritis who presents with joint pain, but no skin changes to suggest psoriasis. Clubbing of the fingers may occur in association with a wide range of diseases including carcinoma of the lung, cystic fibrosis, chronic infective endocarditis and inflammatory bowel disease (Crohn's disease and ulcerative colitis). Koilonychia (spoon shaped nails) suggests iron deficiency.

RADIOLOGICAL ANATOMY

Imaging of the bones and joints

When there are symptoms and/or signs of joint problems or a fracture, an X-ray is usually the first imaging investigation to be performed. Two X-rays are taken at 90° to each other. The joints above and below the injury may also be x-rayed, especially if the forearm or lower leg are involved. X-rays can provide information not only on bones or joints, but also on surrounding soft tissues, e.g. calcification may indicate a tumour or endocrine problem.

Normal radiographic anatomy

Normal bone has a smooth cortex which is thicker along the shaft of a long bone, e.g. humerus, compared with a small bone, e.g. carpal. The smooth cortex is interrupted

at the sites of tendon or ligament insertions, and at entry points of the nutrient arteries supplying bone. Medullary trabeculae appear as thin white lines along the planes of weight-bearing forces within a bone. Figures 3.35, 3.36 and 3.37 demonstrate the normal appearances of the shoulder, elbow and hand/wrist joints.

CLINICAL NOTE

Shoulder dislocation

In shoulder dislocation the humeral head most commonly dislocates anteriorly, coming to lie in front of the glenoid fossa. On examination there is squaring of the shoulder, i.e. it loses its smooth convex profile and Hamilton's ruler test is positive (a ruler joins the acromion to the lateral epicondyle and the arm appears to bow medially). On X-ray the continuity of the humeral head and the glenoid fossa is lost. In the rare posterior dislocation of the joint a lateral X-ray demonstrates the 'light bulb sign'; this describes the appearance of the humeral head and is diagnostic of the underlying condition. A shoulder dislocation has a high chance of recurrence – in patients under 20 years of age, the likelihood of recurrence is over 80%.

Interpretation of an X-ray

There are many ways to interpret X-rays. However, by following the same system each time you look at an X-ray, you are much less likely to miss pathology.

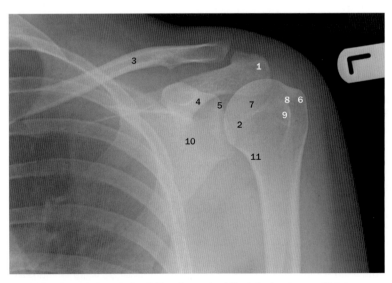

1. Acromion of scapula
2. Anatomical neck
3. Clavicle
4. Coracoid process
5. Glenoid fossa
6. Greater tubercle
7. Head of humerus
8. Intertubercular groove
9. Lesser tubercle
10. Scapula
11. Surgical neck

Fig. 3.35   An anterioposterior (AP) radiograph of the left glenohumeral joint.

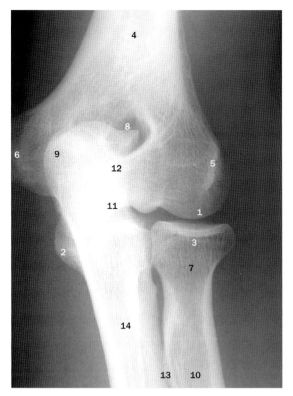

1. Capitulum of humerus
2. Coronoid process of ulna
3. Head of radius
4. Humerus
5. Lateral epicondyle
6. Medial epicondyle
7. Neck of radius
8. Olecranon fossa of humerus
9. Olecranon process of ulna
10. Radius
11. Trochlea of humerus
12. Lateral margin of the trochlear notch of ulna
13. Tuberosity of radius
14. Ulna

Fig. 3.36 An anteroposterior (AP) radiograph of the left elbow.

The following method applies to interpretation of orthopaedic X-rays, but much of it can be applied to any X-ray:

- Check that the name, date of birth, date and time of the X-ray, and the type of X-ray (including which side) are correct.
- Particularly in orthopaedic X-rays, ensure that there is more than one view available.
- Ensure that the area of concern is fully visible.
- Check the alignment of each bone and joint. Examine the joint for narrowing of the joint space, loss of the smooth joint surface, osteophytes, bone cysts and erosions.
- Examine each bone, looking at the cortex for any breaks in continuity. Study bones, looking for lytic lesions, areas of sclerosis (bone thickening) or rarefaction (bone loss).
- Examine the outline of the skin and soft tissues, looking for wasting or areas of swelling. Dense shadows may indicate an abscess, fluid or solid mass. Translucency may represent gas or fat.
- If you have found one abnormality, e.g. a fracture, keep looking because there may be more.
- Always check to see if the patient has any previous X-rays of the same area of the body. Changes in X-rays over time are often more important than one-off findings.

CLINICAL NOTE

Fractures of the hand

A scaphoid fracture is not always evident on first X-ray. Imaging for a second time 10 days later will reveal the fracture line through the scaphoid bone because the fracture ends undergo calcification (sclerosis) as the fracture begins to heal. A fracture at the base of the first metacarpal that extends into the metacarpophalangeal joint is known as a Bennett's fracture. A fracture of the fifth metacarpal is known as a Boxer's fracture, often sustained by punching.

CT/MRI scanning

These imaging modalities can be used in order to visualize parts of the upper limb. For example MRI scanning of the shoulder is often performed in order to diagnose impingement syndromes and rotator cuff tears (Fig. 3.38).

Angiography of the limbs

Figures 3.39, and 3.40 demonstrate the arterial supply to the thoracic cage, shoulder girdle, upper arm and forearm.

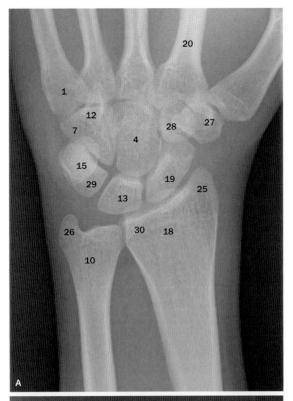

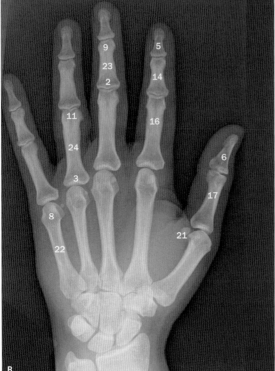

1. Base of fifth metacarpal
2. Base of middle phalanx of middle finger
3. Base of proximal phalanx of ring finger
4. Capitate
5. Distal phalanx of index finger
6. Distal phalanx of thumb
7. Hamate
8. Head of fifth metacarpal
9. Head of middle phalanx of middle finger
10. Head of ulna
11. Head of proximal phalanx of ring finger
12. Hook of hamate
13. Lunate
14. Middle phalanx of index finger
15. Pisiform
16. Proximal phalanx of index finger
17. Proximal phalanx of thumb
18. Radius
19. Scaphoid
20. Second metacarpal
21. Sesmoid bone
22. Shaft of fifth metacarpal
23. Shaft of middle phalanx of middle finger
24. Shaft of proximal phalanx of ring finger
25. Styloid process of radius
26. Styloid process of ulna
27. Trapezium
28. Trapezoid
29. Triquetral
30. Ulnar notch of radius

Fig. 3.37 Dorsolpalmar radiographs of (A) the left wrist and (B) the left hand.

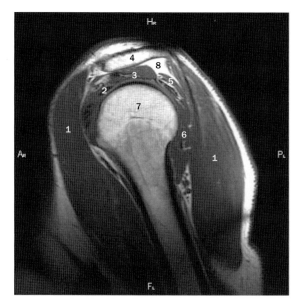

1. Deltoid muscle
2. Biceps brachii tendon
3. Supraspinatus muscle
4. Acromion
5. Infraspinatus muscle
6. Teres minor muscle
7. Humeral head
8. Subacromial bursa

Fig. 3.38   An MRI scan (sagittal section) of the glenohumeral joint.

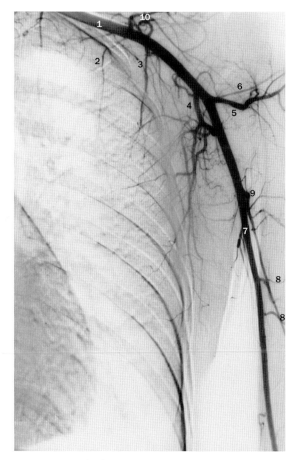

1. Axillary artery
2. Superior thoracic artery
3. Lateral thoracic artery
4. Subscapular artery
5. Posterior circumflex humeral artery
6. Anterior circumflex humeral artery
7. Brachial artery
8. Muscular branches of brachial artery
9. Profunda brachii artery
10. Thoraco-acromial artery

Fig 3.39   Digital subtraction arteriogram of the left axilla

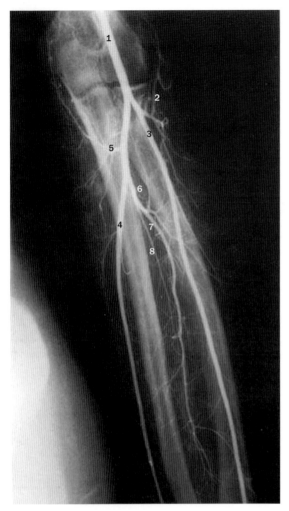

1. Brachial artery
2. Radial recurrent artery
3. Radial artery
4. Ulnar artery
5. Ulnar recurrent artery
6. Common interosseous artery
7. Anterior interosseous artery
8. Posterior interosseous artery

Fig. 3.40 A left brachial arteriogram.

The thorax

Objectives

In this chapter you will learn to:
- Describe the surface markings of the major thoracic viscera (heart, lungs, pleurae and great vessels).
- Discuss the lymphatic drainage of the breast.
- Define the boundaries of the thoracic inlet and state the structures passing through it.
- State the attachments of the diaphragm and name the structures which pass through and peripheral to it.
- Describe the subdivisions of the mediastinum, and be able to state the boundaries and contents of each.
- Describe the major features of each chamber of the heart, and describe the arterial supply and venous drainage of the heart.
- Describe the thoracic sympathetic trunk.
- Describe the structure, course, innervation and blood supply of the oesophagus.
- Name the structures which lie in the hila of the lungs and describe their positions relative to each other.
- Explain the divisions of the bronchial tree and explain the concept of a bronchopulmonary segment.
- Describe the blood supply, innervation and lymphatic drainage of the lungs and pleurae.
- Describe the course and distribution of the vagus and phrenic nerves.
- Outline the mechanics of respiration.
- Review a chest X-ray and recognize the major bony and soft-tissue features.
- Identify the major structures on a transverse CT section of the thorax.

REGIONS AND COMPONENTS OF THE THORAX

The thorax lies between the neck and the abdomen. The thoracic cavity contains the lungs, heart, great vessels, trachea and oesophagus. The lungs lie in the right and left pleural cavities, whilst the remaining structures lie within the more centrally positioned mediastinum. The bony thoracic cage is formed by the thoracic vertebrae, ribs, costal cartilages and sternum. It protects the thoracic viscera and some of the abdominal contents, e.g. the liver and spleen. Superiorly the thorax communicates with the neck via the superior thoracic aperture/thoracic inlet. Inferiorly the diaphragm separates the thorax from the abdominal cavity.

SURFACE ANATOMY AND SUPERFICIAL STRUCTURES

Bony landmarks

The bony landmarks of the thorax are illustrated in Figure 4.1. Clinically, imaginary vertical lines are used to aid description:

- The midsternal line is the equivalent of the midline of the body.
- The midclavicular line lies halfway between the tip of the acromion and the midsternal line.
- The anterior axillary line corresponds to the anterior axillary fold.
- The posterior axillary line corresponds to the posterior axillary fold.
- The midscapular line passes centrally through the inferior angle of the scapula.

Anteriorly, in the midline of the thorax, the sternum can be palpated. However, its full width is not palpable, since its lateral edges are overlapped by pectoralis major muscle. The superior border of the manubrium of the sternum forms the jugular notch. The manubriosternal joint lies between the manubrium and the body of the sternum. At this joint the posterior angulation of the manubrium, relative to the body of the sternum, forms a palpable landmark known as the sternal angle (angle of Louis). The sternal angle is an important landmark as it indicates:

- The level of the transthoracic plane (passes from the sternal angle to the T4/T5 intervertebral disc), which divides the mediastinum into superior and inferior regions (Fig. 4.13).

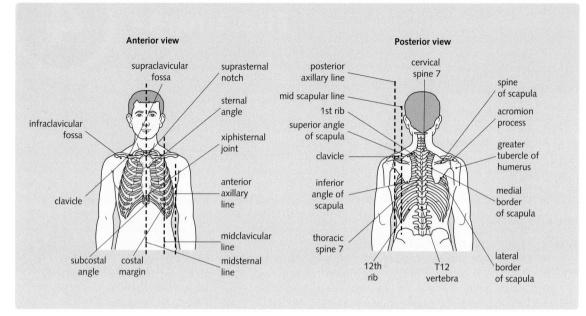

Fig. 4.1 Surface markings of the anterior and posterior thoracic walls.

- The level of the second costal cartilage (palpable on either side of the sternal angle)
- The beginning and end of the aortic arch
- The bifurcation of the pulmonary trunk
- The bifurcation of the trachea into left and right bronchi (the carina)
- The superior border of the pericardium
- The level at which the thoracic duct deviates to the left of the midline
- Entry of the arch of the azygos vein into the superior vena cava.

Inferiorly, the body of the sternum articulates with the xiphoid process, which can be palpated within a triangular depression known as the epigastric fossa. The costal cartilages of ribs 1–7 articulate with the lateral edges of the manubrium and sternum. Ribs 1–6 and their associated costal cartilages are covered anteriorly by pectoralis major. The costal margin begins at the xiphisternum and comprises the costal cartilages of ribs 7–10. Posteriorly the spinous processes of the thoracic vertebrae are palpable inferior to the vertebra prominens – the spinous process of C7 vertebra.

(numbered V1–6) are placed using the sternal angle as the initial landmark: V1 and V2 lie in the 4th intercostal space (ICS) on either side of the sternum. V4 lies in the 5th ICS in the midclavicular line, with V3 equidistant between V2 and V4. V6 lies in the 5th ICS in the midaxillary line, with V5 equidistant between V4 and V6.

Muscles of the thorax

The muscles covering the anterior aspect of the thoracic cage are pectoralis major and minor, subclavius and serratus anterior (Fig. 3.10).

Trachea, lungs and pleurae

The trachea is palpable in the midline, above the jugular notch. It bifurcates behind the sternal angle (at the level of T4) into the right and left main bronchi. Each lung is contained within a pleural cavity, lined with parietal pleura. Superiorly, the dome of the pleura extends approximately 2.5 cm above the medial end of the clavicle (Fig. 4.28). The pleural cavity extends inferiorly, posterior to the sternum, to reach the xiphisternum. At the level of the 4th costal cartilage, the left pleural cavity deviates laterally to form the cardiac notch. Inferiorly, the pleural cavity extends as far as the 8th rib in the midclavicular line, the 10th rib in the midaxillary line and the 12th rib adjacent to the vertebral column.

CLINICAL NOTE

Electrocardiography (ECG)

The sternal angle, with the second ribs lying laterally, is a useful landmark when palpating the intercostal spaces. When performing an ECG, the chest electrodes

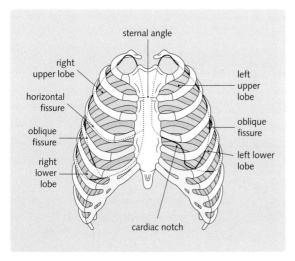

Fig. 4.2 Surface markings of the lungs.

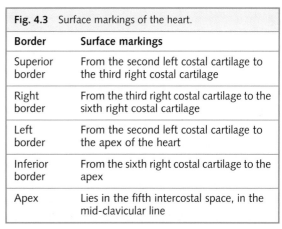

Fig. 4.3	Surface markings of the heart.
Border	**Surface markings**
Superior border	From the second left costal cartilage to the third right costal cartilage
Right border	From the third right costal cartilage to the sixth right costal cartilage
Left border	From the second left costal cartilage to the apex of the heart
Inferior border	From the sixth right costal cartilage to the apex
Apex	Lies in the fifth intercostal space, in the mid-clavicular line

The surface markings of the lungs (Fig. 4.2) during mid-inspiration are similar to those of the pleurae except inferiorly where they lie at the level of the sixth rib in the midclavicular line, eighth rib in the midaxillary line and the 10th rib adjacent to the vertebral column. The oblique fissure corresponds to a line drawn from the T2 spinous process, around to the sixth rib in the midclavicular line. The horizontal fissure (only present in the right lung) corresponds to a line drawn from the fourth costal cartilage, to its intersection with the oblique fissure at the midaxillary line.

Thus the pleural cavities are not completely filled by the lungs. There is a space approximately two ribs deep, known as the costodiaphragmatic recess (costophrenic angle), lying between the junction of the pleura covering the diaphragm and the pleura covering the inner aspect of the thoracic wall. An accumulation of fluid in this space is known as a pleural effusion.

Heart

The surface markings of the heart are outlined in Figure 4.3 and illustrated in Figure 4.4. The apex of the heart lies on the left in approximately in the fifth intercostal space, in the midclavicular line.

Great vessels

The aortic arch, a continuation of the ascending aorta, begins at the sternal angle. It arches posteriorly and to the left of the vertebral column, where, again at the level of the sternal angle, the arch ends to become the descending (thoracic) aorta. The aortic arch, brachiocephalic trunk, left common carotid and left subclavian arteries lie posterior to the manubrium. The brachiocephalic trunk bifurcates into the right common carotid

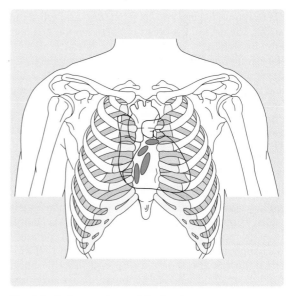

Fig. 4.4 Surface anatomy of the heart.

and subclavian arteries, posterior to the right sternoclavicular joint.

The subclavian artery gives rise to the internal thoracic (or mammary) artery which travels inferiorly, posterior to the costal cartilages and 1 cm lateral to the sternal edge. Upon reaching the 6th intercostal space it divides into musculophrenic and superior epigastric arteries.

The superior vena cava is formed behind the first right costal cartilage by the union of the right and left brachiocephalic veins. It runs inferiorly, posterior to the right sternal border, entering the right atrium of the heart, posterior to the third costal cartilage. The azygos vein drains into the superior vena cava at the level of the second right costal cartilage.

Diaphragm

The central tendon of the diaphragm lies behind the xiphisternal joint. The right dome lies higher than the left, due to the presence of the liver in the right upper quadrant of the abdomen. The diaphragm flattens in inspiration. In full expiration the right dome reaches the 4th intercostal space, whilst the left dome reaches the 5th rib (NB the nipple lies in the 4th intercostal space).

Breasts

The breasts lie in the superficial fascia, superficial to the pectoralis major and serratus anterior muscles. They consist of glandular tissue and fat and fibrous tissue which forms the suspensory ligaments (of Cooper). The adult breast is composed of 15–20 lobules, each drained by a lactiferous duct, which opens onto the nipple. The nipple is surrounded by a circular pigmented area called the areola. The base of the breast lies between the 2nd and 6th ribs vertically, and between the lateral border of the sternum and the midaxillary line horizontally (the upper outer quadrant of the breast extends into the axilla and is known as the axillary tail). The blood supply to the breast is derived from branches of the internal thoracic artery, the lateral thoracic artery, the thoracoacromial artery and the posterior intercostal arteries. Venous drainage is via the axillary and internal thoracic veins.

Lymph from the breast initially drains into the sub-areolar plexus. Lymph from the superior and lateral quadrants of the breast drains to the pectoral group of axillary nodes. This constitutes 75% of the total lymph which is drained from the breast (Fig. 3.15). Lymph from the medial part of the breast drains to the parasternal lymph nodes (which lie in close proximity to the internal thoracic artery) or to the opposite breast. Lymph from the inferior region of the breast may drain to abdominal lymph nodes.

THE THORACIC WALL

The bony thoracic cage is formed by the sternum, the ribs with their associated costal cartilages and the thoracic vertebrae (Fig. 4.5).

Sternum

The sternum has three components:

- The manubrium is the upper part of the sternum. It articulates with the clavicles and with the 1st and upper part of the 2nd costal cartilages.
- The body of the sternum articulates with the manubrium at the manubriosternal joint superiorly and

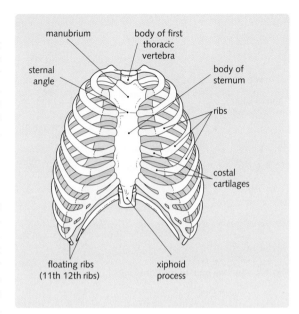

Fig. 4.5 Thoracic cage.

with the xiphisternum inferiorly. These are secondary cartilaginous joints. Laterally the body of the sternum articulates with the 2nd to 7th costal cartilages via synovial joints.
- The xiphoid process is the most inferior part of the sternum.

CLINICAL NOTE

Breast cancer

One in 8 females in the UK will develop breast cancer during their lifetime (breast cancer can also occur in males, although this is rare). Signs of breast cancer include: a lump in the breast, nipple retraction or inversion (due to traction on the lactiferous ducts by a tumour), discharge from the nipple, oedema of the breast tissue secondary to obstruction of lymphatic drainage (referred to as peau d'orange – breast skin resembles the skin of an orange), dimpling of the skin (tumour invasion may lead to shortening or traction of suspensory ligaments) and erythema. Diagnosis is made by 'triple assessment' consisting of history/examination, ultrasonography or mammography (ultrasonography is the technique of choice in women under 35 years of age due to the density of the breast tissue) and fine needle or core biopsy.

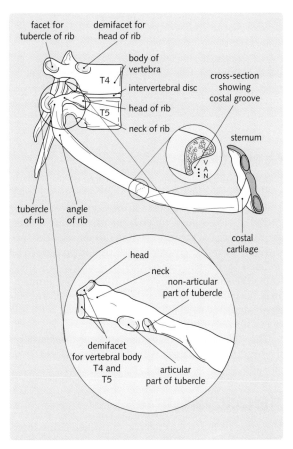

Fig. 4.6 Right 5th rib with the inset showing the posterior surface of the rib.

Ribs and costal cartilages

There are 12 pairs of ribs, all of which articulate with the vertebral column posteriorly. Anteriorly, ribs 1–7 articulate directly with the sternum via their individual costal cartilages. These are so called 'true ribs'. Ribs 8–12 have no direct articulation with the sternum. They are known as 'false ribs'. The costal cartilages of ribs 8–10 articulate with the cartilage above, whilst ribs 11 and 12 have no anterior attachment for their costal cartilages.

Typical ribs

A typical rib has the following features (Fig. 4.6):

- It has a head with two demifacets for articulation with its corresponding vertebral body and that of the vertebra immediately above.
- The neck lies between the head and the tubercle.
- The tubercle lies between the neck and the shaft, and has a facet for articulation with the transverse process of the corresponding vertebra.
- Lateral to the tubercle is the angle of the rib, at which point the shaft curves anteriorly. The shaft is thin, flat and curved. It has a rounded superior border, and a sharp inferior border forming the costal groove (which contains the neurovascular bundle).

most commonly inserted into the 5th intercostal space in the midaxillary line. The chest drain passes through the skin, superficial fascia, the external, internal and innermost intercostal muscles, the endothoracic fascia and parietal pleura, coming to lie in the pleural cavity.

Atypical ribs

Figure 4.7 illustrates the major features of the 1st rib, and its relations, which pass through the thoracic inlet. The 1st rib is the broadest, shortest and most sharply curved rib. The scalene tubercle lies on its inner border, for attachment of the scalenus anterior muscle. The subclavian vein and artery pass anteriorly and posteriorly to the scalene tubercle respectively. The subclavian artery forms the subclavian groove on the rib, and immediately posterior to the artery the lower trunk of the brachial plexus (C8–T1) lies in direct contact with the upper surface of the rib.

The 10th, 11th and 12th ribs have only one facet on the head for articulation with their own vertebra.

Thoracic vertebrae

There are 12 thoracic vertebrae with intervening intervertebral discs (Fig. 2.2).

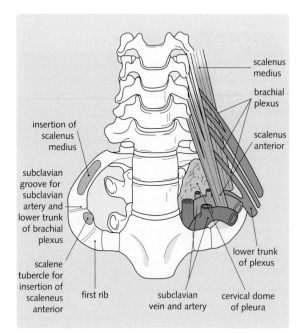

insertion of scalenus medius

scalenus medius

brachial plexus

scalenus anterior

subclavian groove for subclavian artery and lower trunk of brachial plexus

lower trunk of plexus

scalene tubercle for insertion of scaleneus anterior

first rib

subclavian vein and artery

cervical dome of pleura

Fig. 4.7 First rib and its relations to the thoracic inlet.

Openings into the thorax

Thoracic inlet (superior thoracic aperture)

The thoracic inlet (referred to clinically as the thoracic outlet) slopes anteroinferiorly and allows communication between the root of the neck and the thoracic cavity (Fig. 4.7). It is bounded posteriorly by the body of the T1 vertebra, laterally by the medial border of the 1st rib and anteriorly by the superior border of the manubrium. The oesophagus, trachea and the apices of the lungs, together with major blood vessels and nerves, pass through the inlet.

Thoracic outlet (inferior thoracic aperture)

The thoracic outlet lies between the thorax and the abdomen. It is bounded posteriorly by the T12 vertebra and the 12th ribs, anteriorly by the costal margin and xiphoid process and is closed by the diaphragm. Numerous structures pass between the thorax and abdomen, passing either through a hiatus (hole) in the diaphragm or passing peripherally (Figs 4.8 & 4.9).

Intercostal spaces

There are eleven intercostal spaces between adjacent ribs. Each space contains a neurovascular bundle and three layers of intercostal muscles (Fig. 4.10). The innermost intercostals are lined by endothoracic fascia; deep to this lies the parietal pleura. Anteriorly, each external intercostal muscle is replaced by the anterior intercostal membrane, which runs from the costochondral junction to the sternum. Posteriorly, each internal intercostal muscle is replaced by the posterior intercostal membrane.

Intercostal nerves and vessels

The intercostal nerves are the anterior rami of thoracic spinal nerves. The anterior rami of T1–T11 lie in the superior part of the intercostal spaces between the ribs. The anterior ramus of T12 lies below rib 12 and is known as the subcostal nerve. Each intercostal nerve initially passes between the parietal pleura and the posterior intercostal membrane. At the angle of the ribs, it comes to lie in the costal groove of the corresponding rib, between the innermost and internal intercostal muscles. Each nerve has several branches:

- Communicating branches (rami communicates) to the sympathetic trunk
- A collateral branch at the angle of the ribs, which passes along the superior border of the rib below, supplying the intercostal muscles and parietal pleura

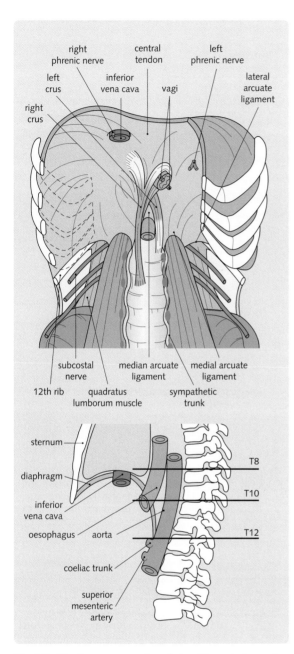

Fig. 4.9   Diaphragmatic apertures and structures passing through them.

Opening	Structures
Aortic hiatus – posterior to the diaphragm at the level of T12	Abdominal aorta, thoracic duct, azygos and hemiazygos veins
Oesophageal hiatus – passes through the right crus of the diaphragm at the level of T10	Oesophagus, left and right vagus nerves, oesophageal branches of the left gastric vessels and lymphatic vessels
Caval opening – through the central tendon at the level of T8	Inferior vena cava, right phrenic nerve
Structures passing posterior to the diaphragm	Splanchnic nerves and sympathetic trunk
Structures passing anterior to the diaphragm	Superior epigastric vessels and lymphatics
Structures passing lateral to the diaphragm	Lower six intercostal vessels and nerves.

Fig. 4.8 Diaphragm as seen from below (the anterior portion of the right side has been removed) and as a sagittal section.

- A lateral cutaneous branch, which divides into an anterior and posterior branch, and innervates overlying skin
- A terminal branch – the anterior cutaneous branch, which divides into a medial and a lateral branch and innervates the skin of the anterior chest wall or the abdomen.

The first intercostal nerve (T1) divides into a superior and inferior branch. The larger superior branch joins the brachial plexus, whilst the inferior branch passes beneath the first rib to run in the 1st intercostal space. At the costal margin the 7th to 11th nerves pass from the intercostal spaces to lie between the muscles of the anterior abdominal wall. They supply the anterior abdominal wall muscles, overlying skin and parietal peritoneum. The subcostal nerve lies between the muscles of the abdominal wall. Its lateral cutaneous branch pierces the internal and external oblique muscle layers, to supply the skin over the lateral aspect of the buttock. The nerve eventually joins the L1 spinal nerve, forming the ilioinguinal and iliohypogastric nerves.

Figure 4.11 shows the arterial supply to the thoracic wall.

HINTS AND TIPS

Each neurovascular bundle consists of (from superior to inferior) an intercostal vein, artery and nerve (VAN – vein, artery, nerve). The bundles lie inferiorly in the costal groove of each rib.

Diaphragm

The diaphragm separates the thoracic and abdominal cavities. It is the primary muscle of respiration and consists of a central tendon and a peripheral muscular part.

Fig. 4.10 Muscles of the thorax.

Name of muscle (nerve supply)	Origin	Insertion	Action
External intercostal (intercostal)	Inferior border of rib above	Superior border of rib below	All the intercostal muscles assist in both inspiration and expiration during respiration ventilation
Internal intercostal (intercostal)	Costal groove of rib above	Superior border of rib below	
Innermost intercostal (intercostal)	Costal groove of rib above	Adjacent rib below	
Diaphragm (phrenic)	Xiphoid process, lower sixth costal cartilages, L1–L3 vertebrae by crura, and medial and lateral arcuate ligaments	Central tendon	Important muscle of inspiration; increases vertical diameter of thorax by flattening the central tendon

Fig. 4.11 Arterial supply to the thoracic wall.

Artery	Origin	Distribution
Anterior intercostal (spaces 1–6)	Internal thoracic artery	Intercostal spaces and parietal pleura
Anterior intercostal (spaces 7–9)	Musculophrenic artery	
Posterior intercostal (spaces 1–2)	Superior intercostal artery (from costocervical trunk of subclavian artery)	
Posterior intercostal (all other spaces)	Thoracic aorta	
Internal thoracic	Subclavian artery	Runs inferiorly, posterior to the costal cartilages and lateral to the sternum terminating by dividing into the superior epigastric and musculophrenic arteries
Subcostal	Thoracic aorta	Abdominal wall

From the front the diaphragm consists of two domes, the right dome being higher than the left. A lateral view shows the diaphragm to resemble an inverted pudding bowl (Fig. 4.8). Figure 4.9 lists the openings in the diaphragm and the structures passing through them. The blood and nerve supply of the diaphragm are shown in Figure 4.12.

HINTS AND TIPS

The sole motor supply to the diaphragm is via the phrenic nerves – root value C3, 4, 5 (C3, 4, 5 keeps the diaphragm alive). Remember that the phrenic nerve also receives sensory input from the mediastinal pleura, diaphragmatic pleura and peritoneum.

Fig. 4.12 Nerves and vessels of the diaphragm.

Innervation	Motor supply: phrenic nerves (C3–C5) Sensory supply: centrally by phrenic nerves (C3–C5), peripherally by intercostal nerves (T5–T11) and subcostal nerve (T12)
Arterial supply	Superior phrenic arteries; musculophrenic arteries; pericardiacophrenic arteries; inferior phrenic arteries
Venous drainage	Musculophrenic and pericardiacophrenic veins drain into internal thoracic vein; superior and inferior phrenic veins
Lymphatic drainage	Diaphragmatic lymph nodes drain to posterior mediastinal nodes eventually to the superior lumbar lymph nodes; lymphatic plexuses on superior and inferior surfaces communicate freely

THE THORACIC CAVITY

The thoracic cavity is filled laterally by the lungs and the pleural cavities. The mediastinum lies centrally within the thoracic cavity.

Mediastinum

For descriptive purposes, the mediastinum is divided into superior and inferior regions by the transverse thoracic plane (a horizontal plane from the sternal angle to the T4 vertebra) (Fig. 4.13).

The superior mediastinum lies between the manubrium anteriorly and the T1–T4 vertebrae posteriorly. It contains the remnants of the thymus, the arch of the aorta and the roots of its major branches – the brachiocephalic trunk, left common carotid artery, left subclavian artery, the brachiocephalic veins, the superior vena cava, the left and right vagus and phrenic nerves, the left recurrent laryngeal nerve, the trachea, the oesophagus and the thoracic duct. The apices of the lungs lie on either side of the superior mediastinum.

The inferior mediastinum lies posterior to the body of the sternum and the pericardium subdivides it into anterior, middle and posterior regions:

- The anterior mediastinum (T4–T8), lying between the sternum and pericardium contains fat, lymph nodes and part of the thymus in children.
- The middle mediastinum (T4–T8) contains the pericardium and heart, the ascending aorta, the arch of the aorta, and the proximal right and left pulmonary arteries.

- The posterior mediastinum, lying between the pericardium and the T4–T12 vertebrae contains the oesophagus, thoracic aorta, thoracic duct, azygos system of veins and the thoracic part of the sympathetic trunk.

Figure 4.14 A and B shows the left and right surfaces of the mediastinum.

The pericardium

The pericardium is a fibroserous sac which encloses the heart and the roots of the great vessels. It is composed of two layers. The strong outer layer, the fibrous pericardium, limits the movement of the heart, and is attached inferiorly to the central tendon of the diaphragm, anteriorly to the sternum (via the sternopericardial ligaments), and superiorly to the tunica adventitia of the great vessels. The inner layer is known as the serous pericardium and is itself divided into two layers – the parietal pericardium, which is firmly adherent to the fibrous pericardium and the visceral pericardium, a serous layer, which reflects onto the great vessels and surface of the heart. The visceral pericardium also forms the outer layer of the heart, known as the epicardium. There is a potential space between the parietal and visceral pericardial layers, which is normally filled with a thin layer of serous fluid, allowing the heart to move smoothly within the pericardium. The main arterial supply to the pericardium is via the pericardiacophrenic artery (a branch of the internal thoracic artery). Venous drainage is via the pericardiacophrenic veins and the azygos veins. The phrenic nerve (C3,4,5) provides sensory innervation to the fibrous and parietal layers of the pericardium (this can lead to referred pain to the skin above the clavicle (C3,4,5 dermatomes)). The visceral layer has no somatic innervation and so it is insensitive to pain.

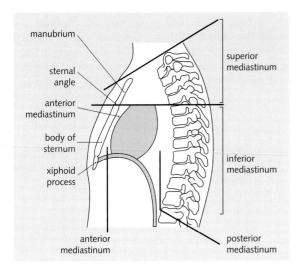

Fig. 4.13 Subdivisions of the mediastinum.

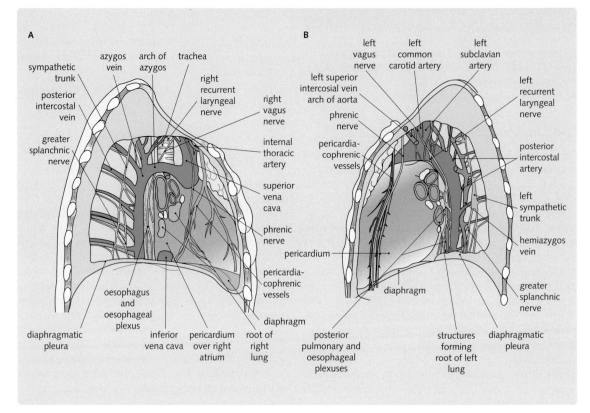

Fig. 4.14 A, Right surface of the mediastinum and the right posterior thoracic wall. B, Left surface of the mediastinum and the left posterior thoracic wall. Mediastinal pleura has been removed.

the indistensible nature of the fibrous pericardium. The result is a heart which cannot contract fully, leading to falling cardiac output, and death if untreated. Treatment is via pericardiocentesis, whereby a needle is inserted into the left 5th intercostal space, allowing aspiration of fluid from the pericardium.

Heart

The heart has four chambers, two atria and two ventricles (Fig. 4.16). The atria receive blood, whilst the right ventricle pumps blood to the lungs, and the left ventricle propels blood throughout the remainder of the body. The heart lies free in the pericardium, connected only to the great vessels. Its walls consist mainly of heart muscle (myocardium), lined internally by endocardium and externally by epicardium (visceral pericardium).

Pericardial sinuses

The reflection of the serous pericardium around the pulmonary veins forms a recess posterior to the left atrium known as the oblique sinus. The oesophagus lies immediately posterior to the oblique sinus. The transverse sinus is formed from a reflection of the serous pericardium around the aorta and the pulmonary trunk anteriorly, and around the superior vena cava and pulmonary veins posteriorly. The transverse sinus separates the arterial outflow and venous inflow of the heart (Fig. 4.15).

Skeleton of the heart

The muscle fibres of the atria and ventricles are attached to a pair of fibrous rings around the atrioventricular orifices. The collagenous rings form the bases of the cusps of the atrioventricular valves, preventing distension during cardiac contraction. They also separate the nerve impulses occurring in the atria and ventricles (the atrioventricular bundle of the conducting system provides the only physiological connection between the atria and ventricles). There are two further fibrous rings supporting the aortic and pulmonary valves.

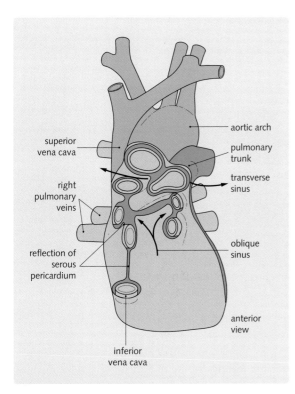

superior vena cava

right pulmonary veins

reflection of serous pericardium

aortic arch

pulmonary trunk

transverse sinus

oblique sinus

anterior view

inferior vena cava

Fig. 4.15 Pericardial sinuses and reflections (the heart has been removed from the pericardial sac). Anterior view. (Adapted from Williams P (ed) (1995) *Gray's Anatomy*, 38th edition, Churchill Livingstone.)

Chambers of the heart

Right atrium

The right atrium forms the right border of the heart. It consists of the right atrium proper and an atrial appendage, the right auricle (Fig. 4.17). The ridged anterior wall of the atrium (composed of pectinate muscles) and the smooth posterior wall are separated internally by a ridge known as the crista terminalis, and externally by a groove known as the sulcus terminalis. The right atrium receives blood from the superior and inferior vena cavae and the coronary sinus.

Interatrial septum

The interatrial septum separates the left and right atria. A depression in the lower part of the septum, known as the fossa ovalis, is a remnant of the foramen ovale of the fetal heart. Failure of the foramen ovale to close after birth results in an atrial septal defect (ASD).

Right ventricle

The right ventricle forms the majority of the anterior surface and inferior border of the heart. Its internal surface has several notable features (Fig. 4.17):

- Trabeculae carneae – irregular muscular bundles which line the wall of the ventricle
- The moderator band – runs from the interventricular septum to the anterior wall of the ventricle, and transmits part of the conducting system of the heart

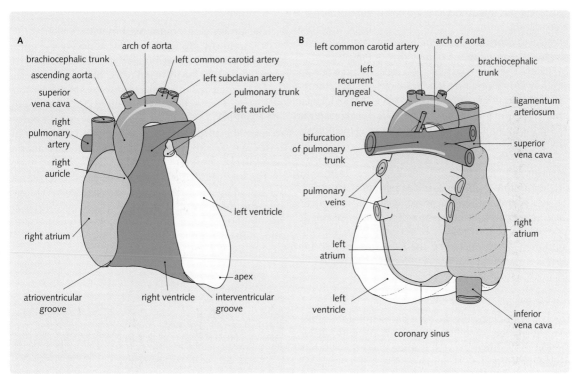

A

brachiocephalic trunk

ascending aorta

superior vena cava

right pulmonary artery

right auricle

right atrium

atrioventricular groove

arch of aorta

left common carotid artery

left subclavian artery

pulmonary trunk

left auricle

left ventricle

right ventricle

interventricular groove

apex

B

left common carotid artery

left recurrent laryngeal nerve

bifurcation of pulmonary trunk

pulmonary veins

left atrium

left ventricle

coronary sinus

arch of aorta

brachiocephalic trunk

ligamentum arteriosum

superior vena cava

right atrium

inferior vena cava

Fig. 4.16 Anterior (A) and posterior (B) surfaces of the heart.

Fig. 4.17 Interior of right atrium and right ventricle.

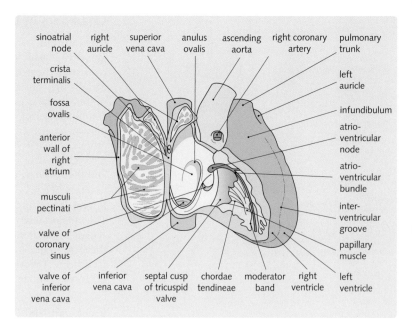

- Chordae tendineae – fibrous cords attached to both the free edges of the tricuspid valve and to the papillary muscles within the wall of the ventricle
- The infundibulum – the outflow tract of the right ventricle.

The right ventricle communicates with the right atrium via the tricuspid valve and with the pulmonary artery via the pulmonary valve. The tricuspid valve has three cusps (anterior, posterior and septal), the bases of which are attached to the fibrous ring of the skeleton of the heart. The free edges of the cusps are attached to papillary muscles via the chordae tendineae. The pulmonary valve has three cusps (anterior, left and right) which project into the pulmonary artery. Above each cusp the wall of the pulmonary artery bulges, forming the pulmonary sinuses.

Left atrium

The left atrium forms most of the base of the heart. It consists of the left atrium proper and the left auricle. The interior of the atrium is smooth, whilst the auricle is ridged due to the presence of pectinate muscles. Four pulmonary veins open into the posterior wall of the atrium. The left atrioventricular orifice is protected by the bicuspid mitral valve.

Left ventricle

The left ventricle forms the apex and left border of the heart. It supplies blood to the entire body, with the exception of the lungs. Its wall is three times thicker than that of the right ventricle and pressures within it are up to six times greater. Its internal surface has several notable features, some of which are similar to those of the right ventricle:

- Well-developed trabeculae carneae
- Chordae tendinae between the free edges of the aortic valve and the papillary muscles
- The aortic vestibule – the outflow tract of the left ventricle.

The left ventricle communicates with the left atrium via the mitral valve and with the aorta via the aortic valve. The mitral valve is bicuspid with anterior and posterior cusps. Like the tricuspid valve, the free edges of the cusps are attached to papillary muscles via the chordae tendineae. The aortic valve has three cusps (posterior, right and left). Above each cusp the aortic wall bulges to form the aortic sinuses. The right and left aortic sinuses give rise to the right and left coronary arteries respectively.

The interventricular septum is of equal thickness to the rest of the left ventricle and, consequently, it bulges into the right ventricle. It is composed of a superior membranous region and an inferior muscular region, and transmits the atrioventricular bundle of the conducting system.

> **CLINICAL NOTE**
>
> **Congenital heart defects**
>
> Failure of the foramen ovale to close results in an atrial septal defect (ASD). This allows oxygenated blood to pass from the left atrium into the right atrium (pressure

in the left atrium is greater than in the right atrium and blood flows from an area of high pressure to an area of lower pressure). This results in enlargement of the right atrium and ventricle, along with dilatation of the pulmonary trunk. The resulting increased blood flow through the pulmonary vasculature can result in pulmonary hypertension. A defect in the interventricular septum (in either its muscular or membranous part) is known as a ventricular septal defect (VSD). The majority of VSDs in the muscular part of the septum will close spontaneously; membranous VSDs are less likely to do so. Failure of a VSD to close leads to a left to right shunt, an increase in pulmonary blood flow and pulmonary hypertension. Defects in the membranous part are likely to be associated with defects in the formation of the valves.

Blood supply of the heart

Figure 4.18 illustrates the blood supply of the heart. The right and left coronary arteries are the first branches of the aorta, arising from the right and left aortic sinuses. They give off a series of important branches, supplying the myocardium and epicardium (the blood supply to the endocardium comes directly from the chambers of the heart). The left coronary artery (LCA) is short and quickly divides into circumflex and anterior interventricular (also known as the left anterior descending artery – LAD) branches. The circumflex branch passes posteriorly in the coronary groove, supplying the left atrium and left ventricle, before anastomosing with the right coronary artery in the coronary groove. The anterior interventricular branch runs in the anterior interventricular groove, supplying both ventricles and the interventricular septum, before anastomosing at the apex of the heart with the posterior interventricular artery.

The right coronary artery (RCA) gives off branches to the right atrium and right ventricle as it descends in the coronary groove. A right marginal branch runs along the inferior border of the heart to supply the right ventricle. On the inferior surface of the heart, the RCA anastomoses with the circumflex artery of the LCA. It also gives off a posterior interventricular (or right posterior descending) branch which runs in the posterior interventricular groove, and supplies both ventricles and the interventricular septum. The RCA supplies the sinoatrial node via a sinoatrial branch in 60% of individuals, and the atrioventricular node in 90% of individuals. It also supplies the atrioventricular bundle (of His) and its right terminal branch. The left terminal branch is supplied by both the RCA and LCA.

Left and right dominance of the heart refers to the coronary artery from which the posterior interventricular branch arises. Right dominance is more common.

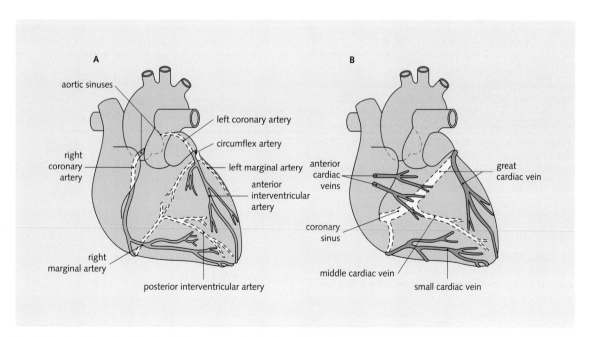

Fig. 4.18   Blood supply of the heart. A, coronary arteries; B, cardiac veins.

Fig. 4.19 Outline of the nerve supply of the heart.

Nerve type	Origin	Action
Sympathetic nerves	Cervical and upper thoracic part of the sympathetic trunk via the cardiac plexuses	Increase the rate and force of contraction
Parasympathetic nerves	Vagus nerves via the cardiac plexuses	Reduce the rate and force of contraction

Venous drainage of the heart

Most of the venous blood from the heart drains into the coronary sinus, which lies in the posterior part of the coronary sulcus, and drains into the right atrium close to the inferior vena cava. The great cardiac vein accompanies and drains the territory of the anterior interventricular artery and empties directly into the coronary sinus. The middle cardiac vein accompanies the posterior interventricular artery and empties directly into the coronary sinus. The small cardiac veins drain the myocardium of the right atrium and empty directly into the coronary sinus, just before it enters the right atrium. The remaining blood is returned to the heart via the anterior cardiac veins, which drain into the right atrium, and other small veins (venae cordis minimae), which open directly into the heart chambers.

Conducting system of the heart

The heart normally contracts rhythmically at about 70 beats per minute. The muscle of the heart is known as the myocardium. All myocardial cells have the ability to contract, and some are specialised, with the ability to conduct electrical impulses, which control the beating of the heart. Conduction of an electrical impulse begins at the sinoatrial node (SA node), also known as the pacemaker of the heart. The SA node lies in the upper part of the sulcus terminalis of the right atrium. Impulses generated here are transmitted through the myocardium of both atria, causing them to contract. Upon reaching the atrioventricular node, which lies in the interatrial septum (superior to the origin of the coronary sinus), impulses are carried by the atrioventricular bundle (of His), which lies in the membranous part of the interventricular septum. Here it divides into a left and right bundle. The right bundle conducts impulses to the right ventricle. The left bundle divides into an anterior and a posterior fascicle, conducting impulses to the left ventricle.

Innervation of the heart arises from the left and right vagus nerves (parasympathetic supply) and branches of the sympathetic trunk (Fig. 4.19).

Great vessels of the thorax

Aorta

Figure 4.20 outlines the course of the thoracic aorta and its branches. Figure 4.21 illustrates the aortic arch and pulmonary trunk.

HINTS AND TIPS

Referred pain from a myocardial infarction is transmitted through the cardiac branches of the cervical sympathetic trunk. Afferent fibres enter the spinal cord of the upper five thoracic nerves and pain is referred to dermatomes that these spinal nerves supply, e.g. the medial surface of the left upper limb is supplied by T1 and 2.

Pulmonary trunk

The pulmonary trunk divides inferior to the arch of the aorta to form the right and left pulmonary arteries, which transport deoxygenated blood to the lungs. The ligamentum arteriosum (Fig. 4.21) is a fibrous band

Fig. 4.20   Aorta and its branches in the thorax.

Artery	Course and origin	Branches
Ascending aorta	Originates from the left ventricle, ascends and becomes the aortic arch at the level of the sternal angle	Right and left coronary arteries
Aortic arch	Begins posterior to the manubrium. Arches posteriorly to the left of the trachea and the oesophagus, and continues as the descending aorta	Brachiocephalic trunk, left common carotid artery, left subclavian artery
Descending aorta	Begins at the level of the sternal angle, to the left of the midline. Travels inferiorly to the left of the vertebral column, moves anteriorly to reach the midline. Exits the thorax by passing posteriorly to the diaphragm (in the midline) through the aortic hiatus opposite vertebra T12.	Posterior intercostal arteries, subcostal arteries and visceral branches (oesophageal, bronchial, superior phrenic)

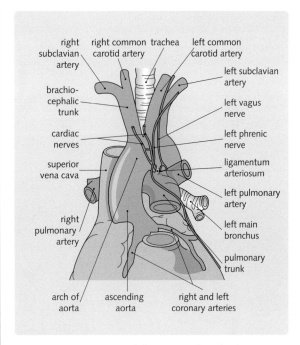

Fig. 4.21   Anterior view of the aortic arch and pulmonary trunk.

that connects the bifurcation of the pulmonary trunk to the aortic arch. It is the remnant of the ductus arteriosus, which in the fetus conducts blood from the pulmonary trunk to the aorta, bypassing the lungs.

Superior vena cava

The superior vena cava is formed by the union of the right and left brachiocephalic veins at the level of the 1st right costal cartilage. It returns blood to the right atrium from the upper limbs, head and neck. Posterior to the 2nd right costal cartilage it receives the azygos vein (see below). The superior vena cava drains into the right atrium, posterior to the 3rd right costal cartilage.

Inferior vena cava

The inferior vena cava pierces the central tendon of the diaphragm opposite the T8 vertebra, along with the right phrenic nerve and almost immediately enters the right atrium. Figure 4.22 shows the superior and inferior venae cavae and their main tributaries.

Pulmonary veins

There are four pulmonary veins. Two pulmonary veins leave each lung, carrying oxygenated blood to the left atrium of the heart.

Azygos system of veins

Figure 4.23 shows the azygos system of veins and the thoracic duct. The azygos system drains the thoracic wall and several thoracic structures, receiving tributaries from the posterior and superior intercostal veins, the vertebral venous plexus, pericardium, mediastinum and oesophagus. The azygos vein passes through the aortic hiatus with the thoracic duct and aorta at the level of T12.

Nerves of the thorax

The phrenic nerves originate from the C3,4,5 nerve roots. The right phrenic nerve descends through the neck on the surface of scalenus anterior muscle and enters the thorax lateral to the right brachiocephalic vein. It continues lateral to the superior vena cava and the pericardium overlying the right atrium (Fig. 4.14A). It then passes anterior to the hilum of the lung, continuing inferiorly on the right side of the inferior vena cava (IVC). It finally passes through the diaphragm with the IVC (Fig. 4.8). The left phrenic nerve descends on the cervical pleura, posterior to the left brachiocephalic vein and anterior to the left subclavian artery. In the thorax,

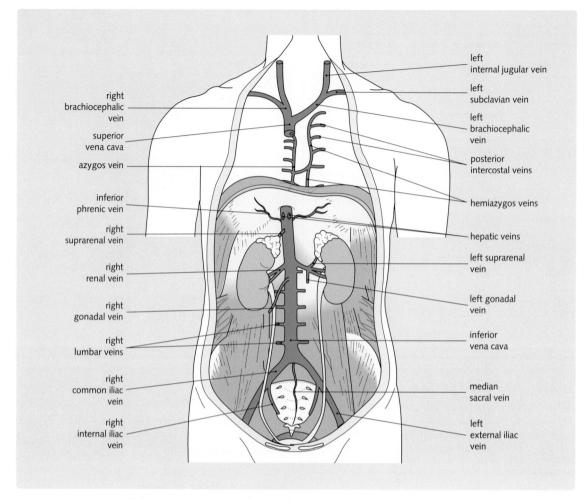

Fig. 4.22 Superior and inferior venae cavae and their main tributaries.

the left phrenic nerve lies between the left common carotid and left subclavian arteries. It lies anterior to the left vagus nerve as it crosses the arch of the aorta, then crosses the left superior intercostal vein (Fig. 4.14B). It passes anterior to the left hilum and the pericardium overlying the left ventricle. Finally, it pierces the left hemidiaphragm (Fig. 4.8). The phrenic nerves provide a motor supply to the diaphragm. They also provide sensory innervation of the central tendon of the diaphragm (the periphery is supplied by the lower six intercostal nerves) and the parietal pleura.

The vagus nerve (cranial nerve X) originates in the brain and exits the skull via the jugular foramen, along with the jugular vein. It descends in the carotid sheath, posterior to the common carotid artery and internal jugular vein, towards the thoracic inlet.

The right vagus nerve descends anterior to the right subclavian artery, coming to lie between the brachiocephalic trunk and right brachiocephalic vein. Within the thorax, the nerve passes behind the brachiocephalic trunk and comes to lie on the lateral side of the trachea (Fig. 4.14A). It gives off cardiac branches in the superior mediastinum to supply the heart. The nerve passes between the arch of the azygos and the trachea, and then posterior to the lung hilum to contribute to the plexuses supplying the lungs and oesophagus. The vagal trunk reforms on the surface of the oesophagus before leaving the thorax with it through the diaphragm (Fig. 4.8).

The left vagus nerve descends into the thorax, posterior to the left brachiocephalic vein, between the left common carotid and left subclavian arteries. As it descends over the aortic arch, it is crossed by the left superior intercostal vein. The nerve gives off cardiac branches in the superior mediastinum, to supply the heart. Its left recurrent laryngeal branch hooks under the aortic arch (Fig. 4.14B) to ascend between the trachea and oesophagus to the larynx. The left vagus nerve passes posterior to the lung hilum to contribute to the plexuses that supply the lungs and oesophagus, before reforming to

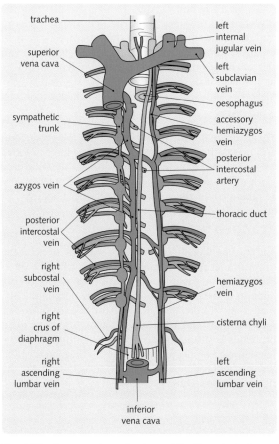

Fig. 4.23 Azygos system of veins and the thoracic duct.

exit the thorax with the oesophagus through the diaphragm (Fig. 4.8).

Figure 4.24 summarizes the major nerves of the thorax.

Thoracic sympathetic trunk

The sympathetic trunks lie on either side of the entire vertebral column. Superiorly the trunks lie over the heads of the ribs, but inferiorly they lie over the vertebral bodies. They pass into the abdomen from the thorax posterior to the medial arcuate ligaments of the diaphragm. There is a sympathetic ganglion associated with every spinal nerve, with the exception of the first ganglion which merges with the inferior cervical ganglion, forming the stellate ganglion. White and grey rami communicates from the sympathetic ganglia between T1 and L2 communicate with the thoracic spinal nerves. Medial branches from the thoracic sympathetic ganglia innervate thoracic viscera. The branches from the upper five to six ganglia form a plexus on the thoracic aorta and supply the heart, lungsx oesophagus and trachea. The branches from the lower ganglia form

Fig. 4.24 Nerves of the thorax.

Nerve (origin)	Course and distribution
Vagus, cranial nerve X (medulla oblongata)	Enters superior mediastinum posterior to the sternoclavicular joint and brachiocephalic vein to contribute to the pulmonary plexus, oesophageal plexus and cardiac plexus
Phrenic (anterior rami of C3–C5)	Enters thorax and runs between mediastinal pleura and pericardium to supply motor and sensory innervation to the diaphragm. It also has a sensory supply to mediastinal pleura, pericardium and diaphragmatic peritoneum (in abdominal cavity)
Intercostal nerves (anterior rami of T1–T11)	Run between internal and innermost layers of intercostal muscles and supply skin, intercostal muscles and parietal pleura. The lower six intercostal nerves also supply the skin, musculature and parietal peritoneum of the abdominal wall
Subcostal nerve (T12)	Follows inferior border of 12th rib and passes into the abdominal wall. Its lateral cutaneous branch pierces the internal and external oblique muscle layers to supply the skin over the hip laterally, between the iliac crest and greater trochanter of femur
Recurrent laryngeal nerve (cranial nerve X)	Loops around subclavian artery on right and arch of aorta on left, and ascends in the tracheoesophageal groove; supplies intrinsic muscles of larynx (except cricothyroid) and sensation below level of vocal folds
Cardiac plexus (cranial nerve X and sympathetic trunks)	Fibres usually pass along the right coronary artery to reach the sinoatrial node; parasympathetic fibres (from vagus nerve) reduce heart rate and force of contraction. Sympathetic nerve fibres (from spinal cord levels T1–T5) increase heart rate and force of contraction
Pulmonary plexus (cranial nerve X and sympathetic trunks)	Plexus forms in hilum (root) of lung and extends along branches of bronchi; parasympathetic fibres (from vagus nerve) constrict bronchioles, sympathetic fibres (from spinal cord segments T2–T6) dilate bronchioles
Oesophageal plexus (cranial nerve X and sympathetic trunks)	Vagus nerve and sympathetic nerves form a plexus around oesophagus to supply smooth muscle and glands.

the greater, lesser and least splanchnic nerves. The greater nerve is formed by branches from the 5th to 9th ganglia. The lesser nerve is formed by branches from the 10th to 11th ganglia, and the least nerve is a branch of the 12th ganglion. These pass into the abdomen behind the diaphragm to relay in the coeliac ganglion and provide a sympathetic supply to abdominal structures.

Lymphatic drainage of the thorax

Figure 4.25 shows the lymphatic drainage of the thoracic cavity. The thoracic duct (Fig. 3.24) receives lymph from:

- The lower half of the body
- The left posterior intercostal nodes
- The left side of the head and neck, and the left upper limb, via the left jugular and subclavian lymph trunks, respectively.

The right lymphatic duct receives lymph from the posterior right thoracic wall. The right side of the head and neck, and the right upper limb drain into the right jugular and subclavian trunks, respectively. These vessels open into the great veins either independently or as a single trunk, the right lymph trunk.

Thymus

This is the major organ responsible for the production and maturation of T lymphocytes. It is a large bi-lobed organ at birth, lying in the superior and anterior divisions of the mediastinum, anterior to the great vessels. In most people, the gland involutes after puberty.

Trachea

The trachea (Fig. 4.26) commences in the neck, at the lower border of the cricoid cartilage (level of C6 vertebral body). It passes into the superior mediastinum, anterior to the oesophagus and slightly right of the median plane. At the sternal angle, the trachea bifurcates into the right and left main bronchi. The right main bronchus is shorter, wider and more vertical than the left – foreign bodies are most likely to lodge in the right lower lobar bronchus, as its direction follows that of the right main bronchus.

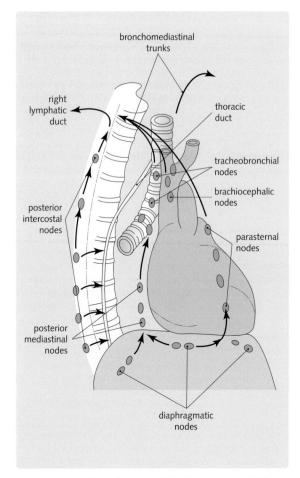

Fig. 4.25 Lymphatic drainage of the thoracic cavity (right hemithorax).

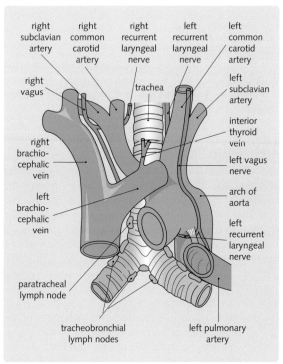

Fig. 4.26 Trachea and its main relations anteriorly and laterally.

Oesophagus

The oesophagus is the continuation of the laryngo-pharynx (at the level of the C6 vertebra). In the thorax the oesophagus lies between the trachea and the vertebral column. It passes through the oesophageal hiatus of the diaphragm, at the level of the T10 vertebra and after 1–2 cm enters the stomach. Fibres from the right crus of the diaphragm form a sling around the oesophagus. The upper oesophageal sphincter, which is primarily composed of the cricopharyngeus muscle, lies at the C5–C6 vertebral level. This is the narrowest part of the oesophagus. There are three further constrictions of the oesophagus – where it is crossed by the aortic arch, by the left main bronchus, and where it pierces the diaphragm. The left atrium is an anterior relation of the oesophagus, and may cause constriction if mitral valve incompetence is present (regurgitation of blood leads to dilatation of the left atrium). Figure 4.27 outlines the muscular composition, blood supply, lymphatic drainage and nerve supply of the oesophagus. The arterial supply and venous drainage is complex as the oesophagus spans the head and neck, thorax and abdomen.

PLEURAE AND LUNGS

Pleurae

Each pleural cavity is lined by pleura. The pleura is composed of an outer parietal layer and an inner visceral layer (Fig. 4.28). A thin layer of loose connective tissue,

known as endothoracic fascia, separates the parietal pleura from the thoracic wall. Parietal pleura lines each pleural cavity, covering the thoracic wall (costal pleura), the thoracic surface of the diaphragm (diaphragmatic pleura) and the lateral aspect of the mediastinum (mediastinal pleura). At the thoracic inlet, it covers the apex of the lungs (cervical pleura). The parietal and visceral pleura are continuous with each other at

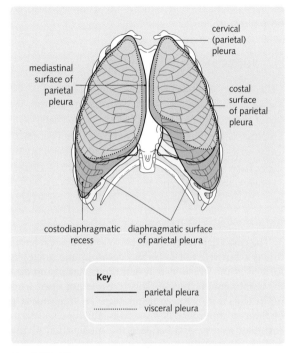

Fig. 4.28 Pleurae.

Fig. 4.27 Muscle composition, blood supply, nerve supply and lymphatic drainage of the oesophagus.

	Superior 1/3rd	Middle 1/3rd	Inferior 1/3rd
Muscle composition of wall	Skeletal	Mixed (skeletal and smooth)	Smooth
Arterial supply	Inferior thyroid artery	Oesophageal branches of the aorta	Left gastric artery
Venous drainage	Brachiocephalic vein	Azygos vein	Oesophageal tributaries of the left gastric veins which drain into the portal vein
Nerve supply	Recurrent laryngeal nerves and sympathetic fibres from cell bodies in the middle cervical ganglion running on the inferior thyroid artery	Fibres from the anterior and posterior oesophageal plexus from the vagus nerves; sympathetic fibres from the sympathetic trunks and greater splanchnic nerves	
Lymphatic drainage	Deep cervical nodes near the origin of the inferior thyroid artery	Tracheobronchial and posterior mediastinal nodes	Preaortic nodes of the coeliac group

Adapted from Hall-Craggs ECB (1995) Anatomy as a Basis for Clinical Medicine, *Williams & Wilkins.*

the hilum of the lung, where the parietal pleura is reflected from the mediastinal surface of the pleural cavity to become the visceral pleura. The visceral pleura is adherent to the lung, covering the outer surface and invaginating into the lung fissures. Between the two layers there is a narrow potential space (the pleural space) containing approximately 4 ml of clear pleural fluid. Inferior to the hilum of the lung, a double fold of pleura hangs downwards. This is known as the pulmonary ligament, which allows the hilum to descend during inspiration.

HINTS AND TIPS

The arrangement of the pleura is often difficult to visualize and a useful analogy is to imagine pushing your fist into a partly inflated balloon – your hand represents the lung, the outer surface of the balloon represents the parietal pleura, the balloon covering your hand represents the visceral pleura, and the space between them represents the pleural space.

The costodiaphragmatic recess (in radiological terms this is often referred to as the costophrenic angle) is formed at the junction between the costal pleura and the diaphragmatic pleura. This recess is not filled with lung except during forced inspiration. An accumulation of fluid in this space is known as a pleural effusion. A similar recess exists between the mediastinal pleura and the costal pleura (costomediastinal recess). The arterial supply, venous and lymphatic drainage, and innervation of the pleura are described in Figure 4.29.

Fig. 4.29 Arterial supply, venous drainage, lymphatic drainage and innervation of the pleura.		
	Parietal pleura	**Visceral pleura**
Arterial supply	Intercostal arteries and branches of the internal thoracic artery	Bronchial arteries
Venous drainage	Intercostal veins	Bronchial and pulmonary veins
Lymphatic drainage	Intercostal, internal thoracic (parasternal), posterior mediastinal and diaphragmatic nodes	Bronchopulmonary (hilar) nodes

Lungs

The lungs in life are light, spongy and elastic. The surface changes from a pink colour at birth, to a mottled darker colour in later life as a result of atmospheric pollution, particularly due to carbon particles. This is more pronounced in city-dwellers and smokers. Each lung lies free in the pleural cavity except at its root, where it is attached to the mediastinum.

Surfaces and borders of the lungs

These are illustrated in Figures 4.30 and 4.31. Each lung has an apex which projects approximately 2.5 cm into the neck, above the medial end of the clavicle, a base which lies on the diaphragm, a costal surface and a mediastinal surface. The hilum of the lung (Fig. 4.31) lies on the mediastinal surface.

Bronchi and bronchopulmonary segments

The trachea divides into the right and left main bronchi at the carina (posterior to the sternal angle). The bronchi are fibromuscular tubes, lined by respiratory epithelium and reinforced by C-shaped rings of cartilage, which are incomplete posteriorly. In the lung, the main bronchus divides into lobar bronchi (there are three on the right and two on the left), which in turn divide into segmental bronchi (there are ten on the right and nine on the left). The latter supply the bronchopulmonary segments, which are the functional units of the lungs (Fig. 4.32). The segments are wedge shaped, with their

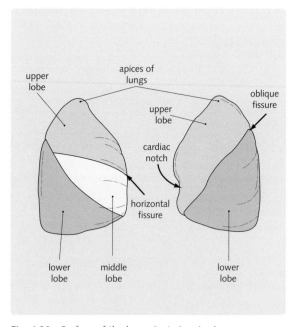

Fig. 4.30 Surface of the lungs (anterior view).

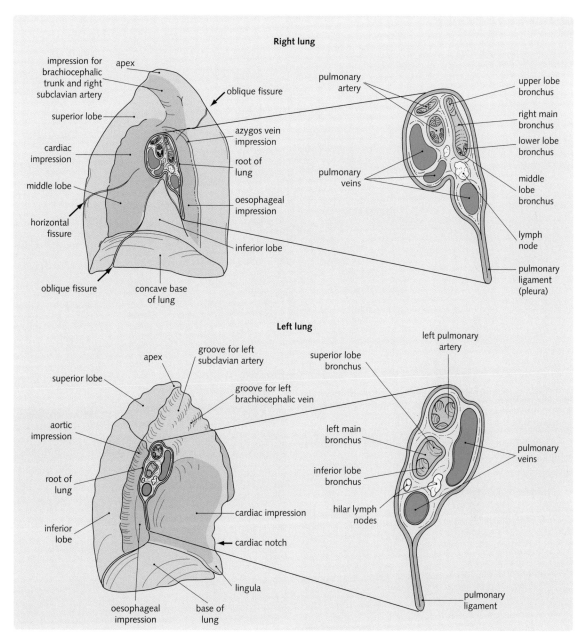

Fig. 4.31 Medial aspect of the right and left lungs and contents of their roots. Impressions are only seen in fixed lungs.

bases lying peripherally and their apices projecting towards the hilum of the lung. Each segment has its own segmental bronchus, artery, lymphatic vessels and autonomic nerve supply. The pulmonary veins run between the bronchopulmonary segments. The segmental bronchi repeatedly subdivide and reduce in diameter with each division. When the airways are no longer supported by cartilage, they are referred to as bronchioles. Bronchioles subdivide, becoming terminal bronchioles (the most distal airways which are lined by respiratory epithelium). They divide in turn into respiratory bronchioles giving rise to millions of alveoli. Alveoli are thin-walled sacs of epithelium surrounded by capillaries, allowing blood to come into close contact with inhaled air, thus allowing gas exchange.

Blood supply of the lungs

The lungs have a dual blood supply:

- Bronchial arteries (branches of the thoracic aorta) supply the walls of the bronchi.

Fig. 4.32 The bronchial tree of the lung.

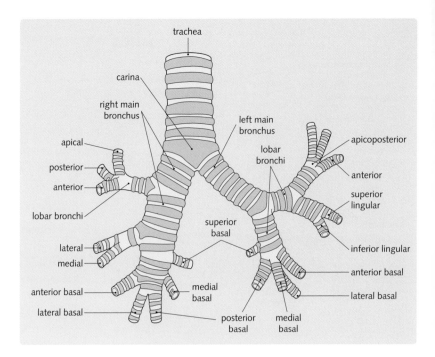

- Pulmonary arteries transport deoxygenated blood to the alveolar capillaries. The pulmonary veins return oxygenated blood to the left atrium.

  There are anastomoses between the pulmonary and bronchial circulations.

CLINICAL NOTE

Pulmonary embolus

A pulmonary embolism occurs when a venous embolus (normally from the lower limbs, where it is known as a deep vein thrombosis (DVT)) becomes lodged in the pulmonary arterial circulation. A recognizable risk factor is present in the majority of patients. They include recent surgery, prolonged immobility, malignancy and pregnancy. Symptoms include dyspnoea, tachypnoea, tachycardia, pleuritic chest pain, hypoxia and haemoptysis (coughing up blood). A massive pulmonary embolus can result in sudden death.

CLINICAL NOTE

Oncology

Bronchial carcinoma accounts for 22% of cancer deaths. Metastasis of tumour cells to the tracheobronchial nodes leads to widening of the carina. The left recurrent laryngeal nerve may be affected by left-sided lung tumours, as it hooks under the aortic arch and lies superior to the left main bronchus. Damage results in paralysis of the left laryngeal musculature (except cricothyroid muscle), and the patient presents with hoarseness and a weak voice. They may also have a bovine cough. The phrenic nerves are also vulnerable, leading to paralysis of the ipsilateral diaphragm.

Lymphatic drainage of the lungs

Figure 4.33 illustrates the lymphatic drainage of the lungs. Lung carcinoma is very common and it is important to have an understanding of where it may spread.

Mechanics of respiration

Respiration consists of an inspiratory and an expiratory phase as the diameters of the thoracic cavity increase and decrease respectively (Fig. 4.34):

- Vertical diameter: lies between the apex of the pleural cavity superiorly and the diaphragm inferiorly

Nerve supply of the lungs

Sympathetic and parasympathetic nerves from the pulmonary plexuses, which lie anterior and posterior to the lung roots, supply the smooth muscle of the bronchial tree, the vessels and the mucous membrane.

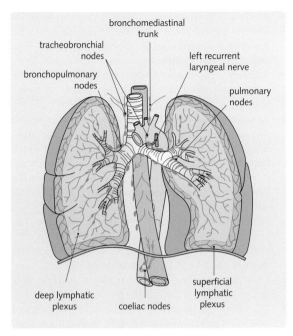

Fig. 4.33 Lymphatic drainage of the lungs.

and superior movement of the upper ribs (resembles the movement of a pump handle). The axis of movement passes through the neck of the rib
- The transverse diameter lies between corresponding right and left ribs.

- The anteroposterior diameter lies between the sternum and costal cartilages anteriorly, and the vertebral column and ribs posteriorly. Its diameter is increased by forward movement of the sternum

Fig. 4.34	Movements and muscles involved in respiration.	
Movements	**Effect**	**Muscles involved**
Quiet inspiration	Increased vertical diameter	Diaphragm contracts causing flattening of the domes
Quiet inspiration	Increased anteroposterior diameter	Scalenus muscles contract and fix the first rib. The upper intercostal muscles contract to elevate the upper ribs at their sternal ends towards the first rib and this pushes the sternum forwards—known as the pump handle movement
Quiet inspiration	Increased transverse diameter	Scalenus muscles contract fixing the first rib. The intercostal muscles contract raising the lower ribs along an anteroposterior axis that runs through the costochondral joint (anteriorly) and costovertebral joint (posteriorly). The lower ribs are raised upward and outward in a bucket handle movement
Forced inspiration	Increase of all three diameters	In addition to the diaphragm contracting, the scalenus and sternocleidomastoid muscles elevate the ribs and manubrium. The intercostal muscles forcefully contract elevating the ribs. Quadratus lumborum lowers and fixes the twelfth rib. This allows a forceful diaphragmatic contraction. The erector spinae muscles arch the back and increase the thoracic volume. With the humerus and scapula fixed the pectoral and serratus anterior muscles raise the ribs
Quiet expiration	Decrease of all three diameters	Elastic recoil of the lungs and controlled relaxation of the intercostal and diaphragmatic muscles causes this passive movement
Forced expiration	Decrease of all three diameters	Contraction of the anterior abdominal wall muscles depresses the ribs and reinforces the elastic recoil of the lungs. The abdominal contents are pushed up forcing the diaphragm upwards. The intercostal muscles contract and prevent bulging of their intercostal spaces

RADIOLOGICAL ANATOMY

Imaging of the thorax

Chest X-ray

A chest X-ray (radiograph) is commonly requested to assess the heart, lungs, blood vessels and bones. A typical chest X-ray view reflects the direction in which the X-ray beam is projected, e.g. posteroanterior (PA) and lateral.

The normal radiographic anatomy of a PA chest X-ray is illustrated in Figure 4.35.

How to examine a PA chest X-ray methodically

It may be tempting to focus on any obvious abnormality observed on a chest X-ray, but there may be other areas of less obvious, but more important, pathology. Therefore, it is essential to develop a system and follow this each time you interpret an X-ray. The following is one method of how to examine a chest x-ray (although there are many):

- Patient identity – name and date of birth, and date and time of X-ray (patients may have more than one X-ray in a day).

- Projection – posteroanterior (PA), anteroposterior (AP) or lateral. Most films are PA. In patients who are unable to stand, an AP film is taken. An AP film will artificially enlarge the heart.
- Rotation – the medial ends of the clavicle should be equidistant from an intervening thoracic vertebral spinous process. If not, rotation is present.
- Inspiration – X-rays of the chest are taken during full inspiration in order to obtain an image of the entire lung field, and prevent the false appearance of an enlarged heart (cardiomegaly), or pulmonary oedema. If 5–7 anterior ribs are visible in the mid-clavicular line, or ten posterior ribs, then inspiration is adequate.
- Penetration – the thoracic vertebral bodies should be just visible through the cardiac shadow. If the vertebral bodies cannot be seen through the cardiac shadow the film is under-penetrated.
- Look for any obvious abnormality – describe this, then continue to examine the remainder of the X-ray.
- Trachea – the trachea should be central. Causes of deviation include pneumothorax, mediastinal mass, lung collapse or fibrosis.
- Mediastinum – the right heart border is formed by the right atrium. The superior vena cava lies above

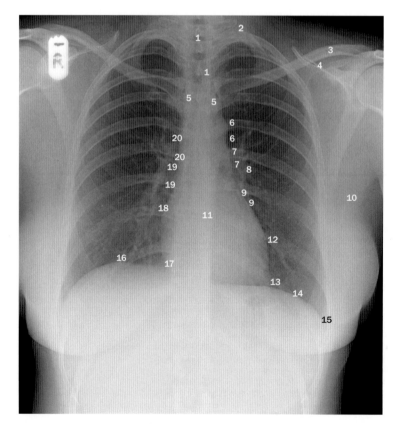

1. Trachea
2. First rib
3. Clavicle
4. Spine of scapula
5. Sternum
6. Arch of aorta
7. Pulmonary trunk
8. Left pulmonary artery
9. Region of tip of auricle of left atrium
10. Anterior axillary fold
11. Descending aorta
12. Border of left ventricle
13. Left cardiophrenic angle
14. Left dome of diaphragm
15. Left costophrenic angle
16. Right dome of diaphragm
17. Inferior vena cava
18. Right atrial border
19. Right pulmonary artery
20. Superior vena cava

Fig. 4.35 A posteroanterior chest radiograph – adult female.

this. The aortic arch is the first structure on the left, followed by the left pulmonary artery. The left heart border is made up by the left atrium and left ventricle. The transverse diameter of the heart should occupy no more than 50% of the transverse diameter of the chest (the cardiothoracic ratio). A cardiothoracic ratio > 0.5 (i.e. the heart occupies more than 50% of the diameter of the chest, is defined as cardiomegaly).

- Hilar structures – the site of the main bronchi, pulmonary arteries and lymph nodes. Hilar enlargement may be due to enlarged nodes, or a tumour.
- Lungs – examine the entire lung fields, particularly the apices. Look for abnormal opacities, masses, infiltrates and calcifications. Examine the vascular patterns – prominent vasculature may be due to heart failure, myocardial infarction, mitral valve disease, etc.
- Costophrenic and cardiophrenic angles – these should be well defined. They may be blunted if an effusion is present.
- Diaphragm – the right diaphragm is higher than the left due to the position of the liver. Free air under the hemidiaphragm, suggests perforation of an intra-abdominal viscus.

- Soft tissues – e.g. breast tissue, neck (for subcutaneous emphysema).
- Bones – examine the clavicles, scapulae, ribs and vertebrae for fractures, sclerotic or lytic lesions. Examine the joints (e.g. narrowing of joint space suggesting osteoarthritis).

CLINICAL NOTE

Radiology

In pneumonia, inflammation causes the alveoli to become filled with exudate (consolidation). Consolidation appears white on a chest X-ray. Bronchi are not normally visible on a chest X-ray – the outline of patent (open) bronchi within an area of consolidation is known as an air bronchogram.

CT scanning of the thorax

CT scanning of the thorax is often and undertaken to follow up an abnormality found on a chest X-ray (Fig. 4.36). Scans are commonly requested when diseases such as tumours, pulmonary fibrosis,

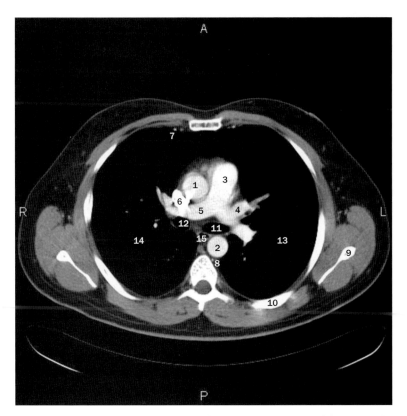

1. Ascending aorta
2. Descending aorta
3. Pulmonary trunk
4. Left pulmonary artery
5. Right pulmonary artery
6. Superior vena cava
7. Internal thoracic artery
8. Posterior intercostal arteries
9. Scapula
10. Rib
11. Left main bronchus
12. Right main bronchus
13. Left lung
14. Right lung
15. Oesophagus

Fig. 4.36 A CT scan (transverse section) of the thorax at the level of the T4 vertebra.

pulmonary emboli and tuberculosis are suspected. The radiation exposure resulting from a CT scan of the thorax (approximately equivalent to 2 years of background radiation) is greater than that of a chest X-ray (approximately equivalent to 10 days of background radiation). Traditional CT scans can be enhanced by reconstruction of CT slices, to produce 3D images of body structures, e.g. viscera, blood vessels and bones (Fig. 4.37A&B).

Angiography of the great vessels

Figure 4.38 shows the branches of the aortic arch and their subsequent divisions to form the arterial supply of the head, neck and thoracic cage.

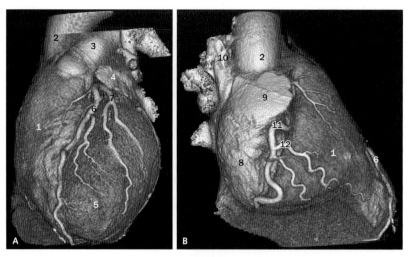

1. Right ventricle
2. Aorta
3. Pulmonary trunk
4. Left atrial appendage
5. Apex of left ventricle
6. Left anterior descending artery
7. Left marginal artery
8. Right atrium
9. Right atrial appendage
10. Superior vena cava
11. Right coronary artery
12. Right marginal artery

Fig. 4.37   3D CT angiogram of left (A) and right (B) coronary arteries.

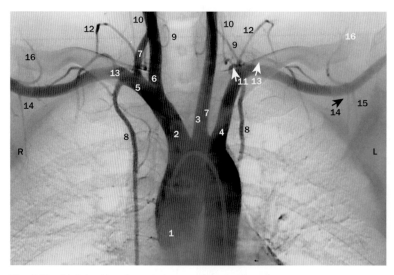

1. Ascending aorta
2. Brachiocephalic trunk
3. Left common carotid artery
4. Left subclavian artery
5. Right subclavian artery
6. Right common carotid artery
7. Vertebral artery
8. Internal thoracic artery
9. Inferior thyroid artery
10. Ascending cervical artery
11. Thyrocervical trunk
12. Suprascapular artery
13. Costocervical trunk
14. Superior thoracic artery
15. Lateral thoracic artery
16. Deltoid branch of the thoraco-acromial artery

Fig. 4.38   Digital subtraction arteriogram of the aortic arch.

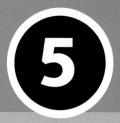

The abdomen 5

REGIONS AND COMPONENTS OF THE ABDOMEN

The abdominal cavity is separated from the thoracic cavity by the diaphragm. The domes of the diaphragm arch above the costal margin, therefore some of the abdominal organs (liver, spleen, upper poles of the kidneys and suprarenal glands) are protected by the bony thoracic cage. The bony pelvis surrounds the lower part of the abdominal cavity.

Posteriorly, the vertebral column protects the contents of the abdomen. The anterolateral wall is muscular and is, therefore, more vulnerable to injury.

Over the anterior abdominal wall, the superficial fascia is composed of two layers. The outer layer (Camper's fascia) is continuous with the superficial fascia of the thigh. Deep to Camper's fascia lies Scarpa's fascia – a thin membranous layer. The arrangement of these two layers allows Camper's fascia to move freely, allowing the abdomen to expand. Scarpa's fascia fades over the thoracic wall superiorly, and inferiorly it fuses with the fascia lata of the thigh. In males it continues into the scrotum and penis as the superficial perineal fascia (of Colles) and the superficial fascia of the penis respectively. In the female the superficial perineal fascia lines the labia majora and is perforated by the vagina.

The anterolateral abdominal wall is composed of three layers of muscle. These form an aponeurosis anteriorly to surround the rectus abdominis muscle.

The abdominal cavity is lined by parietal peritoneum, with visceral peritoneum covering many of the organs. The cavity contains most of the gastrointestinal tract, together with its accessory organs (liver, gallbladder and pancreas).

Abdominal pain is very common—knowledge of embryology and anatomy will help in diagnosis (Fig. 5.1).

SURFACE ANATOMY AND SUPERFICIAL STRUCTURES

To aid description, the abdomen is divided into regions. The simplest method is to divide the abdomen into four quadrants by a vertical and a horizontal line through the umbilicus; however, for more accurate description, it is divided into nine regions (Fig. 5.2) by:

- Two vertical lines – extending inferiorly from the midpoint of each clavicle
- Two horizontal lines: **the transtubercular plane** (passing horizontally between the two tubercles of the iliac crest) and **the transpyloric plane** (passing

Fig. 5.1 Origin and blood supply of the abdominal viscera and sites of referred pain.

Part of fetal gut	Organs	Blood supply	Site of abdominal pain
Foregut	Oesophagus, stomach, first and half of the second part of duodenum, liver, gallbladder, spleen and pancreas	Coeliac trunk	Epigastric region
Midgut	Remainder of duodenum, jejunum, ileum, caecum, appendix, ascending colon, and proximal two-thirds of transverse colon	Superior mesenteric artery	Umbilical region
Hindgut	Distal one-third of transverse colon, descending colon, sigmoid colon, rectum, and part of the anal canal	Inferior mesenteric artery	Suprapubic region

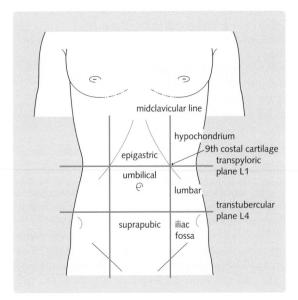

Fig. 5.2 Regions of the abdomen.

horizontally midway between the pubic symphysis and suprasternal notch).

The linea alba is a midline depression running from the xiphisternum to the pubis. The linea semilunaris is a slightly curved line which represents the lateral margin of the rectus abdominis muscle on each side.

The inguinal ligament lies between the anterior superior iliac spine and the pubic tubercle. The deep inguinal ring lies at the midinguinal point (halfway between the anterior superior iliac spine and the pubic symphysis). The umbilicus lies at approximately the level of the L3 vertebra.

Liver

The inferior border of the liver extends from the 10th costal cartilage on the right, in the midclavicular line, to the 5th rib on the left, in the midclavicular line.

The upper border runs between the left and right 5th ribs; both in the midclavicular line.

Fundus of the gallbladder

The fundus of the gallbladder lies posterior to the 9th right costal cartilage, at the intersection of the transpyloric plane with the costal margin.

Spleen

The spleen lies deep to the left 9th, 10th and 11th ribs, posterior to the midaxillary line. It is not palpable unless enlarged, in which case the spleen extends inferiorly and anteriorly below the costal margin.

Pancreas

The head of the pancreas lies in the 'C' shaped concavity of the duodenum at the level of the L2 vertebra. The neck lies in the transpyloric plane (at the level of the L1 vertebra). The body of the pancreas extends left, curving upwards towards the hilum of the spleen.

Kidneys

The hilum of each kidney lies in the transpyloric plane. The upper pole of the kidneys lie deep to the 12th rib posteriorly. They lie opposite the L1–L4 vertebrae (the right lies slightly lower than the left due to the presence of the liver).

Ureters

Each ureter begins at the hilum of the kidney, in the transpyloric plane. The ureter runs inferiorly over psoas major muscle, anterior to the tips of the transverse processes of the lumbar vertebrae, as far as the sacroiliac joint, where it enters the pelvis.

THE ABDOMINAL WALL

Osteology

Figure 5.3 shows the skeleton of the abdominal and pelvic cavities (see Chapter 6).

The costal margin and floating ribs have been described previously (see Chapter 4). The characteristics of a typical lumbar vertebra are illustrated in Figure 2.3E.

The pelvic bones articulate with the sacrum at the sacroiliac joint (a modified synovial joint) and with each other at the pubic symphysis (a secondary cartilaginous joint). Each pelvic bone is formed from the ilium, ischium and pubis.

The ilia protect underlying structures and provide a site for muscle attachment. The superior border of the ilium – the iliac crest – runs from the anterior superior iliac spine (ASIS) to the posterior superior iliac spine (PSIS). The ASIS is often visible and the PSIS is marked by a dimple on the skin of the back. The iliac tubercle is the highest point of the crest. The three muscle layers of the anterolateral abdominal wall originate from the iliac crest, as do latissimus dorsi, quadratus lumborum and the thoracolumbar fascia.

The pectineal line lies on the superior ramus of the pubic bone, and medial to it lie the pubic tubercle and pubic crest. The pectineal line continues posteriorly as the arcuate line, which forms part of the pelvic brim.

Thoracolumbar fascia

The lumbar part of this fascia arises from the vertebrae in three layers:

- The anterior layer – from the anterior aspect of the lumbar transverse processes
- The middle layer – from the tips of the lumbar transverse processes
- The posterior layer – from the tips of the lumbar spinous processes.

The anterior and middle layers enclose quadratus lumborum; the middle and posterior layers enclose the erector spinae muscles. The three sheets fuse laterally and provide attachment for the internal oblique and transversus abdominis muscles. The thoracic part of the fascia consists of the posterior layer only. This attaches to the thoracic spinous processes and angles of the ribs (Fig. 4.6).

Muscles of the anterolateral abdominal wall

Figure 5.4 outlines these muscles. The conjoint tendon is formed by the lowest fibres of internal oblique and transversus abdominis, inserting into the pubic crest and most medial part of the pectineal line.

Rectus sheath

Each rectus abdominis muscle is enclosed in a fibrous sheath, formed by the aponeuroses of the three muscles of the abdominal wall (Fig. 5.5). The composition of the rectus sheath changes at three points:

- Above the costal margin the sheath is composed of an anterior layer only – formed by the aponeurosis of external oblique. The posterior aspect of the rectus muscle lies on the costal cartilages.
- Between the costal margin and a point midway between the umbilicus and pubic symphysis, the internal oblique splits into an anterior and posterior layer. The anterior part of the sheath is formed by the aponeurosis of external oblique along with the anterior layer of internal oblique. The posterior part of the sheath is formed by the aponeurosis of transversus abdominis, along with the posterior layer of internal oblique. The lower limit of the posterior part of the sheath is known as the arcuate line.
- Inferior to the arcuate line, all three aponeuroses pass anterior to the rectus muscle, and the posterior wall of the sheath is composed only of transversalis fascia and peritoneum.

The inferior epigastric artery and vein enter the sheath at the level of the arcuate line and pass superiorly, deep to the rectus abdominis, to anastomose with the superior epigastric vessels.

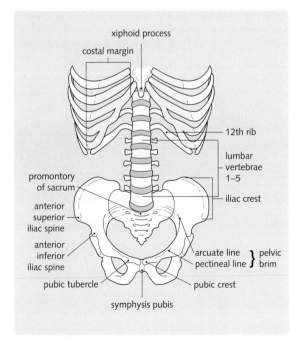

Fig. 5.3 Skeleton of the abdomen and pelvis.

Fig. 5.4 Muscles of the anterolateral abdominal wall.

Name of muscle (nerve supply)	Origin	Insertion	Action
External oblique (outermost layer) (T6–T12 spinal nerves)	Lower eight ribs	Becomes aponeurotic and attaches to the xiphoid process, linea alba, pubic crest, pubic tubercle, and iliac crest	Flexes and rotates trunk; pulls down ribs in forced expiration
Internal oblique (spinal nerves T6–T12, iliohypogastric and ilioinguinal nerves)	Thoracolumbar fascia, iliac crest, lateral two-thirds of inguinal ligament	Ribs 10–12 and costal cartilages, linea alba, pubic symphysis; forms conjoint tendon with transversus abdominis	Assists in flexing and rotating trunk; pulls down ribs in forced expiration
Transversus abdominis (innermost layer) (spinal nerves T6–T12, iliohypogastric and ilioinguinal nerves)	Lower six costal cartilages, thoracolumbar fascia, iliac crest, lateral third of inguinal ligament	Xiphoid process, linea alba, pubic symphysis: forms conjoint tendon with internal oblique	Compresses abdominal contents with external and internal oblique
Rectus abdominis (spinal nerves T6–T12)	Symphysis pubis and pubic crest	Costal cartilages 5–7 and xiphoid process	Compresses abdominal contents and flexes vertebral column

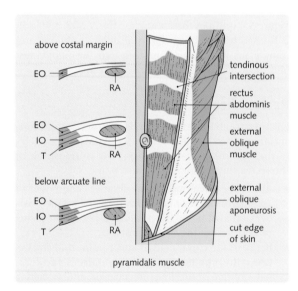

above costal margin

EO
RA

tendinous intersection
rectus abdominis muscle

EO
IO
T
RA

external oblique muscle

below arcuate line

EO
IO
T
RA

external oblique aponeurosis

cut edge of skin

pyramidalis muscle

Fig. 5.5 Rectus sheath and rectus abdominis muscle. EO, external oblique; IO, internal oblique; T, transversus abdominis; RA, rectus abdominis.

Nerve and blood supply of the anterolateral abdominal wall

The principal nerves and arteries of the anterolateral abdominal wall are shown in Figure 5.6. Nerves run in a 'neurovascular plane' between the transversus abdominis and internal oblique muscles. All the nerves give off anterior and lateral cutaneous branches, except for the ilioinguinal nerve, which gives off an anterior branch only.

Venous drainage of the anterolateral abdominal wall

The superficial veins of the abdominal wall include the superficial epigastric and thoracoepigastric veins, which ultimately drain into the femoral vein and axillary veins respectively.

The superior and inferior epigastric veins and the deep circumflex iliac veins follow the course of the arteries and drain into the internal thoracic and external iliac veins.

Of the four lumbar veins, the lower two drain into the inferior vena cava. The upper two join to form the ascending lumbar vein and, with the subcostal vein, drain into the azygos vein on the right and hemiazygos vein on the left.

CLINICAL NOTE

Abdominal incisions
- A midline incision passes through the linea alba: this allows rapid access with minimal blood loss.
- A paramedian incision passes through the anterior wall of the rectus sheath, the rectus muscle is displaced laterally and the posterior sheath is then divided. Postoperatively, the rectus muscle covers and strengthens the scar on the posterior layer of the sheath.
- A subcostal incision is made 2.5 cm below and parallel to the costal margin (on the right for biliary surgery and on the left to expose the spleen).
- A gridiron incision is made centred at McBurney's point. Each muscle layer is incised individually in line

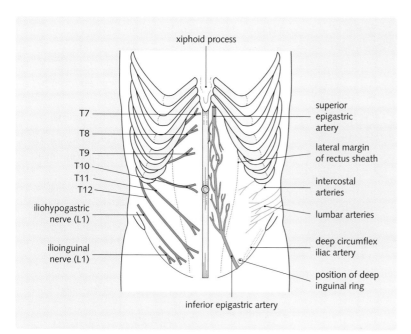

Fig. 5.6 Innervation (left) and arterial supply (right) of the anterolateral abdominal wall.

xiphoid process

T7
T8
T9
T10
T11
T12

iliohypogastric
nerve (L1)

ilioinguinal
nerve (L1)

superior
epigastric
artery

lateral margin
of rectus sheath

intercostal
arteries

lumbar arteries

deep circumflex
iliac artery

position of deep
inguinal ring

inferior epigastric artery

with its fibres, so the strength of the wall is virtually unaffected, although there is a risk of damaging the iliohypogastric and ilioinguinal nerves.
• Transverse incisions are made across the rectus abdominis muscle – it is supplied segmentally, so there is no danger of denervation.

Inguinal region

Inguinal ligament

The inguinal ligament is formed from the lower edge of the aponeurosis of external oblique. It extends from ASIS to the pubic tubercle. It gives origin to the internal oblique and transverse abdominis muscles, and the fascia lata of the thigh.

Inguinal canal

This is a narrow passage, approximately 4 cm long, which lies superior and parallel to the medial half of the inguinal ligament. It runs inferomedially and extends from the deep inguinal ring (DIR) to the superficial ring (SIR) (Fig. 5.7). The DIR is an opening in the transversalis fascia approximately 1 cm superior to the midinguinal point, and lateral to the inferior epigastric artery. The spermatic cord in males, the round ligament in females and the genitofemoral nerve in both sexes, pass through the DIR to enter the inguinal canal. The ilioinguinal nerve also passes through the inguinal

canal, but enters it by piercing the transversalis fascia, i.e. it does not pass through the DIR. The superficial inguinal ring is a triangular opening in the external oblique aponeurosis, superolateral to the pubic tubercle. The contents of the inguinal canal exit through this ring. It has an anterior wall, a posterior wall, a roof and a floor (Fig. 5.8).

CLINICAL NOTE

Inguinal hernias

An inguinal hernia occurs when bowel, omentum or another organ protrudes either through the deep inguinal ring (DIR) (indirect hernia) or the transversalis fascia (direct hernia) of the abdomen.
• An indirect hernia is congenital. It occurs secondary to a patent processus vaginalis. Herniation occurs through the DIR and may extend along the inguinal canal, through the superficial inguinal ring (SIR) (lateral to the inferior epigastric artery) and into the scrotum.
• A direct hernia normally occurs in older males. The hernia passes through Hesselbach's triangle (its boundaries are the rectus sheath, inferior epigastric vessels and the inguinal ligament), located in the posterior wall of the inguinal canal, medial to the inferior epigastric artery. It then continues through the inguinal canal and exits the superficial inguinal ring.

A hernia can normally be reduced back into the abdominal cavity with gentle pressure or manipulation. If a hernia cannot be reduced it is referred to as an incarcerated hernia and may produce symptoms of bowel obstruction, i.e. pain, nausea and vomiting. The blood supply to an incarcerated hernia is normally not compromised. If the blood supply to a hernia becomes compromised, it is referred to as a strangulated hernia. The patient may present with symptoms similar to that of an incarcerated hernia. However, they are generally more unwell (tachycardic and pyrexial). Strangulated hernias require emergency surgery to prevent necrosis of the bowel.

Fig. 5.8	Boundaries of the inguinal canal.
Region	**Components**
Anterior wall	External oblique aponeurosis; lateral one-third reinforced by internal oblique
Floor	Lower edge of the inguinal ligament; reinforced medially by the lacunar ligament, which lies between the inguinal ligament and the pectineal line
Roof	Lower edges of the internal oblique and transversus muscles: the muscles fibres arch over the front of the spermatic cord laterally, and behind the cord medially, where their joint tendon – the conjoint tendon – is inserted into the pubic crest and pectineal line of the pubic bone
Posterior wall	Conjoint tendon medially and the transversalis fascia laterally

Spermatic cord

The structures entering the deep inguinal ring pick up a covering from each layer of the abdominal wall as they pass through the canal to form the spermatic cord (Fig. 5.9). The spermatic cord is not complete until it emerges from the superficial inguinal ring with all of its coverings.

The coverings from superficial to deep are:

- External spermatic fascia – derived from the aponeurosis of external oblique muscle
- Cremasteric fascia – derived from internal oblique and the transversus abdominis muscles
- Internal spermatic fascia – derived from the transversalis fascia.

The contents of the spermatic cord are:

- The ductus deferens
- Arteries – testicular artery (from the abdominal aorta), the artery to the ductus deferens (from inferior vesical arteries) and the cremasteric artery (from the inferior epigastric artery)
- Veins – the pampiniform plexus of veins
- Lymphatics – accompany the veins from the testis to the para-aortic nodes
- Nerves – the genital branch of the genitofemoral nerve supplies the cremaster muscle and sympathetic nerves supply arteries and smooth muscle of the ductus deferens
- The processus vaginalis – the obliterated remains of the peritoneal connection with the tunica vaginalis of the testis.

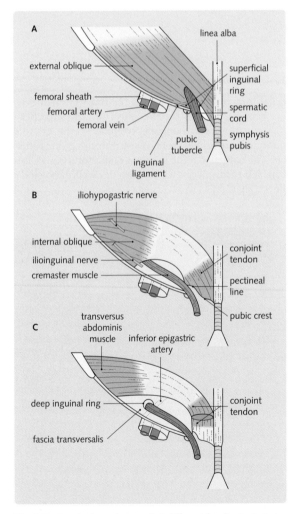

Fig. 5.7 Inguinal canal viewed at different levels: A, Anterior view of the inguinal canal; B, Anterior view of the inguinal canal with external oblique removed; C, Anterior view of the inguinal canal with external and internal oblique removed.

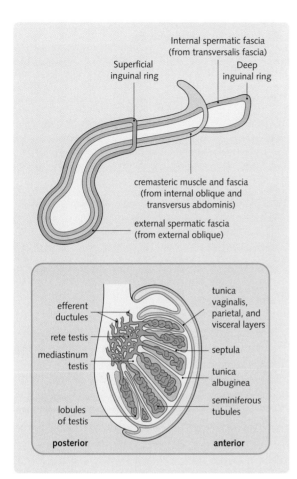

Fig. 5.9 Left testis and coverings of the spermatic cord.

Scrotum

The scrotum contains the testes, epididymis, vas deferens and the distal part of the spermatic cord. The wall of the scrotum is composed of several layers:

- Skin
- Superficial fascia containing the dartos muscle. The dartos muscle receives sympathetic innervation, and contracts in response to cold, pulling the testes closer to the body and wrinkling the skin. The scrotum is divided into two compartments by the median raphe (composed of superficial fascia), separating the testes. Deep to the dartos muscle lies Colles' fascia – a continuation of Scarpa's fascia of the abdomen
- External spermatic fascia
- Cremasteric fascia
- Internal spermatic fascia
- Parietal layer of the tunica vaginalis

Blood supply, lymphatic drainage and nerve supply of the scrotum

The arterial supply of the scrotum arises from anterior and posterior scrotal arteries (branches of the external pudendal artery and internal pudendal artery respectively). Venous drainage occurs via scrotal veins, which drain into the external pudendal artery and, eventually, into the great saphenous vein. Innervation of the scrotum occurs via the genitofemoral, ilioinguinal, pudendal nerves and the posterior cutaneous nerve of thigh. The ilioinguinal nerve supplies the anterior third of the scrotum. The posterior two-thirds is innervated by the posterior scrotal branch of the perineal nerve (medially) and the perineal branch of the posterior cutaneous nerve of thigh (laterally). Lymph vessels drain to the medial superficial inguinal lymph nodes of the thigh.

> **CLINICAL NOTE**
>
> **Cremasteric reflex**
>
> In the male, the genital branch of the genitofemoral nerve supplies the cremaster muscle. Its femoral branch supplies a small area of skin on the thigh. Stimulation of this skin causes the cremaster muscle to contract, raising the testis towards the inguinal canal – testing L1. This reflex is very active in children, often leading to a misdiagnosis of undescended testes.

Testis

The testis is suspended in the scrotum by the spermatic cord (Fig. 5.9) and is surrounded by three layers (tunics). The outermost layer is the tunica vaginalis, composed of a parietal and visceral layer. Testicular development begins at approximately 6 weeks' gestation, on the posterior abdominal wall. In the third month of fetal development, a sock-like evagination of the fetal peritoneum (processus vaginalis) passes through the abdominal wall, into the developing scrotum. At 7–9 months' gestation the testis descends retroperitoneally into the scrotum (preceded by the gubernaculum) coming to lie posterior to the processus vaginalis. After testicular descent is complete, the proximal part of the processus vaginalis is obliterated, leaving a double layered, serous sac at the distal end – the tunica vaginalis. The tunica vaginalis covers the epididymis and the testis except for its posterior surface, where it reflects onto the wall of the scrotum.

Deep to the tunica vaginalis lies the tunica albuginea, a tough fibrous capsule, which gives rise to numerous septa, dividing the testis into 200–300 lobules. Within the lobules lie the seminiferous tubules (the site of spermatogenesis). The seminiferous tubules open into the rete testis (a network of channels lying on the posterior aspect of the testis). The rete testis converge upon the efferent ducts, which in turn connect to the first part of the epididymis (Fig. 5.9). Deep to the tunica albuginea lies the tunica vasculosa, containing blood vessels and areolar tissue.

HINTS AND TIPS

It is important to remember that the scrotum is part of the body wall and receives a local arterial and nerve supply, while the testis develops in the abdomen during fetal life and retains its vascular supply and abdominal lymphatic drainage. In the female, the ovaries are retained within the abdominal cavity.

Epididymis

The epididymis lies on the posterolateral border of the testis. It is a tightly coiled single tube, the site of sperm storage and maturation. It is composed of a head (lying at the upper poles of the testis), a body and a tail. The efferent ducts drain into the head of the epididymis. At its tail the epididymis becomes less coiled, wider and becomes known as the ductus (vas) deferens.

Ductus deferens

Muscular contractions of the ductus transmit sperm from the epididymis to the prostatic urethra during ejaculation (sympathetic innervation). Its arterial supply arises from a small branch of the superior vesical artery.

Blood supply and lymphatic drainage of the testis

The testicular artery (a branch of the abdominal aorta at the level of the T2 vertebra) enters the spermatic cord and supplies the testis and epididymis. The pampiniform plexus of veins drains these structures. In the inguinal canal, the plexus forms four veins. As they emerge through the DIR, they merge to form two veins, which subsequently join to form a single testicular vein. The left testicular vein drains into the left renal vein and the right directly into the inferior vena cava. The plexus surrounds the testicular artery and cools the arterial blood, thereby providing the cooler environment required for spermatogenesis in the testis. Lymphatic drainage of the testes is to the para-aortic nodes in the abdomen.

CLINICAL NOTE

Conditions affecting the testes

Undescended testis
- The testis may not descend completely, stopping at any point along its descent. Undescended testes carry a higher than normal risk of malignant change.

Testicular torsion
- Testicular torsion occurs when the spermatic cord becomes twisted. This compromises the blood supply to the testicle. It results in acute, severe unilateral testicular pain, often with nausea and vomiting. The testicle is swollen, elevated within the scrotum and extremely tender. This is a medical emergency and requires immediate treatment, usually involving surgery.

Testicular swellings
- A hydrocele is an accumulation of serous fluid within the tunica vaginalis, usually secondary to a persistent processus vaginalis. It results in a painless enlarged scrotum.
- A haematocele is an accumulation of blood within the tunica vaginalis, usually as a result of trauma. It results in an enlarged scrotum, which may be painful.
- A varicocele is an abnormal dilatation of the veins of the pampiniform plexus, usually secondary to failures of valves in the testicular vein, or due to compression of the venous drainage of the testicle (e.g. from a pelvic or abdominal malignancy). It causes a dragging sensation or ache within the scrotum and may be visible or palpable (often described as 'a bag of worms').
- A spermatocele is a cystic structure which arises from the epididymis and contains spermatozoa. It is normally asymptomatic. It lies superior and posterior to the testis but is separate from it.

The cause of most testicular swellings can be diagnosed by ultrasound examination.

THE PERITONEUM

The peritoneum lines the abdominal and pelvic cavities. It consists of a parietal and visceral layer. Parietal peritoneum lines the anterior, posterior and lateral walls of the abdomen, the inferior surface of the diaphragm and the walls of the pelvic cavity. It reflects off the body wall, to surround some of the abdominal viscera. The peritoneum extending from the body wall to the organs forms mesenteries and ligaments. Between the parietal and visceral peritoneum lies a potential space, the peritoneal cavity, filled with a small amount of serous fluid, to allow free movement of viscera. In males the peritoneal cavity is completely closed; in females the uterine (Fallopian) tubes open into the peritoneal cavity and provide a connection to the exterior through the uterus and vagina.

Embryology of the gut

In the embryo the gut begins development as a simple tube-like structure. It develops into the foregut, midgut and hindgut, and invaginates into the peritoneal cavity (in a similar way to the lungs in the pleural cavity). The gut tube is then suspended from the posterior abdominal wall by the dorsal mesentery – the double layer of peritoneum connecting it to the body wall. Between the two layers of peritoneum are blood vessels, lymphatics and nerves (Fig. 5.10). The dorsal mesentery eventually forms the dorsal mesentery of the small intestine and other named mesenteries e.g. the greater omentum. Organs suspended from these mesenteries (and so almost entirely covered by visceral peritoneum) are termed intra-peritoneal. Some organs develop or come to lie upon the posterior abdominal wall, posterior to the visceral peritoneum and are, therefore, termed retroperitoneal.

The foregut is also connected to the body wall via the ventral mesentery. Growth of the liver divides the ventral mesentery into the falciform ligament anteriorly and the lesser omentum posteriorly (Fig. 5.11).

Nerve supply of the peritoneum

The parietal peritoneum is supplied segmentally by the nerves supplying the overlying muscles and skin. The peritoneum covering the inferior surface of the diaphragm is supplied by the intercostal nerves peripherally and by the phrenic nerve (C3,4,5) centrally. The parietal peritoneum in the pelvis is supplied by the obturator nerve. The visceral peritoneum does not have a somatic innervation, so is insensitive to pain. However, it receives sympathetic innervation and so it is sensitive to stretch, tension and ischaemia.

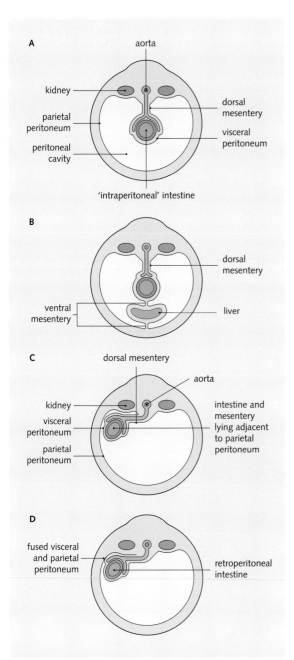

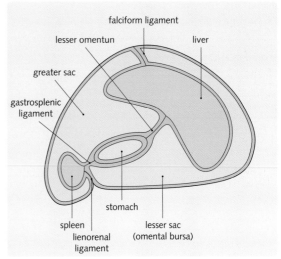

Fig. 5.10 The embryonic (A) dorsal and (B) ventral mesenteries (C and D) and the formation of the retroperitoneal part of the intestines.

Fig. 5.11 Division of the ventral mesentery, forming the falciform ligament and the lesser omentum.

Peritoneal folds of the anterolateral abdominal wall

Peritoneal folds are reflections of peritoneum, forming ridges on the body wall. They are produced by an underlying vessel or duct, or the remnant of a fetal vessel. There are five peritoneal folds on the abdominal wall (Fig. 5.12):

- Median umbilical fold – contains the remnant of the urachus (median umbilical ligament)
- Two medial umbilical folds – containing remnants of the umbilical arteries (medial umbilical ligaments)
- Two lateral umbilical folds – containing the inferior epigastric vessels.

The falciform ligament is an anterior peritoneal fold (originally the ventral mesentary), lying between the diaphragm and the umbilicus, which contains the ligamentum teres (the remnant of the umbilical vein) in its free margin.

Greater and lesser sacs

During development, the peritoneal cavity is divided into greater and lesser sacs, by growth of the liver (which rotates the stomach and duodenum to the right), and elongation of the dorsal mesentery. The lesser sac (omental bursa) is a sac of peritoneum lying posterior to the stomach. The remainder of the abdominal cavity forms the greater sac. The lesser sac communicates with the greater sac through the epiploic foramen. The boundaries of the epiploic (omental) foramen are:

- Superiorly – caudate process of liver
- Anteriorly – portal vein, hepatic artery and bile duct, in the free edge of the lesser omentum
- Inferiorly – first part of the duodenum
- Posteriorly – inferior vena cava.

For descriptive purposes, the greater sac is divided into compartments. The supracolic compartment lies superior to the transverse mesocolon (containing the stomach, liver and spleen). It is divided into left and right regions by the falciform ligament. The infracolic compartment lies inferior to the transverse mesocolon (containing the small bowel, the ascending and descending colon) (Fig. 5.13A). The infracolic compartment is further subdivided by the mesentery of the small intestine into right and left divisions. The supracolic and infracolic compartments communicate via the paracolic gutters, lying lateral to ascending and descending colon.

Fig. 5.12 Peritoneal folds of the anterior abdominal wall, viewed from the posterior aspect.

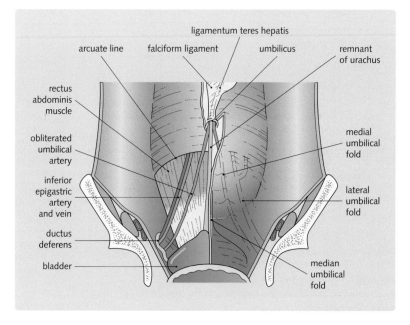

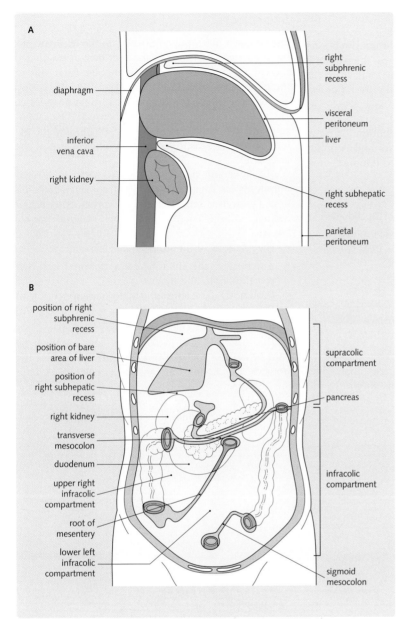

Fig. 5.13 A, Sagittal section of the upper abdomen to show recesses of the right supracolic compartment. B, Posterior abdominal wall showing lines of peritoneal reflection and the compartments of the greater sac (liver, stomach, small intestine, caecum, transverse and sigmoid colons have been removed). (Adapted from Williams P (ed.) (1995) *Gray's Anatomy*, 38th edition, Churchill Livingstone.) B, Sagittal section of the upper abdomen to show the recesses of the right supracolic compartment.

Between the upper surface of the liver and the diaphragm lies the subphrenic recess, divided into left and right halves by the falciform ligament. Inferior to the liver and superior to the right kidney lies the right subhepatic recess (the hepatorenal recess or Morrison's pouch), which communicates with the right paracolic gutter (Fig. 5.13B). The left subhepatic recess forms part of the lesser sac.

In the pelvic compartment the peritoneum lies over and between pelvic viscera. The peritoneal pouches formed differ between genders. Males have a rectovesical pouch. Females have vesicouterine and rectouterine pouches (Ch. 6).

Greater and lesser omenta

The greater omentum is the largest peritoneal fold, arising from the greater curvature of the stomach. It hangs like an apron over the intestines and is filled with fat.

It is fused with the transverse mesocolon and with the anterior aspect of the transverse colon.

The lesser omentum extends from the inferior border of the liver to the lesser curvature of the stomach (known as the hepatogastric ligament), and from the proximal part of the duodenum to the liver (known as the hepatoduodenal ligament).

Peritoneal folds, sacs, recesses and omenta are important as they determine the distribution of intraperitoneal fluid and act as boundaries and conduits for disease (e.g. infection, tumours and trauma).

HINTS AND TIPS

The greater omentum is the 'policeman' of the abdomen - it has the ability to wall off areas of infection within the abdominal cavity, thereby preventing free peritonitis.

THE ABDOMINAL ORGANS

Oesophagus

After passing through the diaphragm, accompanied by the vagal trunks, the oesophagus turns anteriorly and left to enter the stomach. Its blood and nerve supply are shown in Figure 4.27.

Stomach

The stomach lies intraperitoneally, in the left hypogastric and epigastric regions of the abdomen. It is a dilated muscular bag, which is relatively mobile, fixed only to the oesophagus and duodenum (Fig. 5.14). It is composed of the cardia, fundus, body, antrum and pylorus. The gastro-oesophageal junction (between the oesophagus and the cardia) lies at the level of T10 and the pyloric sphincter (gastroduodenal sphincter) lies at the level of L1.

The mucosal lining of the stomach is thrown into folds or rugae, which allow considerable dilation. The wall is muscular and comprises outer longitudinal, middle circular and inner oblique muscle layers.

The relations of the stomach are:

- Anteriorly – the anterolateral abdominal wall, left costal margin, and diaphragm
- Posteriorly – the left suprarenal gland, upper pole of the left kidney, pancreas, spleen, splenic artery and left colic flexure (forming the stomach bed).

The stomach and oesophagus are supplied by branches of the coeliac trunk. Venous drainage of the stomach accompanies the arteries. Smaller veins drain into the superior mesenteric vein (SMV) and the splenic vein, which combine to form the hepatic portal vein (some veins drain directly into the portal vein).

Fig. 5.14 Arterial supply and lymph nodes of the stomach.

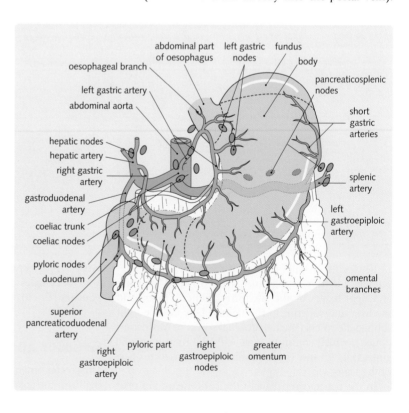

The hepatic portal vein carries blood to the liver. Lymph from the stomach drains to the coeliac nodes and eventually into the thoracic duct.

Innervation of the stomach is via the coeliac plexus (part of the autonomic nervous system): sympathetic supply arises from the greater and lesser splanchnic nerves. Parasympathetic innervation arises from the anterior and posterior vagal trunks.

Duodenum

The duodenum is approximately 40 cm long and C-shaped, curving around the head of the pancreas. It is divided into four parts (the first part is intraperitoneal, the remainder is retroperitoneal):

- The first part passes anterolateral to the L1 vertebra, and travels superiorly and posteriorly.
- The second part passes inferiorly. The major duodenal papilla (the opening of the bile duct and main pancreatic duct) opens into this part at the level of L2 vertebra.
- The third part lies horizontally and crosses the vertebral column at the level of L3. It is crossed by the superior mesenteric artery (SMA) and SMV.
- The fourth part travels superiorly to the level of the L2 vertebra and joins with the jejunum.

Figure 5.15 shows the relations of the duodenum. Its blood supply arises from the superior and inferior pancreaticoduodenal arteries, branches of the gastroduodenal artery (a branch of the hepatic artery) and SMA respectively. Venous drainage occurs via the SMV and the splenic vein. Lymphatic drainage of the duodenum is via the coeliac and superior mesenteric nodes. Its nerve supply arises from the vagus and sympathetic nerves via the coeliac and superior mesenteric plexuses.

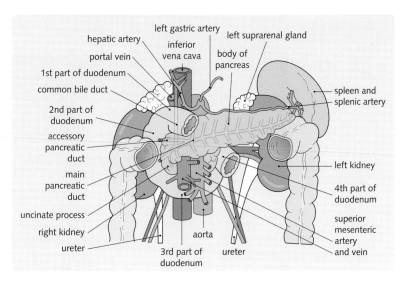

Fig. 5.15 Relations of the duodenum. Note the splenic vein runs posterior to the pancreas and is, therefore, not visible. The inferior mesenteric vein has been omitted for clarity.

Gastric and duodenal ulcers

A gastric ulcer in the posterior stomach wall may erode into the splenic artery, causing massive haemorrhage into the lesser sac. It may also erode into the pancreas, causing referred pain in the back.

95% of duodenal ulcers occur in the posterior wall of the first part of the duodenum. Perforation causes the duodenal contents to enter the abdominal cavity causing peritonitis. An ulcer may also erode the gastroduodenal artery causing major haemorrhage. An anterior ulcer may be sealed off by the greater omentum.

Jejunum and ileum

The jejunum and ileum are intraperitoneal. They are attached to the posterior abdominal wall by the mesentery of the small intestine. The root of the mesentery extends along the posterior abdominal wall from the left of the L2 vertebra to the right sacroiliac joint and contains blood vessels, fat, lymph nodes and nerves.

Figure 5.16 outlines the differences between the jejunum and ileum. Of note are lymphoid nodules known as Peyers patches, found mostly, but not exclusively, in the ileum. They play a role in generating the immune response, containing many of the cells of the immune system.

Fig. 5.16 Distinguishing characteristics of the jejunum and ileum.

Characteristic	Jejunum	Ileum
Colour	Deep red	Paler pink
Wall	Thick and heavy	Thin and light
Vascularity	Greater	Less
Vasa recta	Long	Short
Arcades	A few large loops	Many short loops
Peyer's patches (aggregated lymphoid follicles)	No	Yes
Plicae circulares (mucosal folds increasing surface area)	More and larger	Less and smaller/absent
Fat	Less – stops at the mesenteric border with the jejunum	More – encroaches onto the ileum

The jejunum and ileum are supplied by jejunal and ileal arteries (branches of the SMA) which form anastomotic loops known as arterial arcades. Vasa recta (straight arteries) arise from the arcades to supply the walls of the intestine. The vasa recta are end arteries – occlusion may result in infarction. Venous drainage occurs via the SMV. Lymphatic drainage of the jejunum and ileum is to the superior mesenteric nodes.

Innervation arises from the posterior vagal trunks (parasympathetic) and the greater and lesser splanchnic nerves (sympathetic).

Large intestine

This consists of the caecum and appendix, colon, rectum and upper part of the anal canal.

Caecum and appendix

The caecum and the vermiform appendix lie in the right iliac fossa. The caecum is a blind ending pouch invested by peritoneum. It is the first part of the large intestine, continuous with the ascending colon. The ileum enters the caecum at the ileocaecal valve (not a true valve).

The appendix is a blind-ending tube, 6–9 cm long, and rich in lymphoid tissue. It opens into the posteromedial wall of the caecum, 2 cm inferior to the ileocaecal junction. It is suspended by a mesentery (the mesoappendix). The taeniae coli (bands of smooth muscle which correspond to the outer, longitudinal layer of muscle elsewhere in the gastrointestinal tract) of the caecum merge at the base of the appendix – this is a useful landmark during surgery. The position of the body of the appendix varies – the majority are retrocaecal (65%) or pelvic (30%), with the remainder (5%) occupying a variety of positions. Swelling of the appendix may obstruct the artery, resulting in necrosis and perforation. The arterial supply, venous and lymphatic drainage, and nerve supply of the caecum and appendix are detailed in Figure 5.17A and B.

Appendicitis

Appendicitis occurs when the appendix is obstructed by faecoliths or by swelling of lymphoid tissue (often after a viral infection). As the appendix becomes inflamed it produces periumbilical pain (the appendix is part of the midgut and visceral pain from this region is felt around the umbilicus). Pain subsequently becomes sharper and localized to the right iliac fossa, due to irritation of the parietal peritoneum. Treatment is appendicectomy.

Untreated appendicitis can result in rupture, peritonitis (with increased pain, nausea/vomiting and abdominal rigidity), the formation of an appendix abscess and sepsis.

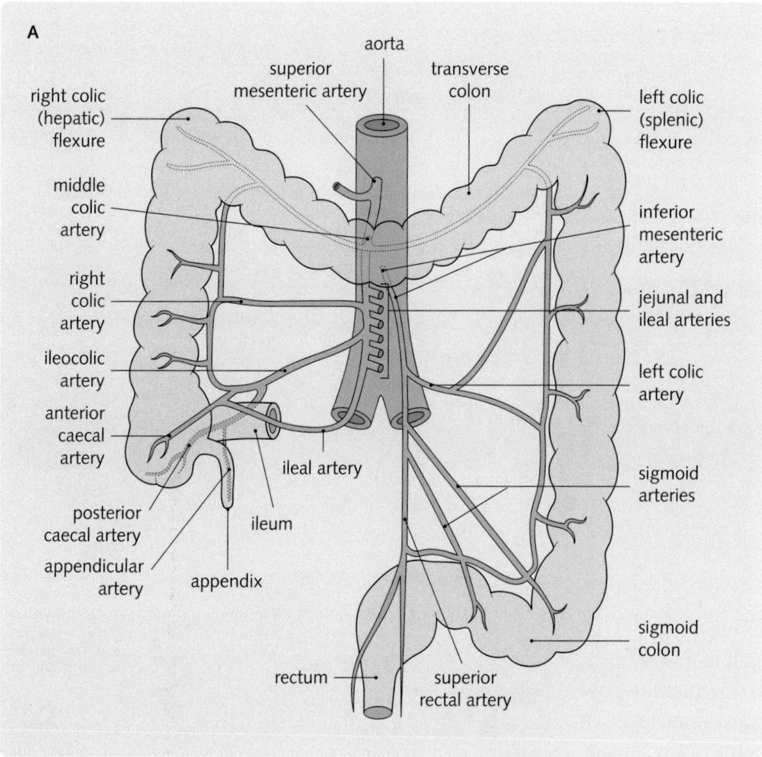

Fig. 5.17A Colon and its blood supply.

Fig. 5.17B Arterial supply, venous and lymphatic drainage and innervation of the colon.

	Arterial supply	Venous drainage	Nerve supply	Lymphatic drainage
Caecum	SMA → ileocolic artery → anterior and posterior caecal arteries	Ileocolic veins → SMV → portal vein		Superior mesenteric nodes
Appendix	SMA → ileocolic artery → appendicular artery	Appendicular vein → SMV → portal vein	Parasympathetic fibres from the vagus nerves and sympathetic fibres from the superior mesenteric plexus	
Ascending colon	SMA → ileocolic and right colic arteries	Ileocolic and right colic veins → SMV → portal vein		
Transverse colon	Proximal two-thirds: SMA → middle colic artery Distal one-third: SMA→ left colic artery	Proximal two-thirds: middle colic vein → SMV → portal vein Distal one-third: left colic vein → IMV → portal vein	Proximal two-thirds: sympathetic and vagus nerves in the superior mesenteric plexus Distal one-third: sympathetic via inferior mesenteric ganglion, parasympathetic via pelvic splanchnic nerves	
Descending colon	IMA → left colic and sigmoid arteries	Superior rectal veins → IMV → portal vein	Sympathetic via inferior mesenteric ganglion, and parasympathetic pelvic splanchnic nerves	Inferior mesenteric nodes
Sigmoid colon	IMA → sigmoid arteries and superior rectal arteries	Superior rectal veins → IMV → portal vein		

IMA, inferior mesenteric artery; IMV, inferior mesenteric vein, SMA; superior mesenteric artery; SMV superior mesenteric vein; → branches of, with regard to arterial supply and tributary of, with regard to venous drainage

CLINICAL NOTE

Meckel's diverticulum

This is a remnant of the vitelline duct (a connection between the gut tube and the embryonic yolk sac). It projects from the ileum, approximately 2ft from the ileocaecal junction in roughly 2% of people. It is twice as common in males compared with females. It may contain ectopic mucosa (gastric, pancreatic or colonic). It may cause ulceration with pain, bleeding or diverticulitis, producing symptoms similar to those of appendicitis.

CLINICAL NOTE

Diverticulae

Outpouchings of mucous membrane may herniate through the perforations in the muscle layer of the colon made by the blood vessels between the taeniae coli. The outpouchings are known as diverticulae and are most common in the sigmoid colon. The presence of diverticulae is known as diverticulosis. Inflammation of the diverticulae, resulting in pyrexia, and pain in the left iliac fossa, is known as diverticular disease.

Colon

The colon has several characteristic features:

- Three bands of smooth muscle which run longitudinally along the wall of the colon – the taeniae coli. They correspond to the outer longitudinal layer of the muscularis externa in other regions of the gastrointestinal tract
- Haustra – pouches along the length of the colon, formed by the taeniae coli, which 'bunch together' the colonic wall
- Appendices epiploicae – pouches of peritoneum filled with fat project from the external surface of the colon.

The colon is composed of the following regions:

- Ascending colon: this occupies a retroperitoneal position, and extends from the ileocolic junction to the right colic (hepatic) flexure. The right paracolic gutter lies on its lateral side.
- Transverse colon: this extends from the right colic (hepatic) flexure to the left colic (splenic) flexure, the former being lower due to the right lobe of the liver. It is intraperitoneal suspended by the transverse mesocolon.
- Descending colon: this extends from the left colic (splenic) flexure to the sigmoid colon. It lies retroperitoneally. The left paracolic gutter lies on its lateral side.
- Sigmoid colon: this extends from the descending colon and becomes continuous with the rectum inferiorly. It hangs free from the sigmoid mesocolon. The mesocolon is an inverted V-shape (Fig. 5.13B), the base of which lies over the sacroiliac joint. From here, one part runs to the midinguinal point along the external iliac vessels and the other runs to the level of the S3 where the rectum begins.

The arterial supply, venous and lymphatic drainage, and nerve supply of the colon is illustrated and detailed in Figure 5.17 A and B.

CLINICAL NOTE

Ischaemic bowel and Hirschprung's disease

The terminal branches of the superior mesenteric artery (SMA) and inferior mesenteric artery (IMA) form an anastomotic network (important in the event of arterial occlusion), known as the marginal artery. Vasa recta arise from the marginal artery to supply the colon. The splenic flexure is the watershed area between the arterial supply of the SMA and IMA. Anastomoses here are often weak or absent, and so this region is an area particularly prone to ischaemia and infarction.

Hirschsprung's disease generally presents in infancy or childhood. It arises due to an absence of nerve plexuses within the wall of the gut, most commonly in the rectosigmoid region. This results in constipation, bowel obstruction and vomiting. It is normally confirmed by biopsy. Treatment consists of surgical removal (resection) of the affected area of the colon.

Spleen

The spleen is a large lymphoid organ, located in the left hypochondrium, inferior to the diaphragm. It is only palpable when enlarged. It removes damaged or antibody-coated cells from the blood and assists in mounting immunological responses against blood-borne pathogens. It is a site of haematopoeisis in the fetus and a potential site of haematopoeisis in the adult. It has a convex diaphragmatic surface and on its concave visceral surface lies the hilum – the site of entry and exit of the splenic vessels. The visceral surface is also related to the stomach, kidney, colon and the tail of the pancreas. Its anterior and superior borders are notched and sharp, but its posterior and inferior borders are rounded.

It is connected to the greater curvature of the stomach by the gastrosplenic ligament, and to the posterior abdominal wall at the left kidney, by the splenorenal (lienorenal) ligament. It is completely enclosed by peritoneum except at the hilum.

Its arterial supply arises from the splenic artery (a branch of the coeliac trunk), a tortuous vessel which passes along the superior border of the pancreas and anterior to the left kidney. As it does so the splenic artery gives off short gastric and left gastroepiploic arteries to the stomach and branches to the pancreas. Between the layers of the splenorenal ligament, the splenic artery divides into terminal branches which enter the hilum of the spleen.

Venous drainage occurs via the splenic vein, which runs along the posterosuperior aspect of the pancreas, and is joined by the inferior mesenteric vein posterior to the body of the pancreas. Posterior to the neck of the pancreas, the vein unites with the SMV to form the hepatic portal vein.

Lymphatic drainage is to the splenic nodes and, subsequently, the coeliac trunk. Its nerve supply arises from the coeliac plexus.

CLINICAL NOTE

Ruptured spleen and splenectomy

The spleen can be damaged by blunt trauma or rib fractures (particularly of the 9th to 11th ribs). Splenic rupture can lead to massive blood loss and hypovolaemic shock. Emergency splenectomy is required. Patients who have undergone a splenectomy are vulnerable to infection (due to the role of the spleen in immunity) and so they must ensure that they are vaccinated against appropriate diseases. They may also be advised to take lifelong antibiotics.

Liver

The liver is a wedge-shaped organ, surrounded by a fibrous capsule, which lies inferior to the right hemidiaphragm. It spans the right hypochondrium, the epigastrium and the left hypochondrium. It lies largely under the cover of the ribs and it is invested by peritoneum except for the 'bare area', on the diaphragmatic surface of the liver.

The liver has four lobes, although this is a purely anatomical description and does not reflect functional subdivisions (Fig. 5.18). Anteriorly, the falciform ligament (visible on the anterior surface of the liver) attaches the liver to the anterior abdominal wall and also divides the liver into right and left lobes. Posteriorly, the caudate lobe lies superiorly, between the fissure for the inferior vena cava and the fissure for the ligamentum venosum. Inferior to this lies the quadrate lobe, between the gallbladder fossa and the ligamentum teres. The transverse fissure separates the caudate lobe from the quadrate lobe. Functionally, the quadrate and caudate lobes are part of the left lobe as they are supplied

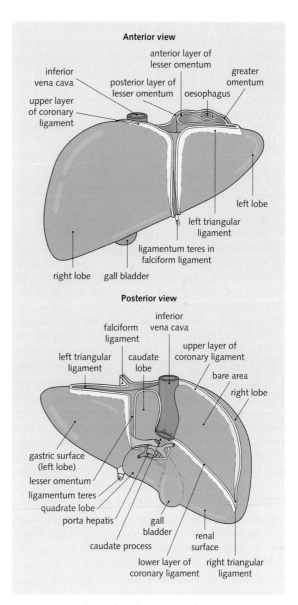

Fig. 5.18 Anterior and posterior views of the liver.

by the left hepatic artery, left branch of the portal vein and deliver bile to the left bile duct.

The falciform ligament is the remnant of the embryonic ventral mesentery. On the superior surface of the liver the falciform ligament forms the left and right triangular ligaments. The right layer forms the upper layer of the coronary ligament, the right triangular ligament and the lower layer of the coronary ligament (Fig. 5.18).

The area between the upper and lower parts of the coronary ligament is the bare area of the liver that lies in contact with the diaphragm. The right and left layers of peritoneum meet on the visceral surface of the liver to form the hepatogastric and hepatoduodenal ligaments, part of the lesser omentum. Between the caudate and quadrate lobes, the two layers surround the porta hepatis. The porta hepatis, the inferior vena cava, the gall bladder and the fissures of the ligamentum venosum and ligamentum teres form an H-shaped pattern. The ligamentum venosum is the remnant of the fetal ductus venosus, which transported blood from the portal and umbilical veins to the hepatic veins.

The porta hepatis contains the following structures (Fig. 5.18):

- The hepatic artery proper (a branch of the coeliac trunk) splits into right and left hepatic arteries and supplies oxygenated blood to the liver. The right hepatic artery gives off the cystic artery, which supplies the gallbladder.
- The hepatic portal vein carries the products of digestion from the gut to the liver. This blood is also partially oxygenated.
- The right and left hepatic ducts drain bile into the common hepatic duct, which joins the cystic duct to form the bile duct.
- These three structures form the portal triad that lies in the right free margin of the lesser omentum. The porta hepatis also contains lymph nodes and nerves.

Venous drainage of the liver occurs via the hepatic veins which pass directly from the posterior surface of the liver into the inferior vena cava, draining the liver.

Lymphatic drainage of the liver is to the hepatic nodes around the porta hepatis and on into the coeliac nodes. Lymphatics of the bare area drain into the posterior mediastinal nodes. Innervation is provided via sympathetic and parasympathetic nerve fibres (via the vagus nerves) in the hepatic plexus, a branch of the coeliac plexus.

The functions of the liver include :

- Production of bile, cholesterol, albumin and clotting factors
- Detoxification of drugs and chemicals
- Homeostasis of blood glucose levels
- Metabolism of carbohydrates, proteins and fats
- Storage of vitamins, cholesterol, fats, proteins, copper and iron

- Destruction of erythrocytes
- Production of heat

Gallbladder and biliary tract

The gallbladder lies in a fossa on the visceral surface of the liver. It has a fundus, a body and a neck (Fig. 5.19). Bile secreted by the liver is concentrated and stored in the gall bladder (its capacity is approximately 50 ml). After fat- or protein-rich food, cells of the duodenum release cholecystokinin (CCK), which stimulates the smooth muscle of the gallbladder wall and relaxes the hepatopancreatic sphincter (sphincter of Oddi – a layer of circular muscle surrounding the ampulla, controlling the flow of bile and pancreatic secretions), releasing bile into the duodenum.

The cystic duct drains the gallbladder and joins the common hepatic duct to form the common bile duct (CBD). The CBD passes through the free margin of the lesser omentum, posterior to the first part of the duodenum. It then enters the second part of the duodenum with the pancreatic duct at the hepatopancreatic ampulla (of Vater). The ampulla opens at the major duodenal papilla.

Blood supply to the gallbladder is via the cystic artery, a branch of the right hepatic artery. Venous drainage occurs via the cystic veins, which drain into the right

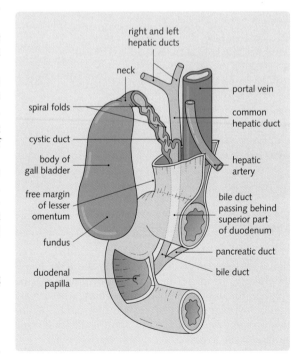

Fig. 5.19 Gall bladder and biliary tract.

hepatic vein. The majority of lymph drains to the hepatic nodes and ultimately into the coeliac nodes. The nerve supply arises from the coeliac plexus, the vagus nerve and the right phrenic nerve.

> **CLINICAL NOTE**
>
> **Jaundice**
>
> Jaundice results from an increased level of bilirubin in the blood. It accumulates in the skin, and mucous membranes, including the conjunctiva of the eye. The causes of jaundice may be classified as pre-hepatic, usually related to increased breakdown of bilirubin; hepatic, disease within the liver; and post-hepatic, disruption to the flow of bile. Obstruction of the biliary tree is most commonly due to gallstones, but may occur secondary to carcinoma of the head of the pancreas. If the biliary tree is obstructed, causing post-hepatic jaundice, bilirubin cannot enter the intestine (bile pigments give stools their brown colour) therefore it is reabsorbed into the blood, filtered by the kidney and excreted in the urine. This produces the characteristic features of obstructive jaundice; dark urine and pale stools.

Pancreas

The pancreas has both exocrine and endocrine functions. It is a retroperitoneal organ, lying posterior to the stomach (Fig. 5.15). It spans the epigastrium and left hypochondrium. It has a head, neck, body and tail:

- The head lies in the concavity of the duodenum, anterior to the inferior vena cava and left renal vein. The bile duct travels through it.
- The uncinate process is an extension of the head; the SMA and SMV pass anterior to the uncinate process.
- The neck lies anterior to the point at which the SMV and splenic vein join to form the portal vein.
- The body is related to the stomach anteriorly, and to the aorta, splenic vein, left kidney and renal vessels, and left suprarenal gland posteriorly.
- The tail passes into the splenorenal ligament, reaching the hilum of the spleen, accompanied by the splenic vessels and lymphatics.

The main pancreatic duct begins in the tail of the pancreas. In the head of the pancreas it joins with the common bile duct to form the ampulla of Vater. This then opens into the duodenum at the major duodenal papilla. Approximately 2 cm proximal to this, the accessory pancreatic duct opens into the duodenum at the minor duodenal papilla. It drains the head of the pancreas.

The splenic artery (a branch of the coeliac trunk) supplies the neck, body and tail of the pancreas. The superior and inferior pancreaticoduodenal arteries supply the head. The splenic and SMV drain the pancreas. Lymphatics drain into superior and inferior pancreatic nodes then to coeliac and superior mesenteric nodes. Nerve supply to the pancreas arises from the vagus nerves (parasympathetic) and the splanchnic nerves (sympathetic) arising from the coeliac and superior mesenteric plexuses.

Arterial supply of the gut

The foregut, midgut and hindgut (Fig. 5.1) are supplied by the branches of the coeliac trunk, the SMA and the IMA, respectively.

The coeliac trunk arises from the abdominal aorta at the level of T12. It gives off the left gastric, common hepatic and splenic arteries (Fig. 5.14).

The SMA arises from the abdominal aorta at the level of L1 (transpyloric plane). It gives off the inferior pancreaticoduodenal, jejunal and ileal, ileocolic, right colic and middle colic arteries. The IMA arises from the abdominal aorta, opposite L3. It gives off the left colic, sigmoid and superior rectal arteries (Fig. 5.17A).

Venous drainage of the gut

Venous drainage of the intestine occurs via the hepatic portal system (Fig. 5.20). The hepatic portal vein is formed by the union of the SMV and the splenic vein, posterior to the neck of the pancreas. The IMV drains into the splenic vein.

The hepatic portal vein passes posterior to the first part of the duodenum, in the free edge of the lesser omentum. At the porta hepatis, the vein divides into left and right branches, supplying left and right lobes of the liver. Within the sinusoids of the liver, hepatic portal blood and oxygenated blood from the hepatic artery mix together and come into contact with hepatocytes, where metabolites, such as the products of digestion, are exchanged. Blood from the sinusoids empties into hepatic veins draining the liver, they in turn drain into the inferior vena cava and blood is returned to the heart.

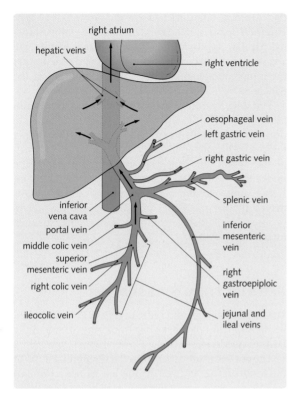

Fig. 5.20 Hepatic portal venous system.

CLINICAL NOTE

Portal hypertension and areas of portosystemic anastomosis

In portal hypertension, the pressure within the portal vein is elevated. This is usually due to either increased blood flow or increased resistance to blood flow through the liver (e.g. in cirrhosis, where the liver becomes fibrosed destroying the blood vessels within the liver). The consequence is that a large amount of the blood which would normally pass through the portal vein into the liver, is shunted into the systemic circulation, via collateral vessels, which provide an alternative route for the blood to return to the inferior vena cava. Dilatation of these vessels increases the risk of rupture and bleeding. There are several sites at which the portal circulation meets the systemic circulation (i.e. where shunting occurs). These are known as portosystemic anastomoses:

• Lower end of the oesophagus – between the oesophageal tributary of the left gastric vein and the oesophageal tributaries of the azygos vein – enlargement results in oesophageal varices, which may rupture, causing massive haematemesis

• Anal canal – between the superior and middle/inferior rectal veins – enlargement results in rectal varices
• Peri-umbilical region of the abdominal wall – between the para-umbilical veins and the superficial and inferior epigastric veins – enlargement causes caput medusae: visible, enlarged, systemic veins radiating outwards from the umbilicus
• Retroperitoneal anastomoses and anatomoses of the bare area of the liver – these are not clinically significant.

Nerve supply of the gut

The gut tube receives sympathetic and parasympathetic nerves that travel with the gut arteries. See the section on nerves of the posterior abdominal wall for more detail.

Lymphatic drainage of the gut

The majority of lymph from the gastrointestinal tract drains to nodes close to the viscera in question (usually of the same name), then into either the para-aortic nodes (coeliac nodes, superior or inferior mesenteric nodes) if the viscera is intraperitoneal, or to the lumbar nodes if the viscera is retroperitoneal. In the case of organs which are secondarily retroperitoneal (the pancreas, the ascending and descending colon) drainage is to the pre-aortic nodes. Lymph from the pre-aortic nodes drains to intestinal trunks, lymph from lumbar nodes drains to lumbar trunks. Lymph from the intestinal and lumbar trunks then drains into the cisterna chyli and into the thoracic duct.

THE POSTERIOR ABDOMINAL WALL

The posterior abdominal wall offers protection to the abdominal contents, houses components of the abdominal cavity and serves as a passageway for structures travelling to other regions of the body (Fig. 5.21). It is composed of:

• Bony structures: the bodies of the five lumbar vertebrae (and their intervertebral discs), which project forwards into the abdominal cavity, the medial region of the ilia, and ribs XI and XII.
• Muscular structures: the psoas major, iliacus and quadratus lumborum muscles (Fig. 5.22). The iliolumbar ligament is a ligament passing from the transverse process of L5 vertebra to the posterior part of the iliac crest.

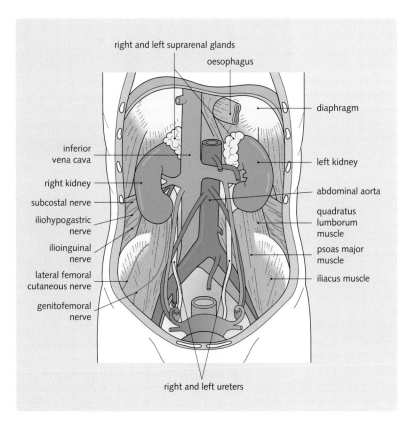

Fig. 5.21 Structures of the posterior abdominal wall.

right and left suprarenal glands

oesophagus

diaphragm

inferior vena cava

left kidney

right kidney

abdominal aorta

subcostal nerve

quadratus lumborum muscle

iliohypogastric nerve

psoas major muscle

ilioinguinal nerve

iliacus muscle

lateral femoral cutaneous nerve

genitofemoral nerve

right and left ureters

Fig. 5.22 Muscles of the posterior abdominal wall.

Name of muscle (nerve supply)	Origin	Insertion	Action
Psoas major (L1–L3)	Bodies, transverse processes and intervertebral discs of T12 and L1–L5 vertebrae	Lesser trochanter of femur	Flexes thigh on trunk
Quadratus lumborum (T12–L3)	Iliolumbar ligament, iliac crest, transverse processes of lower lumbar vertebrae	12th rib	Depresses 12th rib during respiration; laterally flexes vertebral column
Iliacus (femoral nerve)	Iliac fossa	Lesser trochanter of femur	Flexes thigh on trunk

(Adapted from Snell RS (1996) *Clinical Anatomy. An Illustrated Review with Questions and Explanations,* 2nd edn. Little Brown & Co.)

Fascia of the posterior abdominal wall

Fascia covers the muscles of the posterior abdominal wall: psoas fascia covering psoas major and thoracolumbar fascia already mentioned.

The superior edge of the thoracolumbar fascia forms the lateral arcuate ligament slung between the middle of the 12th rib and the transverse process of L1 vertebra. From here, the medial arcuate ligament (the superior edge of psoas fascia) extends to the side of L1 or L2 vertebra.

Tendinous fibres of the diaphragm pass in front of the aorta in the midline to form the median arcuate ligament.

Vessels of the posterior abdominal wall

Abdominal aorta

The abdominal aorta passes through the diaphragm at the level of T12. It passes inferiorly on the bodies of the lumbar vertebrae. Anterior to the L4 vertebrae it

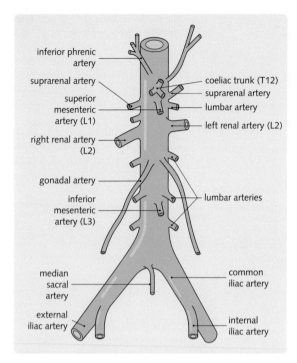

inferior phrenic artery

suprarenal artery

superior mesenteric artery (L1)

right renal artery (L2)

gonadal artery

inferior mesenteric artery (L3)

median sacral artery

external iliac artery

coeliac trunk (T12)

suprarenal artery

lumbar artery

left renal artery (L2)

lumbar arteries

common iliac artery

internal iliac artery

Fig. 5.23 Branches of the abdominal aorta.

divides into the right and left common iliac arteries. The branches of the abdominal aorta are illustrated in Figure 5.23.

CLINICAL NOTE

Abdominal aortic aneurysm

An abdominal aortic aneurysm most commonly occurs infrarenally (distal to the branching of the renal arteries). Aneurysms are most common in males. They may be detected as an incidental finding, felt as an expansile mass on the left of the midline. Symptoms include pain in the abdomen or back, and a pulsing sensation in the abdomen.

Patients suspected to have an aneurysm undergo assessment, to confirm the diagnosis, and to assess risk. Assessment is based upon the age of the patient, the size of the aneurysm (assessed via ultrasound or CT scanning), the rate of enlargement of the aneurysm, family history of aneurysm rupture and the level of a chemical known as MMP-9 in the blood (associated with weakening of the wall of the aorta).

Aneurysms less than 5 cm in diameter are generally monitored by means of regular ultrasound scans. Aneurysms over 5.5 cm normally require surgery – either open surgery or endovascular aortic repair

(EVAR), to place a graft within the weakened area. Management of patients with aneurysms between 5 and 5.5 cm depends upon the presence of risk factors and symptoms.

Aneurysm rupture results in back or abdominal pain, hypotension and shock. The degree of blood loss is usually fatal.

Inferior vena cava

The inferior vena cava (IVC) is formed by the joining of the left and right common iliac veins (Fig. 4.22) at the level of the L5 vertebrae. The IVC ascends to the right of the aorta, passes posterior to the liver and pierces the diaphragm at the level of T8 with the right phrenic nerve. It then almost immediately enters the heart.

Nerves of the posterior abdominal wall

Somatic nerves

The L1–L4 spinal nerves emerge from their intervertebral foramina and enter psoas major, which they supply. The ventral (anterior) rami of the nerves form the lumbar plexus (Fig. 5.24), which is mostly concerned with sensory and motor innervation to the lower limb. However, some branches are motor and sensory to the anterior abdominal wall, e.g. iliohypogastric nerve, and sensory to the parietal peritoneum, e.g. obturator nerve. The lumbosacral trunk joins the first three sacral nerves to contribute to the sacral plexus.

Autonomic nerves

The autonomic nerve supply of the abdomen is composed of the following:

- Parasympathetic supply from the vagal trunks and pelvic splanchnic nerves (S2,3,4)
- Sympathetic supply from the lumbar sympathetic trunks and the thoracic and lumbar splanchnic nerves
- Prevertebral autonomic plexuses surrounding the aorta (coeliac, aortic and superior hypogastric), which distribute the nerve fibres.

Sympathetic nerves

The lumbar sympathetic trunk comprises preganglionic fibres from the lower thoracic trunk and from L1 and L2 nerves (via white rami). This trunk enters the abdomen posterior to the medial arcuate ligament of the diaphragm. It lies on the bodies of the lumbar vertebral bodies, along the medial border of psoas major.

There are usually four lumbar ganglia. These give somatic branches (grey rami communicantes) to all five

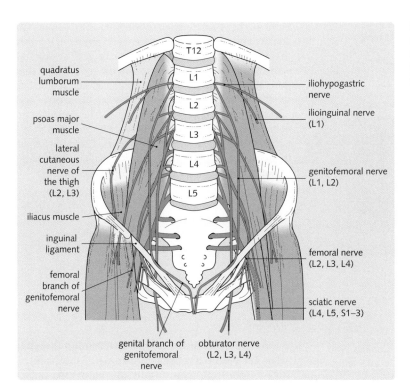

quadratus lumborum muscle

psoas major muscle

lateral cutaneous nerve of the thigh (L2, L3)

iliacus muscle

inguinal ligament

femoral branch of genitofemoral nerve

genital branch of genitofemoral nerve

obturator nerve (L2, L3, L4)

iliohypogastric nerve

ilioinguinal nerve (L1)

genitofemoral nerve (L1, L2)

femoral nerve (L2, L3, L4)

sciatic nerve (L4, L5, S1–3)

lumbar nerves, supplying the body wall and lower limb, and visceral branches (lumbar splanchnic nerves) that join the prevertebral plexuses. Fibres from the third and fourth lumbar ganglia join with fibres from the aortic plexus in front of L5 vertebra to form the superior hypogastric plexus. The superior hypogastric plexus divides into the right and left hypogastric nerves, which run into the pelvis to join the inferior hypogastric plexus. The sympathetic trunks in the abdomen do not give branches to the abdominal viscera, which are supplied by the greater, lesser and least splanchnic nerves.

The greater and lesser splanchnic nerves are preganglionic – they pierce the crura of the diaphragm to synapse in the coeliac ganglion. The least splanchnic nerves relay in a small renal ganglion close to the renal artery.

From the coeliac ganglion, postganglionic fibres form the coeliac plexus around the origin of the coeliac trunk. Fibres either pass directly or via superior and inferior mesenteric plexuses along branches of the aorta to supply all abdominal viscera.

The suprarenal gland also receives preganglionic fibres directly from the lesser splanchnic nerve – stimulation of which causes the release of adrenaline.

Functions of the sympathetic nerves include vasomotor, motor to the sphincters and inhibition of peristalsis, and carrying sensory fibres from all of the abdominal viscera.

Parasympathetic nerves

The vagal trunks supply foregut, midgut and hindgut: they enter the abdomen on the surface of the oesophagus, directly supplying the stomach. Branches to the coeliac plexus then supply the remainder of the gut as far as the distal two-thirds of the transverse colon. Branches to the renal plexus pass to the kidneys.

The pelvic splanchnic nerves (from S2 to S4) join the inferior hypogastric plexus. Some fibres pass up into prevertebral plexuses to be distributed to the distal part of the transverse colon and descending and sigmoid colons (hindgut). Parasympathetic activation of the gut causes stimulation of peristalsis and secretomotor activity of glands (remember 'rest and digest').

Kidneys

The kidneys are involved in removal of toxins, control of blood pressure, stimulation of red blood cell production, maintenance of fluid and electrolyte balance and maintenance of calcium and phosphate levels. They are retroperitoneal organs lying mostly under cover of the costal margin in the paravertebral gutters of the posterior abdominal wall. They extend from approximately the T12 vertebrae to the L3 vertebrae. The right kidney lies slightly lower than the left kidney due to the

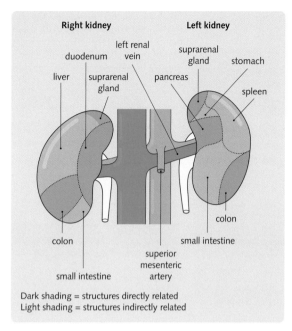

Dark shading = structures directly related
Light shading = structures indirectly related

Fig. 5.25 Kidneys and their main anterior relations.

presence of the liver (Fig. 5.25). Their structure is illustrated in Figure 5.26.

Each kidney is surrounded by three layers. From superficial to deep they are: the renal fascia (encloses both the kidney and the suprarenal gland, and is attached to the renal vessels and the ureter at the hilum of the kidney), the perinephric fat and the renal capsule.

The renal arteries supply the kidneys (Fig. 5.26). They arise from the aorta, inferior to the SMA and divide into anterior and posterior branches at the hilum of the kidney. These are further subdivided into segmental, arcuate and interlobular arteries (end arteries). Venous drainage is via interlobular, arcuate and segmental veins, which join together to form the renal vein – this joins the inferior vena cava at the level of L2. The left renal vein is longer because it passes in front of the aorta to reach the inferior vena cava. The sympathetic nerve supply to the kidneys arises from the coeliac, renal and superior hypogastric plexuses. The parasympathetic nerve supply is from the vagus. Lymphatic drainage is to renal nodes then lumbar nodes.

Ureters

The ureters are muscular tubes which connect the renal pelvis (at the ureteropelvic junction) to the bladder. They descend retroperitoneally on the medial aspect of the psoas major muscle and cross the pelvic brim at the bifurcation of the common iliac artery. At the level of the ischial spine, the ureters pass anteriorly and medially towards the bladder, where they pass through the bladder wall at an oblique angle (this prevents reflux of urine).

There are three points of narrowing within the ureters – these are the sites at which renal calculi are most likely to become impacted:

- At the ureteropelvic junction
- Where the ureter crosses the pelvic brim
- As the ureter passes through the bladder wall.

Blood supply is segmental and arises from the renal artery, abdominal aorta, gonadal and vesical arteries, common and internal iliac arteries, and the middle rectal artery. Venous drainage is to the renal, testicular and ovarian veins. Lymphatic drainage occurs via the para-aortic and common iliac nodes. The ureters receive a sympathetic nerve supply from the coeliac, mesenteric and hypogastric plexuses. Parasympathetic fibres come from the pelvic splanchnic nerves. The pain afferents accompany the sympathetic nerves.

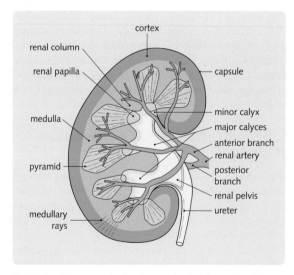

Fig. 5.26 Macroscopic structure and arterial supply of the kidney.

the kidney to the bladder. This normally presents as colicky flank pain, which radiates to the groin, often accompanied by vomiting. Patients with renal colic are restless, moving around frequently (in contrast to patients with peritonitis for whom any movement is very painful). The most effective analgesics are NSAIDs and opiates. Diagnosis is made by X-ray or CT scan. Treatment ranges from allowing the stone to pass spontaneously to extracorporeal shock wave lithotripsy (ESWL) or surgery.

An important differential diagnosis of suspected left-sided renal colic, particulary in older males, is a ruptured or leaking abdominal aortic aneurysm.

Suprarenal gland

The suprarenal gland lies on the medial aspect of the superior pole of each kidney, separated from it by a thin layer of fibrous tissue. The left suprarenal gland lies posterior to the stomach (lesser sac intervening) and the right lies posterior to the inferior vena cava, liver and hepatorenal pouch. The glands consist of a central medulla which secretes adrenaline, and a peripheral cortex which secretes aldosterone, cortisol and sex hormones.

Each suprarenal gland is supplied by three main vessels:

- The superior suprarenal artery – a branch of the inferior phrenic artery
- The middle suprarenal – a branch of the abdominal aorta
- The inferior suprarenal – a direct branch of the renal artery.

The gland is drained by the medullary veins, which merge to form the suprarenal vein. On the right the suprarenal vein drains directly into the inferior vena cava directly. On the left the suprarenal vein drains into the left renal vein. Lymphatic drainage is to the para-aortic lymph nodes. The nerve supply of the suprarenal gland is from the coeliac plexus and splanchnic nerves.

RADIOLOGICAL ANATOMY

Imaging of the abdomen

Ultrasound

Ultrasound examination is quick and simple to perform, therefore it is often a first-line investigation in the diagnosis of abdominal diseases, e.g. testicular swellings, inflammation of the gallbladder, gallstones and abdominal aortic aneurysm.

X-rays

Abdominal X-rays (AXRs) are most commonly requested for patients who present with an 'acute abdomen'. AXRs are normally anteroposterior (AP) films, taken with the patient in a supine position. They are **not** generally used to diagnose a perforated viscus; this is normally diagnosed by an erect chest X-ray, where air will be visible under the diaphragm (usually more easily seen on the right side).

Normal radiographic anatomy of an AP abdominal X-ray

A normal abdominal X-ray is illustrated in Figure 5.27.

How to examine an AP abdominal X-ray methodically

The initial assessment of an AXR is the same as for a chest X-ray, confirming the identity of the patient, date and time of X-ray, and projection, as well as looking for any obvious abnormalities. As with any X-ray it is then important to examine the film in a systematic way. Below is one example:

- Gas: this appears black. Normal sites for gas are the stomach (seen as a 'gastric bubble', particularly if the film is an erect AXR), the large bowel and rectum
- Bowel: the small bowel lies centrally in the film, with large bowel around the periphery. Small bowel has a maximum diameter of 3 cm with valvulae conniventes visible across the width of the bowel wall. Large bowel has a maximum diameter of 6 cm (9 cm for the caecum) and features folds known as haustra, which do not extend across the full diameter of the bowel wall. The large bowel may also contain faeces, giving it a mottled appearance. Gas outwith the bowel or within the bowel wall is not normal.
- Viscera and muscles:
  - Liver: in the right upper quadrant; enlargement pushes the intestines inferiorly
  - Spleen: in the upper left quadrant; enlargement pushes the splenic flexure inferiorly
  - Kidneys: have a smooth outline. Their position varies with inspiration
  - Bladder (and uterus): looking for any calcification
  - Psoas major muscle: its outline can be traced inferiorly into the pelvis to its insertion into the lesser trochanter of the femur. If this outline is lost or not visible it may indicate that fluid, e.g. blood, is present within the abdomen.
- Bones: look at the lower ribs, lumbar vertebrae and pelvis for continuity of the cortex areas of

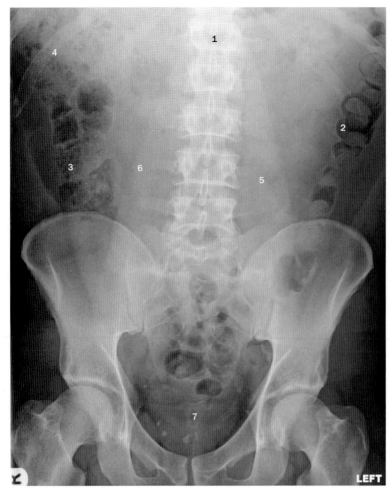

1. L1 vertebra
2. Gas in the descending colon
3. Faeces in the ascending colon
4. Hepatic flexure
5. Left psoas muscle
6. Right psoas muscle
7. Bladder

Fig. 5.27 Abdominal radiograph – supine projection.

darkness (i.e. fracture) or white lesions (i.e. metastatic deposits). Costal cartilages may be calcified. Examine the hip joint for narrowing of the joint space, loss of the smooth joint surface, formation of bone (osteophytes) and loose bodies.

- Calcification: there are areas of the body in which calcification is normal, such as the costal cartilages (above), the mesenteric lymph nodes and the prostate (however, calcification may also occur in carcinoma of the prostate). Calcification is not normal in the pancreas, kidneys, blood vessels, gallbladder and bladder. Calculi (particularly renal) may also appear as calcified masses on X-ray.

Abdominal contrast studies

The use of contrast medium (barium sulphate) enhances images produced by plain abdominal X-ray. Depending upon the area of the gut to be assessed, one of the following may be performed:

- Barium swallow: barium is swallowed in order to detect problems in the oesophagus
- Barium meal: barium is swallowed in order to detect problems in the stomach and duodenum
- Barium follow through: barium is swallowed in order to detect problems in the small intestine (Fig. 5.28)

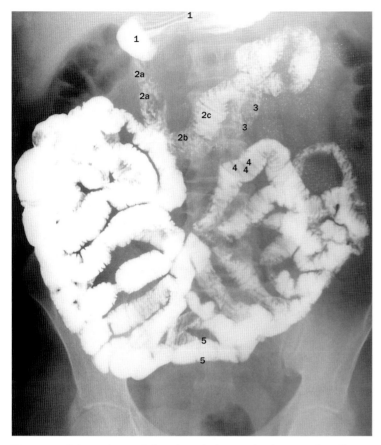

1. Stomach
2. a. Descending (second) part duodenum
2. b. Horizontal (third) part of duodenum
2. c. Ascending (fourth) part of duodenum
3. Proximal jejunum
4. Valvulae conniventes
   (plicae circulares) of jejunum
5. Proximal ileum

Fig. 5.28   Abdomen barium follow-through showing duodenum and small intestine.

- Barium enema – barium is introduced via the rectum in order to detect problems in the colon (Fig. 5.29).

Both a barium meal and a barium enema can be further enhanced by the introduction of air into the gastrointestinal tract (a double contrast barium meal/enema).

CT/MRI scanning of the abdomen

CT or MRI scans of the abdomen are performed to diagnose or provide more detail of diseases within the abdomen, such as tumours, inflammatory bowel diseases, vessel disease (e.g. abdominal aortic aneurysm) and trauma. CT is also used to guide biopsies (e.g. a liver biopsy) or drainage of abscesses. A transverse CT scan of the abdomen at the level of L1 is shown in Figure 5.30.

Angiography of the abdominal aortic branches

Figures 5.31, 5.32 and 5.33 show the branches of the abdominal aorta and their subsequent divisions, forming the arterial supply of the foregut (coeliac trunk) and midgut (superior mesenteric artery).

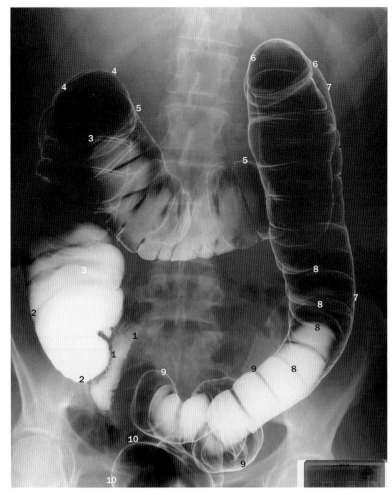

Fig. 5.29 Abdomen double-contrast barium enema of colon.

1. Terminal ileum
2. Caecum
3. Ascending portion
4. Right colic (hepatic) flexure
5. Transverse portion
6. Left colic (splenic) portion
7. Descending portion
8. Sacculations (haustrations)
9. Sigmoid colon
10. Rectum

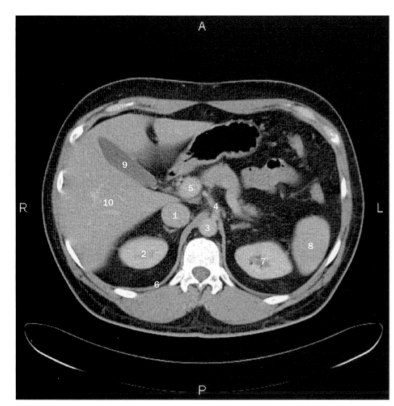

Fig. 5.30 CT scan (transverse section) of the abdomen at the level of L1.

1. Inferior vena cava
2. Right kidney
3. Descending aorta
4. Coeliac trunk
5. Portal vein
6. Right crura of diaphragm
7. Left kidney
8. Spleen
9. Gallbladder
10. Liver

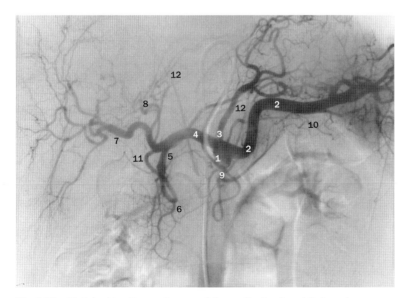

Fig. 5.31 Digital subtraction angiogram of the coeliac trunk and its branches.

1. Tip of catheter in coeliac trunk
2. Splenic artery
3. Left gastric artery
4. Hepatic artery
5. Gastroduodenal artery
6. Superior pancreaticoduodenal
   artery
7. Right hepatic artery
8. Left hepatic artery
9. Dorsal pancreatic artery
10. Left gastro-epiploic artery
11. Right gastro-epiploic artery
12. Phrenic artery

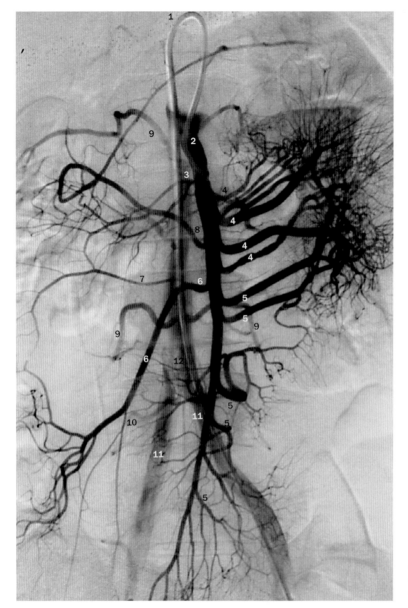

1. Tip of catheter in superior mesenteric artery
2. Superior mesenteric artery
3. Inferior pancreaticoduodenal artery
4. Jejunal branches of superior mesenteric artery
5. Ileal branches of superior mesenteric artery
6. Ileocolic artery
7. Right colic artery
8. Middle colic artery
9. Lumbar arteries arising from abdominal aorta
10. Appendicular artery
11. Common iliac artery
12. Aorta

Fig 5.32 Digital subtraction angiogram of the superior mesenteric artery and its branches

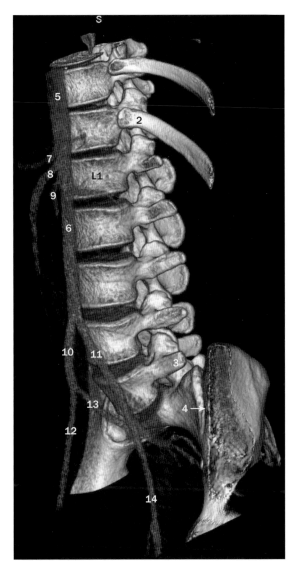

1. L1 vertebra
2. 12th rib
3. Transverse process of L5 vertebra
4. Sacroiliac joint
5. Thoracic aorta
6. Abdominal aorta
7. Coeliac trunk
8. Superior mesenteric artery
9. Inferior mesenteric artery
10. Right common iliac artery
11. Left common iliac artery
12. Right external iliac artery
13. Right internal iliac artery
14. Left external iliac artery

Fig. 5.33 3D CT angiogram of the abdominal aorta and its major branches.

The pelvis and perineum 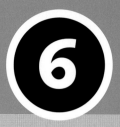 6

● Objectives

In this chapter you will learn to:
- Describe the main features of the pelvic bones, including surface landmarks and sex differences.
- Understand the arrangement of the muscles of the walls and floor of the pelvis, and understand the importance of the perineal body.
- Describe the arrangement of the peritoneum in the pelvis.
- Describe the anatomy of the rectum and anal canal.
- Discuss the anatomy of the bladder and the course of the ureters in the pelvis.
- Describe the anatomy of the male and female reproductive tracts.
- Understand the blood supply, innervation and lymphatic drainage of the pelvis.
- Appreciate that the perineum is divided into an anterior and posterior triangle, and state the contents of each.
- Describe how the superficial perineal space is formed and state its contents in males and females.
- Describe the male and female external genitalia.

REGIONS AND COMPONENTS OF THE PELVIS

The pelvis lies inferior to the abdomen. Its walls are composed of bones, muscles and ligaments. The bony pelvis is formed by the ilia, the sacrum and coccyx. It is open superiorly (pelvic inlet) and inferiorly (pelvic outlet). The greater pelvis (false pelvis) lies superior to the pelvic brim and is flanked by the ilia, whilst the lower pelvis (true pelvis) lies inferior to the pelvic brim (Figs 6.1 & 5.3).

The pelvic and abdominal cavities are continuous with each other, as is the peritoneum lining both cavities. The pelvic cavity is limited inferiorly by the pelvic diaphragm. The perineum lies inferior to the pelvic diaphragm.

The contents of the pelvis include:

- Small intestine
- Sigmoid colon and rectum
- Ureters and bladder
- Ovaries, uterine tubes, uterus and vagina in females
- Ductus deferens, seminal vesicles and prostate in males
- Lumbosacral trunk, obturator nerve, sympathetic trunks and sacral plexus
- Common iliac arteries, gonadal arteries and superior rectal arteries.

SURFACE ANATOMY AND SUPERFICIAL STRUCTURES

Bony landmarks

The iliac crest can be palpated along its entire length. It stretches from the anterior superior iliac spine (ASIS) to the posterior superior iliac spine (PSIS). The ASIS lies at the anterior border of the iliac crest, in the fold of the groin superiorly. The PSIS lies at the posterior border of the iliac crest, deep to a dimple visible on the skin of the back, at the level of the S2 vertebra.

The pubic tubercle is palpable on the upper border of the pubic bone. The pubic symphysis joins the two pubic bones and is also palpable. The pubic crest is a ridge of bone on the superior surface of the pubic bone, medial to the pubic tubercle. The ischiopubic ramus runs from the pubic symphysis to the ischial tuberosity (Fig. 6.2A).

The spinous processes of the sacrum fuse to form the median sacral crest. The crest can be felt deep to the skin in the buttock cleft. The sacral hiatus is found at the lower end of the sacrum, about 5 cm above the coccyx. The coccyx is palpable approximately 2.5 cm posterior to the anus, in the natal cleft.

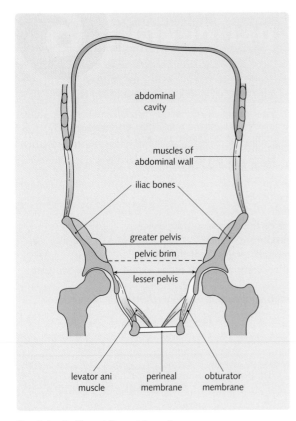

Fig. 6.1   Outline of the pelvic cavity.

Viscera

The adult bladder lies in the pelvis. When full it extends superiorly into the abdominal cavity.

The non-pregnant uterus is not usually palpable. In pregnancy the fundus becomes palpable from about week 12 and at term will lie at the level of the xiphisternum.

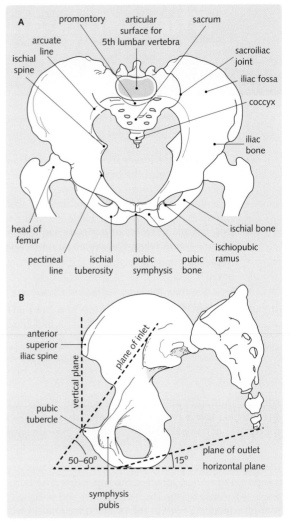

Fig. 6.2   A, Pelvic girdle. B, Pelvic inlet and outlet.

THE BONY PELVIS AND PELVIC WALL

Bony pelvis

The bones of the pelvis consist of two hip bones which articulate with the sacrum and coccyx (Fig. 6.2) thus forming a bony ring which protects the contents of the pelvis. Each hip bone develops from three bones, the ilium, ischium and pubis, which fuse at the acetabulum (Fig. 7.41).

The greater pelvis lies superior to the pelvic brim (pelvic inlet) and consists of the ilia, sacrum and coccyx. The ilia are part of the wall of the abdomen. The lesser pelvis lies between the pelvic inlet and pelvic outlet (Fig. 6.3). The pelvic inlet lies at approximately 45° to the pelvic outlet.

Sacrum and coccyx

The sacrum consists of the fused five sacral vertebrae (Fig. 2.3F). There are four anterior and four posterior sacral foramina, for passage of the anterior and posterior rami of the sacral spinal nerves. The median sacral crest represents the fused spinal processes of the sacral vertebrae.

The sacrum articulates with the ilium on either at the sacroiliac joints. The coccyx lies inferior to the sacrum, attached to it by the sacrococcygeal symphysis, a fibrocartilaginous joint.

Fig. 6.3 Boundaries of pelvic apertures.

Pelvic inlet	Pelvic outlet
Superior border of the pubic symphysis	Inferior margin of the pubic symphysis
Posterior border of the pubic crest	Inferior ramus of the pubis and the ischial tuberosities
Pectineal line	Sacrotuberous ligaments
Arcuate line of the ilium	Tip of the coccyx
Anterior border of the ala of the sacrum	
Sacral promontory	

Ilium

The superior border of the ilium is the iliac crest. The ASIS and PSIS lie on the anterior and posterior extremities of the iliac crest, with the anterior and posterior inferior iliac spines lying below (Fig. 6.4). The iliac fossa lies on the internal surface of the ilium and is the origin of the iliacus muscle. The articular surfaces of the ilium and sacrum form the sacroiliac joint. The ilium forms part of the acetabulum and the bony margin of the greater sciatic notch.

> **HINTS AND TIPS**
>
> The three hip bones (ilium, ischium and pubis) form the acetabulum. They form a Y-shaped epiphysis during development, which allows the acetabulum to enlarge as the femur develops.

Pubis and ischium

The pubic bones articulate in the midline at the pubic symphysis (Fig. 6.4). Each pubic bone has a body, a superior ramus and an inferior ramus. The bodies of the pubic bones articulate at the pubic symphysis in the midline. The superior ramus consists of the pubic symphysis, pubic crest, pubic tubercle and pecten pubis. It joins with the arcuate line of the ischium to form the pelvic brim. The obturator foramen is surrounded by the rami of the pubis and the ischium. In life the obturator foramen is closed by the obturator membrane

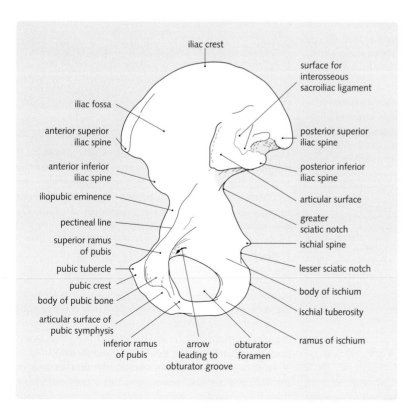

Fig. 6.4 Medial view of the hip bone.

iliac crest

iliac fossa

anterior superior iliac spine

anterior inferior iliac spine

iliopubic eminence

pectineal line

superior ramus of pubis

pubic tubercle

pubic crest

body of pubic bone

articular surface of pubic symphysis

inferior ramus of pubis

arrow leading to obturator groove

obturator foramen

surface for interosseous sacroiliac ligament

posterior superior iliac spine

posterior inferior iliac spine

articular surface

greater sciatic notch

ischial spine

lesser sciatic notch

body of ischium

ischial tuberosity

ramus of ischium

in which there is a canal for the obturator nerves and vessels to exit the lesser pelvis.

The ischium is composed of a body, and superior and inferior rami. Anteriorly, the inferior ramus fuses with the inferior ramus of the pubis, forming the ischiopubic ramus. Posteriorly it fuses with the ilium. The ischial tuberosity, which bears the weight of the body when sitting, projects posteroinferiorly from the body of the ischium.

The posterior border of the ischium contributes to the formation of the greater and lesser sciatic notches. The two notches are separated by the ischial spine. The sacrotuberous and sacrospinous ligaments transform the notches into the greater and lesser sciatic foramina.

The position of the pelvis

When standing, the pelvis lies obliquely in relation to the trunk, with the ASIS and the superior border of the pubic symphysis lying in the same vertical plane. The horizontal plane from the superior border of the pubic symphysis passes through the ischial spine and coccyx.

Male and female pelves

The male and female pelves exhibit sexual dimorphism (Figs 6.5 & 6.6).

Pelvic joints

Pubic symphysis
This is a secondary cartilaginous joint between the two pubic bones (Fig. 6.4). It is usually immobile, reinforced by the superior pubic ligament and the inferior arcuate pubic ligament.

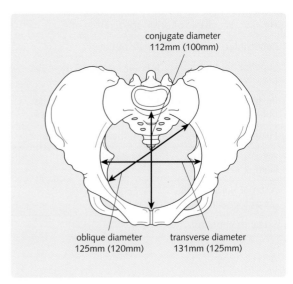

conjugate diameter 112mm (100mm)

oblique diameter 125mm (120mm)

transverse diameter 131mm (125mm)

Fig. 6.6 Female pelvic inlet and its average diameters (male average diameters).

CLINICAL NOTE

Birth

The pelvic inlet is widest transversely, while the pelvic outlet is widest anteroposteriorly (Fig. 6.7). As the fetal head enters the pelvic inlet its widest diameter (the biparietal distance) enters the inlet transversely. As it descends through the birth canal, the head rotates through 90°; its widest diameter then lies anteroposteriorly at the pelvic outlet. Failure of rotation may result in arrest of labour. Instrumental delivery or a caesarean section may then be required.

Sacroiliac joint
This is a specialized synovial joint, which allows only minimal movement. It is strengthened by interosseous and anterior and posterior sacroiliac ligaments. The sacrospinous and sacrotuberous ligaments prevent rotation at the joint. The joint transmits all the body weight to the hip bones.

Pelvic walls and floor

The lateral walls of the pelvis are formed by the hip bones with obturator internus muscles lying deep to the obturator membrane (Fig. 6.7). The posterior wall is formed by the sacrum and coccyx with piriformis lying on the internal surface of the sacrum. Figure 6.8 outlines the muscles of the pelvic wall and floor.

Levator ani takes origin from the tendinous arch (a thickening of the fascia over obturator internus running from the body of the pubis to the ischial spine). Levator

Fig. 6.5	Differences between the male and female pelves.	
	Male	**Female**
Acetabulum	Large	Small
Bones	Robust/ heavier	Lighter/ smoother
Inferior pelvic aperture	Relatively small	Relatively large
Obturator foramen	Round	Oval
Pubic arch	Narrow	Wide
Superior pelvic aperture	Usually heart shaped	Usually oval or rounded

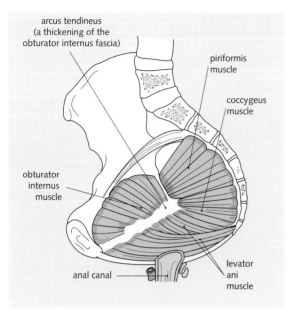

Fig. 6.7 Muscles of the pelvic wall.

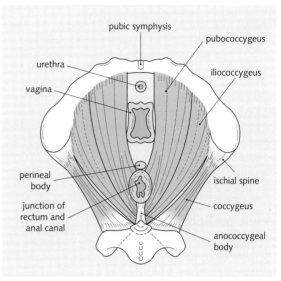

Fig. 6.9 Pelvic floor viewed from below.

ani and coccygeus form a continuous section of muscle known as the pelvic diaphragm, inserting into a series of midline structures. This forms a bowl of muscle around the terminal parts of the rectum, prostate and urethra in the male, and the rectum, vagina and urethra in the female (Fig. 6.9).

Perineal body

The perineal body is a midline knot of fibromuscular tissue which lies at the centre of the line dividing the anal and urogenital triangles. It lies posterior to the prostate or vagina. Parts of levator ani, bulbospongiosus, the external anal sphincter, and the superficial and deep

transverse perineal muscles are attached to, and compose part of the perineal body, thus it has an essential role in supporting pelvic and perineal structures.

Anococcygeal body

The anococcygeal body is a midline raphe running from the anorectal junction to the tip of the coccyx, into which levator ani inserts. It separates the two ischioanal fossae posterior to the anal canal.

Pelvic fascia

Over the internal surface of the pelvic wall the fascia forms a strong covering over obturator internus and piriformis, continuous with that of the abdomen. The

Fig. 6.8	Muscles of the pelvic wall and floor.		
Name of muscle (nerve supply)	**Origin**	**Insertion**	**Action**
Coccygeus (4th and 5th sacral nerves)	Ischial spine	Inferior aspect of sacrum and coccyx	Supports pelvic viscera, flexes coccyx
Levator ani - composed of pubococcygeus, puborectalis, and iliococcygeus (perineal branches of the pudendal nerve, and 4th sacral nerve)	Ischial spine, body of pubis, fascia of obturator internus	Perineal body, anococcygeal body, walls of prostate, vagina, rectum and anal canal	Supports pelvic viscera; sphincter to anorectal junction and vagina Counteracts increased abdominal pressure, e.g. defaecation, parturition
Piriformis (first and second sacral nerves)	Anterior aspect of sacrum	Greater trochanter of femur	Rotates femur laterally at hip and stabilizes hip joint
Obturator internus (nerve to obturator internus; L5, S1, S2)	Obturator membrane and adjacent hip bone	Greater trochanter of femur	Rotates femur laterally at hip and stabilizes hip joint

spinal nerves lie external to the fascia and vessels lie internal to it. The sacral plexus lies between the fascia and piriformis.

Over the pelvic floor, the fascia consists of loose areolar tissue. This condenses around neurovascular bundles to form ligaments, and also gives rise to the puboprostatic and pubovesical ligaments in the male and female respectively. These fibromuscular bands, on either side of the median plane, run from the pubic bone to the bladder neck – immobilizing it and supporting the bladder. The deep dorsal vein of the penis (or clitoris) passes between the ligaments. The fascia varies in thickness over the pelvic viscera.

Pelvic peritoneum

In the male, the peritoneum lines the pelvic walls and the pelvic cavity inferiorly. From the anterior abdominal wall the peritoneum is reflected onto and attaches to the superior surface of the bladder. This means that as the bladder fills and enlarges, it peels the peritoneum away from the anterior abdominal wall. The peritoneum descends on the base of the bladder, before ascending onto the rectum, forming the rectovesical pouch (Fig. 6.10).

In females, the peritoneum leaves the base of the bladder to pass over the uterus, forming the uterovesical pouch. From the superior aspect of the uterus and upper vagina the peritoneum ascends to cover the rectum, forming the rectouterine pouch (pouch of Douglas) (Fig. 6.14). The fold of peritoneum containing the uterus passes to the lateral walls of the pelvic cavity, and is known as the broad ligament of the uterus.

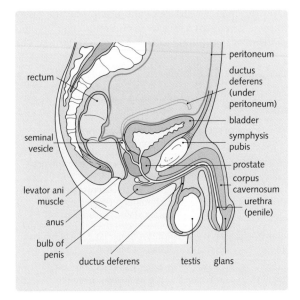

Fig. 6.10 A section through the male pelvis, illustrating the rectum and rectovesical pouch.

124

THE PELVIC CONTENTS

Pelvic organs

Rectum

The rectum commences as a continuation of the sigmoid colon at the level of the S3 vertebra (where the sigmoid mesocolon ends). It is approximately 12 cm long and ends at the anorectal junction, piercing the pelvic floor at the border of puborectalis to become the anal canal. The rectum can be distinguished from the colon by a lack of appendices epiplociae, taeniae coli and haustra.

> ### HINTS AND TIPS
>
> The rectovesical (males) and rectouterine (females) pouches are the lowest part of the peritoneal cavity in the sitting position, and can be a site for collection of pus.

The rectum is concave anteriorly, following the curve of the sacrum – it also has three lateral curves (right, left and right). It contains 3–4 transverse folds containing mucous membrane and circular muscle, which project into the lumen of the rectum. These provide support for faecal material. The most inferior part of the rectum dilates as the rectal ampulla.

The rectum has no mesentery. The upper third is covered by peritoneum on its anterior and lateral surfaces. The middle third is covered by peritoneum on its anterior surface, which reflects onto the posterior surface of the bladder in males (forming the rectovesical pouch), and the posterior surface of the vagina in females (forming the rectouterine pouch). The peritoneum is absent from the lower third of the rectum (Fig. 6.10). Posteriorly the rectum is related to the sacrum, coccyx and pelvic floor.

Vessels and nerves of the rectum

Blood supply to the rectum arises from the superior, middle and inferior rectal arteries. The superior rectal artery is a continuation of the inferior mesenteric artery. The middle and inferior rectal arteries are discussed in the section describing the blood supply to the pelvis.

The rectum drains to the superior rectal vein (into the inferior mesenteric vein, which drains into the portal venous system), and the middle and inferior rectal veins which drain to the internal iliac vein (part of the systemic venous system). The superior rectal vein anastomoses with the middle and inferior rectal veins, forming one of the important sites of porto-systemic anastomosis (page 106). Lymphatics accompany branches of the superior and middle rectal arteries and eventually drain to the preaortic nodes at the origin of the inferior mesenteric vessels.

The nerve supply of the rectum arises from the hypogastric plexus (sympathetic), and pelvic splanchnic nerves (parasympathetic).

Ureters in the pelvis

The ureters (arising in the abdomen) cross the pelvic brim at the bifurcation of the common iliac vessels (Fig. 6.11). In the lesser pelvis they travel posteriorly towards the ischial spines (internal to the obturator nerve and vessels), then turn anteriorly to enter the base of the bladder at an oblique angle through the muscle of the bladder wall. This prevents reflux of urine. Close to the bladder the ductus deferens crosses the ureter in males; in females, the uterine artery crosses the ureter (near the lateral fornices of the vagina).

their left side, in the fetal position, with their knees drawn up to their chest. The perineum and perianal areas are inspected looking for ulceration, warts, bleeding, discharge, etc. A gloved, lubricated finger is inserted, facing posteriorly, into the anus. A brief assessment can be made of anal tone at this point. The walls of the rectum can be examined by rotating the finger 180° clockwise and anticlockwise. The following structures can be palpated:
- Anteriorly: males – the bulb of the penis, the membranous urethra, the prostate; females – the body of the uterus and the cervix
- Posteriorly: the sacrum, the coccyx
- Posterolaterally: the ischial spines.

CLINICAL NOTE

Rectal examination

Rectal examination is performed for various reasons, e.g. as part of examination for prostate or colorectal cancer, in cases of rectal bleeding, or as part of abdominal examination. The patient is asked to lie on

CLINICAL NOTE

Hysterectomy

The close proximity of the ureter and uterine artery may result in damage to the ureter during hysterectomy as the uterine artery is ligated.

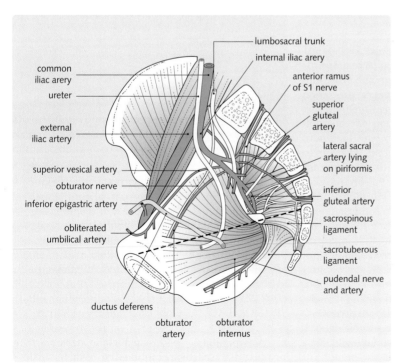

Fig. 6.11 Course of the ureter in the male pelvis.

common iliac arery
ureter
external iliac artery
superior vesical artery
obturator nerve
inferior epigastric artery
obliterated umbilical artery
ductus deferens
obturator artery
obturator internus

lumbosacral trunk
internal iliac arery
anterior ramus of S1 nerve
superior gluteal artery
lateral sacral artery lying on piriformis
inferior gluteal artery
sacrospinous ligament
sacrotuberous ligament
pudendal nerve and artery

Bladder

In adults, the undistended bladder lies in the pelvis (in neonates it lies in the abdomen and descends throughout childhood). It is pyramid shaped, with an apex, a base, two inferolateral surfaces, a superior surface and a neck (Fig. 6.12). The apex faces the pubic symphysis. The median umbilical ligament (a remnant of the urachus) attaches the apex to the umbilicus.

The base of the bladder is triangular and faces posteriorly. In males, the ductus deferens and seminal vesicles are attached to the base. In females, the base lies in contact with the vaginal wall and the upper part of the cervix. In both sexes, the ureters enter the base of the bladder at the posterolateral angles. The interureteric fold (formed by the continuous longitudinal muscle of the ureters) connects the two ureteric orifices. Between the two ureteric orifices and the urethral orifice lies a region known as the trigone (Fig 6.12). The two inferolateral surfaces meet at the inferior angle. The neck of the bladder surrounds the urethra, where the base and the inferolateral surfaces meet. The neck rests on the prostate in males and the pelvic floor in females.

The bladder wall is composed of three layers. The outer layer (serosa) lines the superior surface of the bladder. Deep to the serosa lies a smooth muscle layer (detrusor muscle) composed of muscle and elastic fibres. The detrusor muscle has a parasympathetic nerve supply. A second superficial layer of smooth muscle (with sympathetic innervation) exists in the trigone, extending into the proximal urethra. Here, in males, the muscle is circularly arranged – forming the internal urethral sphincter, which prevents retrograde ejaculation (sperm entering the bladder). This sphincter is not present in females. The external urethral sphincter is present in both sexes, is composed of skeletal muscle, and is under voluntary control. The innermost layer is composed of transitional epithelium (urothelium), which has the ability to stretch to accommodate increasing volumes within the bladder. Within the trigone, the epithelium is firmly attached to the underlying muscular layer. Throughout the remainder of the bladder, the epithelium is only loosely attached to the muscle layer resulting in the trabeculated appearance of the internal surface of the bladder.

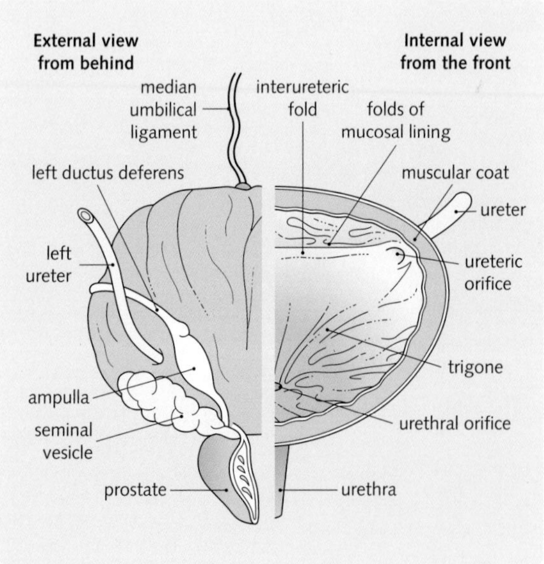

> ### CLINICAL NOTE
>
> **Suprapubic cystostomy**
>
> A distended bladder rises above the pubic symphysis, lifting the peritoneum away from the anterior abdominal wall. This allows a needle to be inserted superior to the pubic symphysis, to drain the bladder (suprapubic cystostomy) without penetrating the peritoneal cavity.

> ### CLINICAL NOTE
>
> **Abnormal insertion of ureters**
>
> The ureters pierce the bladder mucosa obliquely and a valve-like flap of mucosa prevents reflux of urine when the intravesical pressure increases. Abnormal implantation of the ureters in the bladder may lead to reflux of urine into the ureters and into the kidneys (vesicoureteric reflux). This may be diagnosed prenatally by ultrasound scan, showing enlargement of the kidney(s) – hydronephrosis. In infants and children it commonly presents as repeated urinary tract infections. Treatment involves antibiotics and/or ureteric re-implantation.

Vessels and nerves of the bladder

Arterial supply arises from the superior and inferior vesical arteries in males, and the superior vesical and vaginal arteries in females. Venous drainage of the bladder occurs via venous plexuses, which eventually drain into the internal iliac veins. Lymph drains to the internal and external iliac nodes. The nerve supply to the bladder comprises:

- Parasympathetic: pelvic splanchnic nerves – contracts detrusor, relaxes sphincters

Fig. 6.12 Base of the bladder and related structures in the male.

Labels (External view from behind): median umbilical ligament, left ductus deferens, left ureter, ampulla, seminal vesicle, prostate.

Labels (Internal view from the front): interureteric fold, folds of mucosal lining, muscular coat, ureter, ureteric orifice, trigone, urethral orifice, urethra.

- Sympathetic: the superior hypogastric and pelvic plexuses – relaxes detrusor, contracts sphincters
- Pudendal nerve (S2–S4): supplies the external urethral sphincter.

The male urethra

The male urethra is approximately 20 cm long, commencing at the bladder neck and terminating at the external urethral orifice (Fig. 6.13). It is composed of four parts:

- Preprostatic urethra: passes through the wall of the bladder and lies proximal to the prostate gland
- Prostatic urethra: passes through the prostate gland. A central ridge known as the urethral crest, lies on its posterior wall. An elevation on the crest is known as the seminal colliculus. On the surface of the colliculus lies the prostatic utricle. On either side of the utricle lie the orifices of the ejaculatory ducts
- Membranous urethra: begins at the apex of the prostate. It passes through the deep perineal pouch and is surrounded by the external urethral sphincter. It then passes through the perineal membrane, ending at the bulb of the penis. The bulbourethral glands lie lateral to this part of the urethra

- Spongy urethra: passes through the bulb, the corpus spongiosum and the glans of the penis, ending at the external urethral orifice. The bulbourethral glands open into the spongy urethra. There are two expansions of the spongy urethra – the intrabulbar fossa at the bulb, and the navicular fossa at the glans. Numerous urethral glands (Littré glands) open into the spongy urethra.

The female urethra

The female urethra is only 4 cm long. It runs from the bladder neck, through the pelvic floor and the perineal membrane, to open into the vestibule, anterior to the vaginal opening.

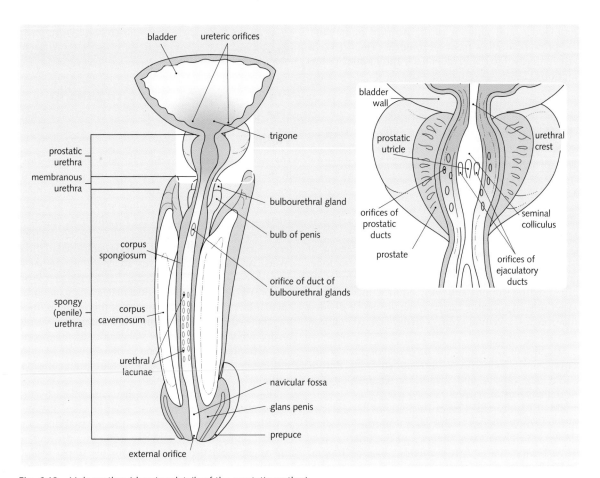

Fig. 6.13 Male urethra (showing details of the prostatic urethra).

Male reproductive organs in the pelvis

Ductus (vas) deferens

The ductus deferens passes from the epididymis to the pelvic cavity via the inguinal canal. At the deep inguinal ring it hooks around the inferior epigastric artery, crossing the external iliac vessels to enter the pelvic cavity. It crosses the ureter and the base of the bladder (see Fig. 6.12). The terminal part dilates, forming the ampulla. It joins the duct of the seminal vesicle to form the ejaculatory duct, which opens into the prostatic urethra on the colliculus.

Seminal vesicles

The seminal vesicles are two elongated lobular sacs lying lateral to the ampulla of the ductus deferens (see Fig. 6.12). They produce seminal fluid.

Prostate

The prostate is a walnut-shaped organ lying inferior to the bladder, and superior to the perineal membrane. The prostatic urethra passes through it (Fig. 6.13). Its base is attached to the bladder neck and its apex points inferiorly.

> **HINTS AND TIPS**
>
> The shorter length of the female urethra, and its proximity to the anus means that urinary tract infections, most commonly caused by gut flora (particularly *Escherichia coli*), are more common in women.

Anatomically, the prostate is described in terms of lobes. It has 5 lobes – two lateral lobes, an anterior lobe, a median lobe and a posterior lobe. The lateral lobes are joined by the isthmus anteriorly and the median lobe posteriorly. In pathological terms the prostate is divided into zones – a central zone, a peripheral zone and a transitional zone.

The fibrous capsule of the prostate completely surrounds the gland. This is surrounded by a fibrous sheath. The capsule and sheath are separated by the prostatic plexus of veins.

Blood supply arises from the inferior vesical and middle rectal arteries. Veins drain to the prostatic plexus, which eventually drains into the internal iliac veins. Lymph drains to the internal iliac and sacral nodes. Parasympathetic innervation of the prostate occurs via the pelvic splanchnic nerves, and sympathetic innervation (stimulates the smooth muscle during ejaculation) occurs via the inferior hypogastric plexus.

> **CLINICAL NOTE**
>
> **Prostatic hypertrophy**
>
> Enlargement of the prostate may be due to benign or malignant disease. Benign enlargement (benign prostatic hypertrophy – BPH) commonly begins after the age of 30, although it may not produce symptoms until 45–50 years of age. BPH commonly affects the lateral lobes or transitional zone. Outward enlargement of the gland is limited by the capsule, therefore the gland enlarges inwards, leading to compression of the urethra, resulting in urinary obstruction. It is detectable on rectal examination, producing an enlarged but smooth prostate.
>
> Malignant disease commonly affects the posterior lobe or peripheral zone, resulting in an enlarged, hard and craggy prostate. Prostate cancer may metastasize to the lumbar vertebrae, due to the communication between prostatic veins and the internal vertebral venous plexus in the vertebral canal.

Female reproductive organs in the pelvis

Vagina

The vagina extends from the vaginal orifice (introitus) in the vestibule, passing superiorly and posteriorly to reach the cervix of the uterus (Fig. 6.14). The fornices of the vagina surround the vaginal portion of the cervix. There are four fornices, namely the anterior, right and left lateral, and posterior fornices. The largest is the posterior fornix. The wall of the vagina is composed of three layers. An outer fibrous layer attaches the vagina to other pelvic viscera. Deep to this lies a muscular layer composed of an external longitudinal layer and an inner circular layer. The internal surface of the vagina is lined by stratified squamous epithelium. Rugae are visible on its surface, which allow distension of the vagina during intercourse. The vagina is related to the bladder and urethra anteriorly, and the rectum and anal canal posteriorly.

The superior part of the vagina is supplied by the uterine artery. The middle and inferior parts are supplied by the vaginal branches of the internal iliac and internal pudendal arteries. Veins drain into the uterine and vaginal plexuses. Lymph from the upper vagina drains to the internal iliac nodes and from the lower vagina to the superficial inguinal nodes.

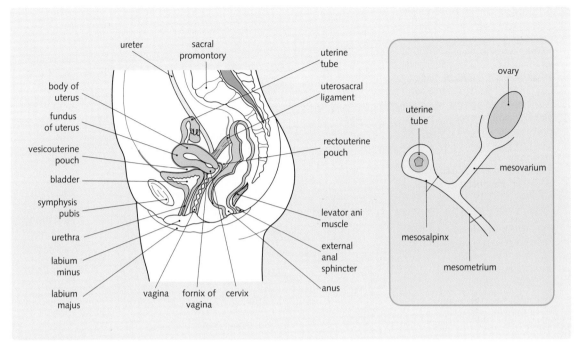

Fig. 6.14 Sagittal section through the female pelvis.

The upper vagina is innervated by the hypogastric plexus. The lower vagina is innervated by the pudendal and ilioinguinal nerves.

Uterus

The uterus is a muscular organ which accommodates the developing embryo. The wall is composed of an outer serosal layer, myometrium (a thick smooth muscle layer) and a lining of endometrium. The thickness of the endometrium varies throughout the menstrual cycle and is shed during menstruation.

The uterus is composed of the following regions (Fig. 6.15):

- The body: this includes the fundus, which lies superior to the openings of the uterine tubes. The cavity of the uterus occupies the body: slit-like in transverse section, triangular in longitudinal section.
- The cervix: this is the narrowest region of the uterus, and is separated from the body by the narrow isthmus. It has a supravaginal part and a vaginal part. The vaginal part is surrounded by the vaginal

fornices. The endocervical canal is continuous with the uterine cavity at the internal os. The endocervical canal opens into the vagina at the external os.

The upper anterior, superior and posterior surfaces of the uterus are covered by a sheet of peritoneum. Laterally, the two layers of peritoneum come into contact with each other, forming the broad ligament, which connects the uterus to the pelvic walls (Fig. 6.16). The broad ligament has three divisions:

- The mesometrium: a mesentery containing the uterus
- The mesosalpinx: a mesentery containing the uterine tubes
- The mesovarium: a mesentery containing the ovaries.

The broad ligament also contains the ovarian and uterine arteries, the ovarian ligament, the round ligament of the uterus and the suspensory ligament of the ovary.

Anteriorly the peritoneum is reflected onto the bladder forming the uterovesical pouch. Posteriorly the peritoneum is reflected onto the rectum to form the rectouterine pouch (Fig. 6.14).

Ligaments

In addition to the broad ligament of the uterus, there are several ligaments which act to stabilize the uterus:

- The round ligament of the uterus: extends from the body of the uterus, through the inguinal canal to the labium majus. It is the female remnant of the gubernaculum

Fig. 6.15 Uterus and its blood supply.

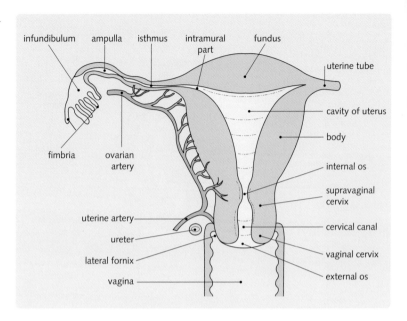

Fig. 6.16 Ligaments of the uterus, viewed from above.

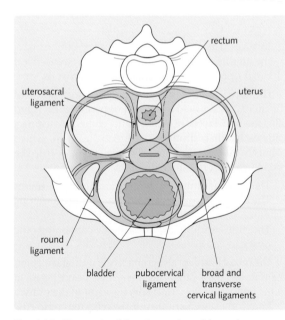

- Transverse cervical (cardinal) ligaments: thickened connective tissue at the base of each broad ligament, extend from the cervix to the lateral walls of the pelvis
- Uterosacral ligaments: extend from the posterior aspect of the cervix to the sacrum
- Pubocervical ligaments extend from the cervix and upper vagina to the posterior aspect of the pubic bones.

Uterine (fallopian) tubes

The uterine tubes extend from the peritoneal cavity close to the ovaries, to the lateral horns of the uterus, at the junction of the body and fundus. They lie in the superior edge of the broad ligament (Fig. 6.15) supported by the mesosalpinx.

The uterine tube is composed of the conical infundibulum, the dilated ampulla (usually the site of fertilization) and the isthmus. The infundibulum, which is open to the peritoneal cavity, bears fimbriae which lie over the medial aspect of the ovary. One fimbria, the ovarian fimbria, is attached to the ovary. When the ovum is shed, it is captured by the fimbriae, enters the infundibulum and travels to the uterus.

CLINICAL NOTE

Ectopic pregnancy

A fertilized ovum which normally implants in the uterus, may implant elsewhere, most commonly in the fallopian tube. This is known as an ectopic pregnancy. It may result in rupture of the uterine tube and haemorrhage into the peritoneal cavity. Ectopic pregnancy is a differential diagnosis of right iliac fossa pain and may be mistaken for appendicitis. Therefore, it is important to perform a pregnancy test in all women of childbearing age who present with pain in the right iliac fossa.

Vessels of the uterus and uterine tubes

The uterine artery, a branch of the internal iliac artery, runs in the broad ligament. It anastomoses with branches of the ovarian artery. Each artery gives rise to tubal branches, which anastomose and supply the uterine tubes (Fig. 6.15). Veins of the uterus form a uterine plexus on either side of the cervix. The plexus empties into the uterine vein, which drains into the internal iliac vein.

Lymphatic drainage of the uterus occurs via the lumbar, superficial inguinal, internal and external iliac, and sacral nodes. Lymphatic drainage of the uterine tubes is to the aortic nodes. Innervation of the uterus arises from the inferior hypogastric plexus. Many postganglionic parasympathetic fibres arise in large pelvic ganglia close to the cervix.

Ovary

The ovary lies in the ovarian fossa (between the internal and external iliac vessels), closely related to the obturator nerve. It contains ova, and produces oestrogen and progesterone.

The ovary is attached to the broad ligament by the mesovarium. It is attached to the uterus by the ligament of the ovary, which runs between the two layers of the broad ligament, and is continuous with the round ligament, both being remnants of the gubernaculum.

It is suspended from the pelvic wall by the suspensory ligament of the ovary. Blood supply arises from the ovarian artery, a branch of the abdominal aorta which runs in the broad ligament, and contributes to the supply of the uterus and uterine tubes by anastomosing with the uterine artery. An ovarian venous plexus communicates with the uterine venous plexus. Two ovarian veins follow the artery: the right ovarian vein drains into the inferior vena cava; the left vein drains into the left renal vein. Innervation of the ovary arises from the ovarian plexus. Lymphatic drainage is to aortic nodes.

CLINICAL NOTE

Positions of the uterus

The normal position of the uterus is anteflexed (the fundus and body point forward relative to the cervix) and anteverted (the uterus is angled forward relative to the vagina). In approximately 20% of women the uterus is retroverted (angled backwards) – this may cause discomfort during intercourse but has no affect on fertility.

HINTS AND TIPS

The ovary is closely related to the obturator nerve in the ovarian fossa – disease of the ovary may cause referred pain to the medial aspect of the thigh and knee.

Vessels of the pelvis

The pelvis is mainly supplied by the internal iliac arteries and the internal iliac veins.

Internal iliac artery

The common iliac artery bifurcates at the pelvic brim, opposite the sacroiliac joint into internal and external iliac arteries (Fig. 6.17). The internal iliac artery passes inferiorly and branches into anterior and posterior divisions. The branches may be divided into those supplying the body wall (iliolumbar, lateral sacral), those leaving the pelvis to supply the lower limb and gluteal region (obturator, superior and inferior gluteal) and visceral branches (superior and inferior vesical, uterine, vaginal, middle rectal, etc.).

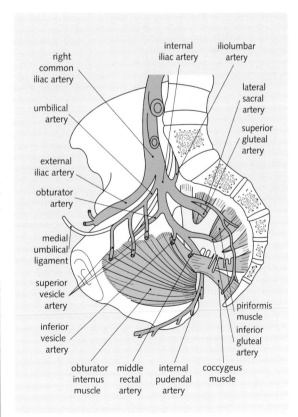

Fig. 6.17 Branches of the internal iliac artery.

Internal iliac vein

The internal iliac vein commences at the greater sciatic notch. It passes superiorly out of the pelvis, posterior to the artery, on the medial surface of psoas major. At the pelvic brim, it joins the external iliac vein to form the common iliac vein.

Tributaries include:

- Veins corresponding to the arteries
- The uterine and vesicoprostatic venous plexuses
- The rectal venous plexuses
- The lateral sacral veins (the internal iliac vein communicates with the vertebral venous plexus via these veins)
- The obturator vein.

Nerves of the pelvis

Obturator nerve

The obturator nerve supplies the adductor compartment of the thigh by piercing the medial border of psoas muscle and passing on the lateral wall of the pelvis to the obturator foramen. It passes through the obturator foramen into the thigh. It supplies the adductor compartment of the thigh and skin on the medial surface of the thigh.

HINTS AND TIPS

If venous drainage of the lower limb becomes obstructed, the pelvic veins enlarge and provide an alternative route for venous return.

Sacral plexus

The sacral plexus lies on piriformis muscle, covered by pelvic fascia. The lateral sacral arteries and veins lie anterior to the plexus. The plexus is formed by the anterior rami of L4 and L5 spinal nerves (the lumbosacral trunk) and the anterior rami of S1–S4 spinal nerves (Fig. 6.18). The sacral nerves and lumbosacral trunk give off branches and then divide into the anterior and posterior divisions.

Autonomic nervous system

See page 10.

Fig. 6.18   Sacral plexus.

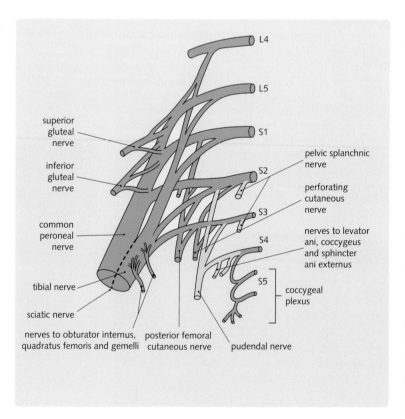

Sacral sympathetic trunk

The sacral sympathetic trunk crosses the pelvic brim behind the common iliac vessels. There are four ganglia along each trunk which unite in front of the coccyx at the ganglion impar. The sacral sympathetic trunk gives somatic branches to all the sacral nerves and visceral branches to the inferior hypogastric plexus.

Inferior hypogastric plexus

The right and left hypogastric plexuses comprise the pelvic plexuses (Fig. 6.19). They lie on the side wall of the pelvis, lateral to the rectum. They receive the right and left hypogastric nerves from the superior hypogastric plexus.

Branches of the plexus are visceral. Functions include the control of micturition, defaecation, erection, ejaculation and orgasm.

Lymphatic drainage of the pelvis

This is summarized in Figure 6.20.

PERINEUM

The perineum describes the area between the superior medial aspects of the thighs. Its superior boundary is the pelvic diaphragm. Its inferior boundary is the skin and superficial fascia. It is a diamond-shaped region, divided into an anterior urogenital triangle and a posterior anal triangle by an imaginary line drawn between the two ischial tuberosities. Its boundaries are illustrated in Figure 6.21.

The blood and nerve supply to the perineum arises from the pudendal artery and nerve (S2, 3, 4).

Anal triangle

The boundaries of the anal triangle are (Fig. 6.21):

* Anteriorly: an imaginary transverse line between the ischial tuberosities
* Laterally: the sacrotuberous ligaments
* Apex: tip of the coccyx
* Base: superficial transverse perineal muscles.

It contains the two ischioanal fossae separated in the midline by the anal canal, the internal and external anal sphincters, the anococcygeal ligament and the perineal

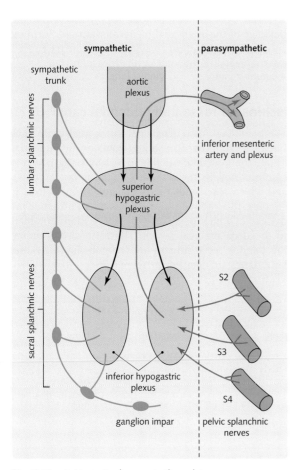

Fig. 6.19 Autonomic plexuses in the pelvis.

Fig. 6.20	Lymphatic drainage of the pelvis.
Structure	**Lymphatic drainage**
Anal canal	Superficial inguinal nodes
Bladder	Internal and external iliac nodes
Ovary	Aortic nodes
Rectum	Inferior mesenteric nodes, internal iliac nodes, pararectal nodes, preaortic nodes
Urethra	Internal iliac nodes, superficial inguinal nodes
Uterus/ uterine tubes	Internal and external iliac nodes, sacral nodes
Vagina	Internal and external iliac nodes, superficial inguinal nodes

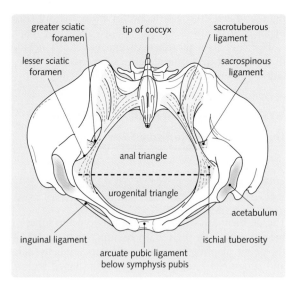

greater sciatic foramen
tip of coccyx
sacrotuberous ligament
lesser sciatic foramen
sacrospinous ligament
anal triangle
urogenital triangle
acetabulum
inguinal ligament
ischial tuberosity
arcuate pubic ligament below symphysis pubis

Fig. 6.21 Boundaries of the perineum.

body. The triangle slopes anteriorly and inferiorly from its apex. Muscles of the anal triangle are outlined in Figure 6.22.

Anal canal

The anal canal is approximately 4 cm long. It commences at the anorectal junction, where it forms a sharp angle with the rectum, due to traction of the puborectalis muscle at the level of the pelvic floor. The anal canal ends at the anus.

Lining of the anal canal

The anal canal is divided into an upper two-thirds and a lower one-third by the dentate line. The upper part is lined by columnar epithelium. It features longitudinal folds known as anal columns. Inferiorly, the columns are linked by horizontal folds, forming the anal valves. The recesses between the columns and valves are known as the anal sinuses, into which the anal glands open.

The lower margins of the anal valves lie at the dentate line. The lower one-third of the canal is lined by stratified squamous epithelium, as is the skin around the anus (Fig. 6.24).

Muscular wall of the anal canal

The anal canal is lined by mucous membrane, which is surrounded by the muscular internal and external anal sphincters (Fig. 6.23).

The internal anal sphincter is a continuation of the circular smooth muscle of the rectum. It surrounds the upper part of the anal canal. It is innervated by the hypogastric and pelvic plexuses (sympathetic) and the pelvic plexus (parasympathetic).

The external anal sphincter is striated and under voluntary control via the perineal branch of S4 spinal nerve, and the inferior rectal nerve (a branch of the pudendal nerve). It is connected to the coccyx via the anococcygeal body. Superiorly, the external anal sphincter blends with puborectalis muscle. In combination with the internal anal sphincter, this forms the anorectal ring. The anorectal ring is the chief muscle of continence.

Figure 6.24 shows the blood supply and lymphatic drainage of the anal canal. Veins anastomose, forming an internal rectal plexus inside the submucosa and an external rectal plexus outside the muscular wall.

Ischioanal fossa and pudendal canal

The ischioanal fossa lies lateral to the anal canal. It is filled with adipose tissue and it contains the pudendal canal. The pudendal canal is roofed by fascia which is continuous with the obturator internus fascia above, and which fuses with the ischial tuberosity below. It contains the internal pudendal vessels and the pudendal nerve, which pass from the lesser sciatic foramen to the deep perineal pouch. The fossa also contains the inferior rectal arteries and nerves (Fig. 6.23). Its boundaries are detailed in Figure 6.25.

Fig. 6.22 Muscles of the anal triangle.			
Name of muscle (nerve supply)	**Origin**	**Insertion**	**Action**
External anal sphincter–subcutaneous part (inferior rectal nerve and perineal branch of fourth sacral nerve)	Encircles anal canal, no bony attachments	Anococcygeal ligament	Voluntary sphincter of anal canal
External anal sphincter–superficial part (inferior rectal nerve and perineal branch of fourth sacral nerve)	Perineal body	Coccyx	
External anal sphincter–deep part (inferior rectal nerve and perineal branch of fourth sacral nerve)	Encircles anal canal	Coccyx	

Adapted from Moore KL (1996) *Essential Clinical Anatomy*. Williams & Wilkins.

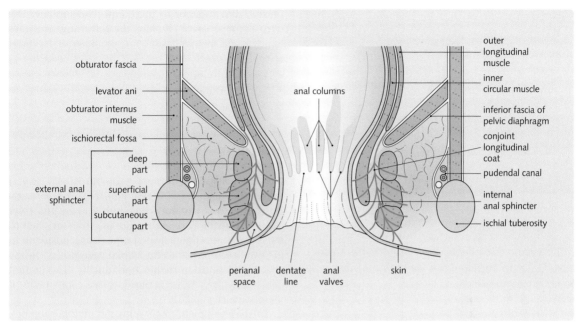

Fig. 6.23 Anal canal and ischioanal fossa.

Fig. 6.24	Blood supply, lymphatic drainage and nerve supply of the anal canal.	
	Above dentate line	**Below dentate line**
Epithelium	Colummar (mucosa)	Stratified squamous
Arteries	Superior rectal (from inferior mesenteric)	Middle and inferior rectal (from internal iliac)
Venous drainage	Superior rectal vein	Middle and inferior rectal veins
Lymphatic drainage	Internal iliac nodes	Superficial inguinal nodes
Nerve supply	Visceral–inferior hypogastric plexus Sensitive to stretch	Somatic–inferior rectal from pudendal (S2, 3, 4) Sensitive to pain, touch, etc.

Fig. 6.25	Boundaries of the ischioanal fossa.
Boundary	**Components**
Base	Skin over anal region of perineum
Medial wall	Anal canal and levator ani
Lateral wall	Ischial tuberosity and obturator internus
Apex	Where levator ani is attached to its tendinous origins over obturator fascia
Anterior extension	Superior to deep perineal pouch

CLINICAL NOTE

Haemorrhoids

Haemorrhoids are dilatations of the internal rectal venous plexus. They normally occur due to straining, secondary to chronic constipation, but may be caused by pregnancy, familial predisposition and, occasionally, by portal hypertension:
• 1st degree haemorrhoids remain inside the anal canal and may cause bleeding

- 2nd degree haemorrhoids prolapse temporarily during defecation
- 3rd degree haemorrhoids prolapse permanently and may strangulate.
  Haemorrhoids appear at 3, 7 and 11 o'clock positions around the anus. They are painless until they extend below the dentate line, into the area of somatic innervation. Haemorrhoids may be treated by injection with a sclerosing material or by ligation with a rubber band.

HINTS AND TIPS

The adipose tissue of the ischioanal fossa has a poor blood supply. Therefore, it is vulnerable to infection and abscess formation.

The male urogenital triangle

The male urogenital triangle is bounded posteriorly by an imaginary transverse line between the two ischial tuberosities. Its lateral boundaries are the ischiopubic rami, which meet anteriorly at the pubic symphysis (Fig. 6.21).

Within the urogenital triangle lies the deep perineal space, lying inferior to the anterior part of the levator ani muscle, and superior to the perineal membrane. The deep perineal space contains the following structures 'sandwiched' between superior and inferior layers of fascia (Fig. 6.26):

- Deep transverse perineal muscles
- Sphincter urethrae
- Membranous urethra
- Bulbourethral glands
- Pudendal vessels (continuing forward from the pudendal canal)
- Dorsal nerve of the penis.

Loose pelvic fascia forms the superior fascial layer of the deep space. The inferior fascial layer forms the inferior boundary of the deep perineal space. This layer is known as the perineal membrane. It is attached to the ischiopubic rami, from immediately posterior to the pubic symphysis to the ischial tuberosities. In the anatomical position, it lies horizontally. The urethra penetrates the deep perineal space and perineal membrane (Fig. 6.26).

The perineal membrane, sphincter urethrae and pelvic fascia together constitute the urogenital diaphragm. The bulbourethral glands are two small glands lying on either side of the membranous urethra (Fig. 6.25) – their ducts pierce the perineal membrane to enter the spongy part of the urethra and their secretions contribute to seminal fluid.

Between the perineal membrane and the superficial perineal fascia (of Colles') lies the superficial perineal space. Figure 6.27 outlines the muscles of the urogenital

Fig. 6.26 Coronal section of the male perineum.

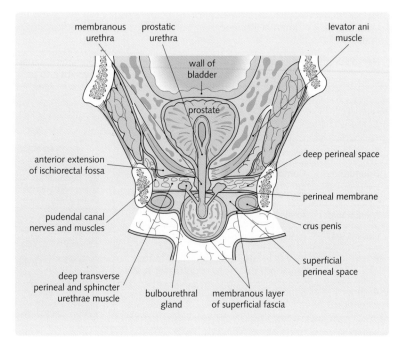

Fig. 6.27 Muscles of the urogenital triangle.

Name of muscle (nerve supply)	Origin	Insertion	Action
Superficial transverse perineal muscle (perineal branch of pudendal nerve)	Ischial tuberosity	Perineal body	Fixes perineal body
Bulbospongiosus (perineal branch of pudendal nerve)	Perineal body and median raphe in male, perineal body in female	Fascia of bulb of penis and corpora spongiosum and cavernosum in male, fascia of bulbs of vestibule in female	In male, empties urethra after micturition and ejaculation, and assists in erection of penis; in female, sphincter of vagina and assists in erection of clitoris
Ischiocavernosus (perineal branch of pudendal nerve)	Ischial tuberosity and ischial ramus in male and female	Fascia covering corpus cavernosum	Erection of penis or clitoris
Deep transverse perineal muscle (perineal branch of pudendal nerve)	Ramus of ischium	Perineal body	Fixes perineal body
Sphincter urethrae (perineal branch of pudendal nerve)	Pubic arch	Surrounds urethra	Voluntary sphincter of urethra, important muscle of urinary incontinence

Adapted from Moore KL (1996) Essential Clinical Anatomy. *Williams & Wilkins.*

triangle. These muscles are involved in micturition, copulation and support of the pelvic viscera.

HINTS AND TIPS

The pudendal nerve supplies levator ani (S2 3 4) – so remember S2, 3, 4 – keep your guts off the floor.

Superficial perineal space

The superficial perineal space is lined inferiorly by Colles' fascia, a continuation of the membranous superficial fascia (Scarpa's fascia) of the anterior abdominal wall, which descends to line the scrotum. It is attached to the ischiopubic rami, the posterior border of the perineal membrane, the perineal body and the fascia lata of the thigh (page 143).

Superiorly the space is limited by the perineal membrane. The contents of the space include the root of the penis, superficial transverse perineal, bulbospongiosus and ischiocavernosus muscles. It also contains the perineal branches of the internal pudendal artery and pudendal nerve.

The male external genitalia

The male external genitalia consist of the penis and the scrotum. The scrotum is described on page 93.

CLINICAL NOTE

Urethral rupture

Rupture of the proximal spongy urethra, inferior to the perineal membrane (often secondary to straddle injuries), leads to extravasation of urine into the superficial perineal pouch and into the fascia around the penis, the scrotum and superiorly into the anterior abdominal wall. Urine will not enter the anal triangle, because the superficial perineal fascia adheres to the perineal membrane along its posterior margin. It will not enter the thigh because the superficial perineal fascia is attached to the fascia lata of the thigh.

Penis

The penis is suspended from the pubic symphysis by the suspensory ligament of the penis. It consists of the root, the shaft and the glans (Fig. 6.28).

The root is composed of three masses of erectile tissue: the bulb of the penis, and the right and left crura. The bulb and crurae are partially surrounded by the bulbospongiosus and ischiocavernosus muscles. The superficial transverse perineal muscle is related to these muscles.

Distally the crura become the corpora cavernosa and the bulb becomes the corpus spongiosum. Cavernous spaces are present in the erectile tissue of the corpus

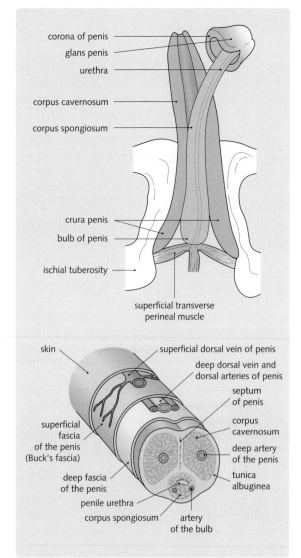

Fig. 6.28 Composition and structure of the penis.

cavernosa. The urethra passes through the corpus spongiosum, which passes from the erectile tissue of the bulb to end at the external urethral orifice. The distal end of the corpus spongiosum expands to form the glans penis. At the proximal part of the glans penis, the skin is reflected upon itself to form the prepuce (foreskin), which covers the glans. The prepuce is attached to the ventral surface of the glans by a fold of skin, the frenulum of the prepuce, which contains a small artery. The shaft is surrounded by thin loose skin.

A tough tunica albuginea surrounds the corpora cavernosa of the penis. Superficial to the corpora cavernosa and corpus spongiosum lies the deep fascia of the penis (Buck's fascia). This is surrounded by the superficial fascia of the penis.

The crura and corpora cavernosa receive blood from the deep arteries of the penis. These vessels allow rapid distension of the cavernous spaces to produce an erection (under the control of parasympathetic nerves). The bulb and corpus spongiosum are supplied by the bulbourethral artery. The dorsal artery supplies the glans, the prepuce and the skin of the penis. Venous drainage is to the deep and superficial dorsal veins. Lymph drains to the superficial inguinal and subinguinal lymph nodes.

Parasympathetic nerves (responsible for erection) and sensory nerves (dorsal nerves supplying the skin) to the penis arise from the pudendal nerves (S2–S4). The dorsal nerve of the penis runs with the dorsal artery of the penis. It passes over the dorsum of the penis lateral to the artery and terminates in the glans.

Vessels of the male urogenital triangle

The internal pudendal artery is a branch of the internal iliac artery. It exits the pelvis via the greater sciatic foramen to enter the pudendal canal, entering the perineum via the lesser sciatic foramen at the ischial spine. At the anterior end of the canal it enters the deep perineal pouch and continues forward on the deep surface of the perineal membrane. It terminates by dividing into the dorsal and deep arteries of the penis or clitoris. Its branches are outlined in Figure 6.29.

The internal pudendal veins are the venae comitantes of the arteries. The deep dorsal vein of the penis drains into the prostatic plexus. The superficial dorsal vein of the penis drains to the superficial pudendal vein which drains to the femoral vein.

Fig. 6.29 Branches of internal pudendal artery.	
Vessel (in female)	**Course and distribution**
Inferior rectal artery	Crosses the ischiorectal fossa to supply the muscles and skin of the anal canal
Perineal branch	Passes to the superficial perineal space to supply its muscles and the scrotum (or labia in female)
Artery to bulb of penis (or clitoris)	Supplies the erectile tissue of the bulb and corpus spongiosum
Deep artery of penis (or clitoris)	Supplies the corpus cavernosum
Dorsal artery of penis (or clitoris)	Passes to the dorsum of the penis (or clitoris). It supplies the erectile tissue of the corpus cavernosum and superficial structures
Urethral artery	Supplies the urethra

The blood supply to the scrotum is described in on page 93.

Lymphatics of the male urogenital triangle

The penis and scrotum drain into the superficial (skin) and deep (glans and corpora) inguinal nodes.

Nerves of the male urogenital triangle

The pudendal nerve (S2–S4) passes with the internal pudendal artery through the lesser sciatic foramen and the pudendal canal, where it gives rise to the inferior rectal nerve. The inferior rectal nerve supplies the external anal sphincter and the skin around the anus. At the posterior border of the perineal membrane the nerve divides into the perineal nerve and the dorsal nerve of the penis. The perineal nerve passes superficial to the perineal membrane. It supplies the scrotum posteriorly and all the remaining striated muscles of the perineum. Spinal segments S2–S4 are therefore essential for continence.

The female urogenital triangle

The muscles, fasciae and spaces of the female urogenital triangle are similar to those of the male urogenital triangle. However, certain features differ because of the presence of the vagina and external female genitalia: the vagina pierces both superficial and deep perineal spaces. The deep perineal space also lacks the female equivalent of the bulbourethral gland.

The superficial perineal space again is similar to that of the male. However, it is lined by a less-defined superficial perineal fascia, it is full of fat, is smaller and it is found within the labia majora.

Perineal membrane

The perineal membrane is wider in the female since the pelvis is wider. It is also weaker than in the male because of the presence of the vagina. As the urethra and vagina pierce the membrane their outer fascial covering fuses with it.

Perineal body

In the female, the perineal body lies between the vagina and the anal canal. The perineal body lacks support from the perineal membrane because of the presence of the vagina, so the perineal body in the female has greater mobility. The superficial and deep transverse perineal muscles, pubovaginalis and bulbospongiosus muscles, and the superficial part of the external anal sphincter are attached to the perineal body.

The female external genitalia

The female external genitalia consist of the following structures, which together comprise the vulva (Fig. 6.30):

- Mons pubis: the mound of coarse-haired skin and fat anterior to the pubic symphysis. The mons pubis extends posteriorly as the labia majora
- Labia majora: two fatty folds of skin, joined anteriorly to form the anterior commissure, and continuous with the mons pubis. The labia pass posteriorly blending into the skin near the anus, forming the posterior commissure, which overlies the perineal body. The round ligament of the uterus ends in the labium majus
- Labia minora: skin folds lying within the labia majora, surrounding the vestibule of the vagina. They enclose the clitoris, by forming the prepuce in front and the frenulum behind
- Clitoris: a homologue of the penis consists of two erectile crura attached to the perineal membrane and ischiopubic rami. Anteriorly, the crura become the corpora cavernosa. These are bound together by fascia to form the body of the clitoris. The external part of the clitoris is known as the glans clitoris, and is covered by the clitoral hood
- Vestibule: contains the openings of the greater vestibular glands, the vagina and the external urethral orifice
- Bulb of the vestibule: the homologue of the penile bulb and corpus spongiosum. Posteriorly these two erectile masses, either side of the vagina, are

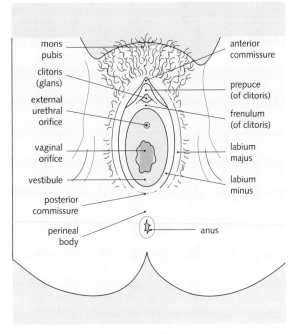

Fig. 6.30 Female external genitalia.

attached to the perineal membrane. Anteriorly they join the glans of the clitoris. Each is covered by the bulbospongiosus muscle

- Greater vestibular glands: homologues of the bulbourethral glands, these are found in the superficial perineal pouch, in contact with the posterior end of the bulb of the vestibule. Their ducts open into the vestibule and lubricate the vagina in sexual arousal
- Vagina: superiorly, the vagina passes through the pelvic floor, surrounded by part of the puborectalis; anteriorly, it is closely related to the urethra; posteriorly, the perineal body separates it from the anal canal; inferiorly it opens into the vestibule at the introitus. This opening is partially occluded by a thin membrane – the hymen – which may be torn by intercourse, internal examination, or sporting activity
- External urethral orifice: this lies in the vestibule posterior to the glans of the clitoris and anterior to the vagina.

Vessels and nerves of the female urogenital triangle

The internal pudendal artery has a similar course and distribution in the female as in the male, except:

- Posterior labial branches replace scrotal branches
- The artery to the bulb and vestibule, and the dorsal arteries of the clitoris replace the arteries to the penis
- The blood supply to the external genitalia mirrors that to the scrotum. It receives the superficial and deep external pudendal arteries (from the femoral artery). Venous drainage occurs via venae comitantes and ends in the great saphenous vein. The pudendal nerve has a similar distribution in both sexes. The only difference is in the naming of the nerves, in which labial replaces scrotal.

The nerve supply to the labia mirrors that of the scrotum:

- The anterior third is supplied by the ilioinguinal nerve.
- The posterior two-thirds are supplied by the posterior labial branch of the pudendal nerve (medially) and by the perineal branch of the posterior femoral cutaneous nerve (laterally).

Lymphatics of the female urogenital triangle

Lymph drains to the superficial inguinal lymph nodes.

RADIOLOGICAL ANATOMY

Pelvic x-rays are most commonly requested after trauma, or when a fracture is suspected (Fig 7.41). Ultrasound is commonly used as a first line imaging modality when investigating potential pathology affecting soft tissues of the pelvis (e.g. ovarian cysts, tumours, bladder disease, ectopic pregnancy, etc.). The use of CT and MRI scanning is helpful in the diagnosis of pelvic malignancies and of complications of diseases such as Crohn's disease (e.g. fistula formation).

The lower limb 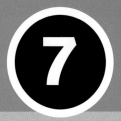 7

Objectives

In this chapter you will learn to:
- Appreciate the major superficial features of each region of the lower limb.
- Describe the venous drainage of the lower limb and understand why varicose veins develop.
- Explain the lymphatic drainage of the lower limb.
- Describe the gluteal region, its contents, and how to identify a safe site for intramuscular injections.
- Name the bones and ligaments which form the hip joint, and state the movements of the hip and the muscles responsible for those movements.
- Explain the blood and nerve supply of the hip joint.
- Describe the compartments of the thigh, the muscles within them and the nerve and blood supply to each.
- List the boundaries and contents of the femoral triangle, femoral canal and adductor canal.
- Describe the sites of the major pulses of the lower limb.
- State the boundaries and contents of the popliteal fossa.
- Understand the anatomy of the knee joint, and the importance of the ligaments supporting it.
- Describe the compartments of the leg, the muscles within them and the nerve and blood supply to each.
- Discuss the osteology of the ankle joint and foot, and the importance of the ankle ligaments.
- Understand the arrangement of structures in the dorsum of the foot.
- List the intrinsic muscles of the foot.
- Describe the blood and nerve supply of the sole of the foot.
- Describe the arches of the foot.
- Recognize the major features of normal x-rays of the lower limb.

REGIONS AND COMPONENTS OF THE LOWER LIMB

The lower limb is designed for support, locomotion and the maintenance of equilibrium. Weight is transferred from the axial skeleton through the bony pelvis, via the hip joint to the lower limb. Propulsive movements are transmitted in a similar way but in the opposite direction. The line of gravity lies posterior to the hip joint, and anterior to the knee and ankle joints.

The hip joint is a ball and socket joint, formed by the acetabulum of the pelvis and the head of the femur. It is a very stable joint, with a good range of movement. The femur articulates with the tibia at the knee joint where flexion and extension movements occur. The proximal fibula is a site of muscle attachment only, it does not

form part of the knee joint, nor is it involved in weight bearing. The distal tibia and fibula articulate with the talus to form the ankle joint, where flexion and extension movements occur. Inversion and eversion occur at the subtalar joint.

The gluteal region is supplied by the superior and inferior gluteal arteries, branches of the internal iliac artery. The external iliac artery supplies blood to the rest of the lower limb. As the artery passes deep to the inguinal ligament, it becomes the femoral artery, which supplies the thigh. The femoral artery enters the popliteal fossa posterior to the knee, where it becomes the popliteal artery which supplies the leg and the foot.

The gluteal region is supplied by the superior and inferior gluteal nerves. The lower limb is innervated by the lumbar and sacral plexuses which give rise to the femoral, obturator and sciatic nerves.

SURFACE ANATOMY

Hip and thigh

The iliac crest, iliac tubercles, anterior and posterior superior iliac spines, and pubic tubercles are palpable (Fig. 6.4). The femur is surrounded by muscles; thus, only the greater trochanter of the femur (the most lateral palpable structure in the hip region) and the femoral epicondyles on either side of the knee joint can be palpated. The lateral epicondyle of the femur is more easily palpated than the medial, due to the position of the vastus medialis muscle; however, the adductor tubercle can be identified on the medial epicondyle.

> **HINTS AND TIPS**
>
> The iliac tubercles (located at the highest point of the iliac crests) are palpable. An imaginary line between them is known as the transtubercular plane. This corresponds approximately to the level of the L3 vertebra.

Knee

The borders of the patella can be palpated, with the apex lying inferiorly and the base superiorly. The quadriceps femoris tendon attaches to the base of the patella. The patellar ligament connects the apex of the patella to the tibial tuberosity, and is tapped when performing the knee jerk tendon reflex. On the lateral side of the knee the head of the fibula is visible and palpable. Immediately anterior to the head of the fibula lies the iliotibial tract, which is most prominent when the knee is fully extended.

Posteriorly, the diamond-shaped popliteal fossa is visible when the knee is flexed against resistance. Its upper borders are formed by the hamstring muscles, and the lower borders by the calf muscles; it contains the popliteal vessels, popliteal lymph nodes, and the tibial and common peroneal nerves.

Leg

The anteromedial surface of the tibia is subcutaneous. The common peroneal nerve exits laterally from the popliteal fossa, and can be palpated as it winds around the neck of the fibula. The peroneal muscles on the lateral aspect of the leg cover the shaft of the fibula.

Ankle

The two prominences at the ankle are known as the medial and lateral malleoli. The distal tibia forms the medial malleolus and the distal fibula forms the lateral malleolus. The malleoli, together with the talus bone, form the ankle joint.

Foot

On the dorsal surface of the foot, the head of the talus is the only tarsal bone which can be individually distinguished on palpation. The metatarsal bones and phalanges are palpable along their length. The tendons of the extensor muscles are visible, together with subcutaneous veins.

On the plantar surface, the calcaneus (heel bone) can be palpated, as well as the navicular tuberosity lying anterior to the medial malleolus. The base of the 5th metatarsal is palpable laterally, but the remaining bones are covered by the plantar aponeurosis, intrinsic muscles and long flexor tendons.

MUSCULATURE

Gluteal region and thigh

The rounded outline of the buttock is formed by subcutaneous fat and the mass of the gluteus maximus muscle. There are three muscular compartments in the thigh. Each compartment has a common nerve supply:

- The femoral nerve supplies the extensor (anterior) compartment.
- The sciatic nerve supplies the flexor (posterior) compartment.
- The obturator nerve supplies the adductor (medial) compartment.

Extensor compartment of the thigh

The large quadriceps muscle mass covers the anterior surface of the thigh. It inserts into the patella and, via the patellar ligament, into the tibial tuberosity. The rectus femoris component of quadriceps is visible when the muscle is contracted. The vastus lateralis and vastus medialis muscles form the lateral and medial borders of the thigh. The vastus intermedius muscle lies deeply between them. Vastus medialis forms a muscular prominence on the medial aspect of the knee. When contracted, the sartorius muscle forms an oblique ridge passing inferiorly on the medial side of the knee. The majority of the gluteus maximus and tensor fasciae latae muscles insert into the iliotibial tract on the lateral surface of the thigh.

Flexor compartment of the thigh

The three hamstring muscles lie in the flexor compartment of the thigh. They arise from the ischial tuberosities inferior to gluteus maximus and can be demonstrated by flexing the knee against resistance. The biceps femoris tendon is palpable and visible laterally where it attaches to the head of the fibula. The semimembranosus and semitendinosus muscles are palpable medially. The tendon of semitendinosus inserts with sartorius and gracilis muscles, into the anteromedial surface of the tibia.

Adductor compartment of the thigh

The adductor muscles form the medial aspect of the thigh.

Leg

There are three muscular compartments in the leg. Each compartment has a common nerve supply:

- The deep peroneal nerve supplies the anterior or extensor compartment.
- The tibial nerve supplies the posterior or flexor compartment.
- The superficial peroneal nerve supplies the lateral compartment.

Extensor compartment of the leg

The anterior extensor muscles lie lateral to the tibia. The tibialis anterior muscle is most easily identified, and its tendon can be traced inferiorly as it crosses the ankle joint and enters the foot. The tendons of the extensor muscles are easily identifiable at the ankle from medial to lateral as tibialis anterior, extensor hallucis longus and extensor digitorum longus.

Flexor compartment of the leg

The two bellies of gastrocnemius are visible on the posterior aspect of the leg during plantarflexion of the foot at the ankle. Deep to gastrocnemius lies the soleus muscle. The tendons of gastrocnemius and soleus join to form the tendocalcaneus (Achilles tendon), which inserts into the calcaneum. Both muscles are powerful plantarflexors of the ankle joint. The tendons of the deep flexor muscles pass posterior to the medial malleolus.

Lateral compartment of the leg

The peroneal muscles are visible on the lateral aspect of the leg. Peroneus longus arises from the fibula superior to peroneus brevis. The peroneus longus tendon passes superficial to peroneus brevis.

Dorsum of foot

On the dorsal surface of the foot, extensor digitorum brevis is visible as a round muscle mass anterior to the lateral malleolus. The dorsal interossei lie between the metatarsal bones.

SUPERFICIAL STRUCTURES

Superficial fascia of the lower limb

The superficial fascia of the lower limb is continuous with the fascia of the abdominal wall anteriorly, the back posteriorly and the perineum medially. It is thickened in the gluteal region and thigh. Anteriorly it is continuous with the membranous superficial fascia (Scarpa's fascia) of the abdomen which extends from the anterior abdominal wall and fuses with the fascia lata of the thigh inferior to the inguinal ligament (this point is visible as the inguinal skin crease) (page 87).

Fascia lata

The fascia lata is the deep fascia of the lower limb. It lies deep to the skin and superficial fascia. It encloses the limb like a stocking, and its attachments, described below, can be traced around the pelvis:

- Posteriorly: the iliac crest, posterior aspect of the ilium and the sacrum, the sacrotuberous ligament
- Inferiorly: the ischial tuberosity ischiopubic ramus and body of the pubic bone
- Anteriorly: the pubic tubercle and pectinate line and inguinal ligament

The fascia is thickened on the lateral aspect of the thigh forming the iliotibial tract. The tract extends from the tubercle of the iliac crest to the lateral tibial condyle, and helps to support the hyperextended knee when standing.

The intermuscular septa which divide the thigh into its muscular compartments (Fig. 7.1) are derived from the fascia lata.

Inferiorly the fascia lata is attached to the tibia and fibula and continues distally as the deep fascia of the calf.

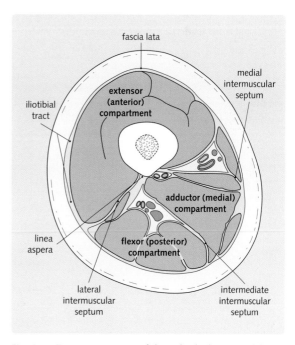

Fig. 7.1 Transverse section of the right thigh - viewed from below.

Superficial veins

Venous blood from the foot drains into the dorsal venous arch, which drains into the great saphenous vein medially, and the small saphenous vein laterally.

HINTS AND TIPS

Fusion of the membranous layer of the superficial fascia (Scarpa's) with the fascia lata of the thigh prevents extravasated fluid (e.g. urine from trauma to the penile urethra) in the superficial perineal pouch from tracking inferiorly in the lower limb (page 143).

Great saphenous vein

The great saphenous vein passes anterior to the medial malleolus and ascends in the superficial fascia on the medial side of the leg, running alongside the saphenous nerve. It passes posterior to the medial condyles of the tibia and femur. In the thigh it passes through the saphenous opening of the fascia lata (perforating the cribriform fascia covering the opening) and joins the femoral vein (Fig. 7.2A and inset) at the saphenofemoral junction (SFJ). It communicates with the deep veins via perforating veins (normally blood flows from the superficial veins to the deep veins). The great saphenous veins contain valves, ensuring that blood flows from distal to proximal. There are more valves in the leg than in the thigh. The vein receives tributaries along

Fig. 7.2   Great (A) and small (B) saphenous veins and their tributaries. Inset shows tributaries of great saphenous vein.

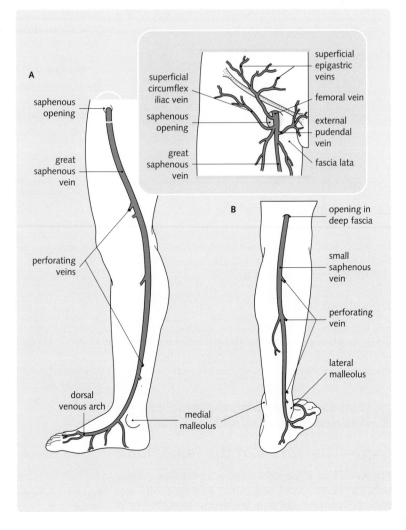

its length. Proximally it receives tributaries from the anterior and medial regions of the thigh and from the anterior abdominal wall. These include:

- The superficial circumflex iliac vein and the superficial epigastric vein, which drain the anterior abdominal wall
- The superficial external pudendal vein which drains the external genitalia.

Small saphenous vein

The small saphenous vein passes posterior to the lateral malleolus and travels superiorly along the posterolateral aspect of the calf with the sural nerve. It pierces the deep fascia of the popliteal fossa, where it joins the popliteal vein (Fig. 7.2B). It drains the lateral part of the leg and communicates with the deep veins of the leg via perforating veins.

CLINICAL NOTE

Clinical examination

Varicose veins normally occur secondary to incompetent valves in the superficial venous system, hence blood passes less effectively from the superficial to deep veins. If valve incompetence occurs at the saphenofemoral junction (SFJ), it may result in saphena varix (a blueish swelling which has a cough impulse and may be mistaken for a femoral or inguinal hernia).

The competence of the SFJ may be assessed by Trendelenburg's test (the tourniquet test). With the patient supine, the affected leg is elevated to empty the veins. The SFJ is occluded by placing two fingers over it (5 cm inferior and medial to the mid-inguinal point) or by applying a tourniquet just distal to the SFJ. The patient is then asked to stand (while the SFJ remains occluded). If the leg veins do not refill this suggests that the site of incompetence is the SFJ. If the leg veins fill it suggests that the SFJ is competent and the level of incompetence lies more distally. The test can then be repeated at more distal levels, usually above and below the knee to determine the site of incompetence. Treatment of varicose veins includes surgery, laser ablation and sclerotherapy (injection of sclerosant which thromboses vessels).

Lymphatic drainage of the lower limb

Lymphatics from the superficial tissues of the lower limb drain into superficial inguinal lymph nodes (Fig. 7.3). These lie superficial to the fascia lata along the inguinal ligament, and around the termination of

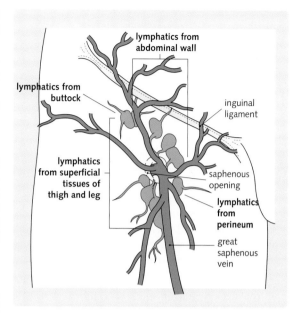

Fig. 7.3 Superficial inguinal lymph nodes.

the great saphenous vein. They also receive lymph from the perineum, the abdominal wall and the buttock.

Superficial nodes drain to deep nodes lying alongside the femoral vessels in the femoral canal. Deep nodes receive lymph from the deep tissues of the lower limb, and eventually drain into the external iliac nodes.

Cutaneous innervation of the lower limb

Figure 7.4 illustrates the dermatomes of the lower limb.

HINTS AND TIPS

The superficial inguinal lymph nodes drain a variety of structures. On palpating enlarged nodes in the groin it is important to consider that they drain the lower limb (cellulitis), perineum (syphilis), buttock (abscess) and the abdominal wall inferior to the umbilicus.

THE GLUTEAL REGION, HIP AND THIGH

Osteology of the hip

Pelvic girdle

The pelvic girdle protects the pelvic cavity and supports the body weight. It transmits load to the lower limbs via the sacrum, hip bone and hip joint (Ch. 6).

sacrospinous ligaments. The piriformis muscle passes through the greater sciatic foramen from the pelvis, and is the key to understanding the relationships of vessels and nerves passing through this region.

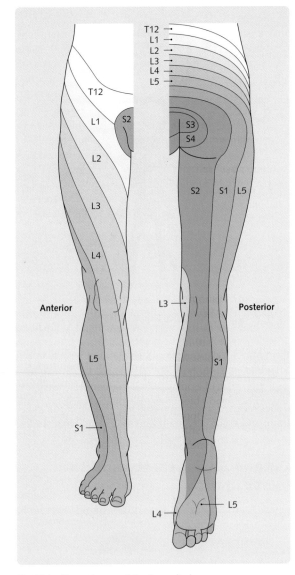

Fig. 7.4 Dermatomes of the lower limb.

CLINICAL NOTE

Neurology

Damage to the superior gluteal nerve results in paralysis of gluteus medius and minimus muscles. These are important abductors of the hip. When walking these muscles contract on the stance (weight bearing) side, elevating the pelvis on the opposite side. This allows the non-weight bearing leg to swing forward, without the foot catching on the ground. To test the function of these muscles, a patient is asked to stand on one leg. Viewing the patient either from in front or behind, the pelvis on the unsupported side should elevate (as above). If the pelvis on the unsupported side drops or does not elevate this indicates a weakness in the abductors on the stance side (positive Trendelenburg sign).

The gluteal region is a common site for intramuscular injection. A safe area for injection, avoiding the sciatic nerve, is the superolateral quadrant of the buttock, as is the area superior and lateral to an imaginary line drawn between the greater trochanter of the femur and the posterior superior iliac spine.

Femur

The femur is the long bone of the thigh (Fig. 7.5).

Gluteal region

The gluteal region (buttock) lies posterior to the pelvis. It extends from the iliac crest to the gluteal fold. The muscles, vessels and nerves which exit and enter this region pass through the greater and lesser sciatic foramina (Figs 7.6–7.9). The foramina are formed anteriorly by the greater and lesser sciatic notches of the pelvic bones, and are completed posteriorly by the sacrotuberous and

Hip joint

The hip joint is a ball-and-socket synovial joint between the acetabulum of the pelvis (which develops from three bones – the ilium, ischium and pubis) and the head of the femur. The C-shaped articular surface of the acetabulum is covered by hyaline cartilage. The edge of the acetabulum is deepened by a rim of fibrocartilage – the acetabular labrum. Inferiorly, the labrum bridges across the acetabular notch forming the transverse acetabular ligament.

The articular surface of the head of the femur is covered by hyaline cartilage. At the centre of the femoral head lies a small non-articular area, known as the fovea capitis which is the site of attachment of the ligament of the head of the femur.

The hip joint is a very stable joint (unlike the shoulder joint) with a good degree of mobility. Stability is mainly achieved from the close apposition of the femoral head and the acetabulum, and by the presence of the acetabular labrum. The femoral neck is much

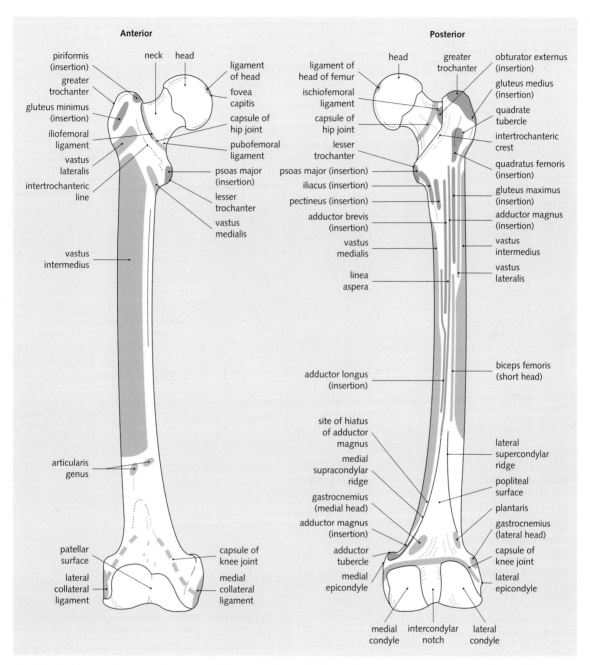

Fig. 7.5 Origins and insertions of muscles and ligaments attached to the anterior and posterior surfaces of the right femur.

narrower than the diameter of the head; this allows considerable movement to occur in all directions before the neck impinges on the labrum.

The joint capsule is loose. It is lined internally by synovial membrane and attaches around the labrum, the transverse acetabular ligament and the neck of femur. Around the neck of the femur, the joint capsule binds down blood vessels supplying the femoral head. A femoral neck fracture can disrupt these vessels. The capsule is reinforced by three strong ligaments extending from the pelvic bone to the femur:

- Inferiorly, the pubofemoral ligament – prevents overabduction and hyperextension
- Posteriorly, the ischiofemoral ligament – prevents excessive medial rotation and hyperextension
- Anteriorly, the iliofemoral ligament – prevents hyperextension and lateral rotation.

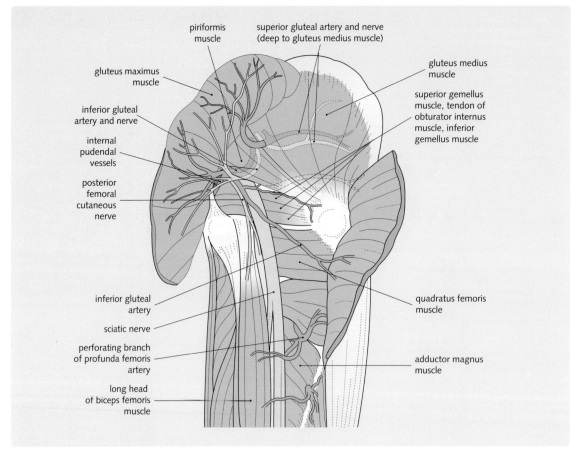

Fig. 7.6 Right gluteal region showing the main nerves and vessels.

Fig. 7.7	Muscles of the gluteal region.		
Name of muscle (nerve supply)	**Origin**	**Insertion**	**Action**
Tensor fasciae latae (superior gluteal nerve)	Iliac crest	Iliotibial tract	Extends knee joint Tenses iliotibial tract
Gluteus maximus (inferior gluteal nerve)	Ilium, sacrum, coccyx, and sacrotuberous ligament	Iliotibial tract and gluteal tuberosity of femur	Extends and laterally rotates thigh at hip joint Extends knee joint
Gluteus medius (superior gluteal nerve)	Ilium	Greater trochanter of femur	Abducts thigh at hip joint and tilts pelvis when walking
Gluteus minimus (superior gluteal nerve)	Ilium	Greater trochanter of femur	As gluteus medius and medially rotates thigh
Piriformis (S1, S2 nerves)	Anterior surface of sacrum	Greater trochanter of femur	
Obturator internus (sacral plexus)	Inner surface of obturator membrane	Greater trochanter of femur	
Gemellus inferior (sacral plexus)	Ischial tuberosity	Greater trochanter of femur	All of these muscles rotate thigh laterally at hip joint and stabilize the hip joint
Gemellus superior (sacral plexus)	Ischial spine	Greater trochanter of femur	
Quadratus femoris (sacral plexus)	Ischial tuberosity	Quadrate tubercle on femur	

Fig. 7.8 Arteries of the gluteal region.

Artery	Course and distribution
Internal pudendal	Passes through the greater sciatic foramen to enter the gluteal region, supplying obturator internus and piriformis, then passes into the perineum via the lesser sciatic foramen; supplies the muscles of the pelvic region and the external genitalia
Superior gluteal	Enters the gluteal region through the greater sciatic foramen; supplies gluteus maximus, medius and minimus, piriformis, obturator internus and tensor fasciae latae
Inferior gluteal	Passes through the greater sciatic foramen to enter the gluteal region; supplies gluteus maximus, piriformis, obturator internus, superior and inferior gemellus, and quadratus femoris

Blood and nerve supply of the hip joint

The blood supply of the hip joint arises from the trochanteric and cruciate anastomoses. The trochanteric anastomosis lies near the trochanteric fossa. Its vessels lie along the femoral neck and supply the head of the femur. It is composed of the following arteries:

- The medial and lateral circumflex femoral arteries
- The superior and inferior gluteal arteries
- The obturator artery.

The cruciate anastomosis is composed of the following arteries:

- The inferior gluteal artery (a branch of the internal iliac artery)
- The medial and lateral circumflex femoral arteries (branches of the profunda femoris artery)
- An ascending branch of the first perforating branch of the profunda femoris artery.

The trochanteric and cruciate anastomoses may provide a collateral circulation if one of the vessels contributing to the anastomoses becomes occluded.

The nerve supply of the hip joint comprises the following:

- Femoral nerve
- Sciatic nerve
- Obturator nerve.

Movements of the hip joint

The muscles involved, and factors that restrict movement of the joint are described in Figure 7.10.

Thigh

The thigh is divided into three compartments by intermuscular septae (derived from the fascia lata). The medial intermuscular septum separates the extensor

Fig. 7.9 Nerves of the gluteal region.

Nerve (origin)	Course and distributions
Inferior gluteal (anterior rami of L5–S2)	Exits pelvis through greater sciatic foramen inferior to piriformis, and supplies gluteus maximus
Superior gluteal (anterior rami of L4–S1)	Exits pelvis through greater sciatic foramen superior to piriformis and passes between gluteus medius and minimus to supply these muscles and tensor fasciae latae
Nerve to quadratus femoris (anterior rami of L4, L5 and S1)	Exits pelvis through greater sciatic foramen inferior to piriformis to supply the hip joint, inferior gemellus, and quadratus femoris
Nerve to obturator internus (anterior rami of L5, S1 and S2)	Enters gluteal region through greater sciatic foramen inferior to piriformis, descends posterior to ischial spine, enters lesser sciatic foramen. It supplies obturator internus and superior gemellus muscles
Posterior cutaneous nerve of thigh (sacral plexus–S1–S3)	Exits pelvis through greater sciatic foramen, inferior to piriformis, and runs deep to gluteus maximus. It emerges from its inferior border to supply skin of buttock (gluteal branches) and then skin over posterior thigh and calf
Pudendal (anterior rami of S2–S4)	Enters gluteal region through greater sciatic foramen inferior to piriformis. Descends posteriorly over the sacrospinous ligament, entering perineum through lesser sciatic foramen. Supplies the perineum, the male and female external genitalia, the external anal sphincter and urethral sphincter
Sciatic (lumbosacral plexus–L4–S3)	Exits pelvis through greater sciatic foramen inferior to piriformis, to enter gluteal region – it has no motor branches in the gluteal region

Fig. 7.10 Movements of the hip joint and the muscles responsible for these movements.

Movement of the thigh on the trunk	Movement at the hip joint	Muscles involved	Factors limiting movement
Flexion	Head of the femur moves about a transverse axis passing through both acetabula and causes the shaft to swing anteriorly	Psoas major, iliacus, tensor fasciae latae, pectineus, sartorius	Thigh touching abdomen, hamstring muscle tension if leg is extended
Extension	As flexion but opposite direction	Gluteus maximus, hamstrings	Iliofemoral ligament, pubofemoral ligament
Abduction	Head of the femur moves in the acetabulum about an anteroposterior axis and causes the femoral neck and shaft to swing laterally	Gluteus medius, gluteus minimus	Abductor muscle tension, pubofemoral ligament
Adduction	As abduction but opposite direction	Adductors, gracillis	Gluteus medius, gluteus minimus, other leg
Medial rotation	Rotation of the femoral head in the acetabulum about a vertical axis that passes through the femoral head and medial condyle The neck of the femur swings anteriorly	Tensor fasciae latae, gluteus medius, gluteus minimus, iliopsoas, pectineus, adductor longus	Ischiofemoral ligament
Lateral rotation	As medial rotation but opposite direction	Obturator internus, obturator externus, piriformis, gemelli, quadratus femoris, gluteus maximus	Iliofemoral ligament

(anterior) and adductor (medial) compartments, and the lateral intermuscular septum separates the extensor and flexor (posterior) compartments (Fig. 7.1).

Extensor compartment of the thigh

The muscles of the extensor compartment are described in Figure 7.11. The blood and nerve supply is described in Figures 7.12 and 7.13.

Factors stabilizing the patella

Due to the width of the pelvis, the distance between the hip joints is wider than the distance between the knees. This means that the femur and the quadriceps muscle lie obliquely in the thigh. When the quadriceps contracts it tends to pull the patella laterally. Patellar dislocation is prevented by three factors:

- The anterior prominence of the lateral condyle of the femur (Fig. 7.18)
- The lowest fibres of vastus medialis insert into the medial border of the patella. When quadriceps contracts, these fibres pull the patella medially
- Tension in the medial patellar retinaculum.

Femoral triangle

The femoral triangle contains (from lateral to medial) the femoral nerve, artery and vein (Fig. 7.14) along with lymph nodes (within the femoral canal – see below). These lie deep to the skin, superficial fascia and fascia lata. The femoral artery, vein and canal are enclosed by the femoral sheath, which is a continuation of the abdominal fascia (transversalis fascia anteriorly and iliac fascia posteriorly). The femoral nerve lies outwith the femoral sheath, separated from it by the iliopsoas fascia.

The boundaries of the femoral triangle are the inguinal ligament (superiorly), the medial border of adductor longus (medially) and the medial border of sartorius (laterally). The floor is formed by iliopsoas, pectineus and adductor longus muscles.

Femoral canal

The femoral canal forms the medial compartment of the femoral sheath. Its boundaries (which form the femoral ring in the abdomen) are: the medial part of the inguinal ligament (anteriorly), the pectineal ligament (posteriorly), the lacunar ligament (medially) and the femoral vein (laterally). It contains efferent lymphatics, passing from the

Fig. 7.11 Muscles of the extensor compartment of the thigh.

Name of muscle (nerve supply)	Origin	Insertion	Action
Quadriceps femoris – rectus femoris; vastus lateralis, medialis, and intermedius (femoral nerve)	Ilium and upper part of femoral shaft	Quadriceps tendon into patella, and via the patellar ligament onto the tibial tuberosity	Extends leg at knee joint Flexes thigh at hip joint
Sartorius (femoral nerve)	Anterior superior iliac spine	Medial surface of tibial shaft	Flexes, abducts, and laterally rotates thigh at hip joint Flexes and medially rotates leg at knee joint
Psoas major (lumbar plexus, L1–L3 nerves)	T12 body, transverse processes, bodies, and intervertebral discs L1–L5	Lesser trochanter of femur (together with iliacus muscle)	Flexes thigh on trunk
Iliacus (femoral nerve)	Iliac fossa of hip bone	Lesser trochanter of femur	Flexes thigh on trunk
Pectineus (femoral nerve and obturator nerve)	Superior ramus of pubis	Upper shaft of femur	Flexes and abducts thigh at hip joint

Fig. 7.12 Arterial supply to the thigh.

Artery	Origin	Course and distribution
Femoral	Continuation of external iliac artery distal to inguinal ligament	Descends through femoral triangle, enters the adductor canal, and ends by passing through the adductor hiatus (where it becomes the popliteal artery) Supplies anterior and anteromedial surfaces of the thigh
Profunda femoris	Femoral artery in the femoral triangle	Passes inferiorly, deep to adductor longus Gives off perforating branches to supply posterior and lateral compartments of thigh
Lateral circumflex femoral	Profunda femoris; may arise from femoral artery	Passes laterally deep to sartorius and rectus femoris Supplies anterior part of gluteal region, the femur and knee joint
Medial circumflex femoral	Profunda femoris	Passes medially and posteriorly between pectineus and iliopsoas, and enters gluteal region Supplies head and neck of femur
Obturator	Internal iliac artery	Passes through obturator foramen and enters medial compartment of thigh Supplies obturator externus, pectineus, adductors of thigh, and gracilis – muscles attached to ischial tuberosity and head of femur

deep inguinal nodes to the abdomen (Fig. 7.12) and provides space for expansion of the femoral vein during times of increased venous return from the lower limb.

Adductor canal

At the apex of the femoral triangle, the femoral vessels pass deep to sartorius, entering the medial aspect of the thigh via the adductor canal. The boundaries of the adductor canal are vastus medialis (laterally), adductor longus and adductor magnus (posteromedially) and sartorius (anteriorly). The contents of the canal are the nerve to vastus medialis, the saphenous nerve, and the femoral artery and vein. The adductor canal ends at the adductor hiatus (an opening in the tendon of adductor magnus muscle). The femoral artery enters the popliteal fossa through the hiatus, where it continues as the popliteal artery. The popliteal vein exits the fossa through the hiatus and continues as the femoral vein.

Fig. 7.13 Nerves of the thigh.

Nerve (origin)	Course and distribution
Ilioinguinal (lumbar plexus – L1)	Supplies skin over the upper and medial part of the thigh, the skin over the root of the penis and upper part of the scrotum, or the skin over the mons pubis and labia majora
Genitofemoral (lumbar plexus – L1–L2)	Descends on anterior surface of psoas major and divides into genital and femoral branches: Femoral branch supplies skin over femoral triangle Genital branch supplies the cremaster muscle and scrotum, or the labia majora
Lateral cutaneous nerve of thigh (lumbar plexus – L2–L3)	Passes deep to inguinal ligament, 2–3 cm medial to anterior superior iliac spine Supplies skin on anterior and lateral aspects of thigh
Medial and intermediate femoral cutaneous (femoral nerve)	Arise in femoral triangle and pierce fascia lata of thigh Supplies skin on medial and anterior aspect of thigh
Posterior cutaneous nerve of thigh (sacral plexus – S2–S3)	Passes through greater sciatic foramen inferior to piriformis Supplies skin over posterior aspect of thigh, buttock and proximal leg
Femoral (lumbar plexus – L2–L4)	Passes deep to inguinal ligament Supplies muscles of the anterior compartment of the thigh, hip and knee joints, and skin on anteromedial side of thigh
Obturator (lumbar plexus – L2–L4)	Enters thigh through obturator foramen and divides: Anterior branch supplies adductor longus, adductor brevis, gracilis, and pectineus Posterior branch supplies obturator externus and adductor magnus
Sciatic (sacral plexus – L4–S3)	Enters gluteal region through greater sciatic foramen inferior to or through piriformis, descends along posterior aspect of thigh, and divides proximal to the knee into the tibial and common peroneal nerves The tibial division innervates the hamstrings (except for short head of biceps femoris – innervated by the common peroneal division) and has articular branches to the hip and knee joints

Flexor compartment of the thigh

The muscles of the flexor compartment are outlined in Figure 7.15 and illustrated in Figure 7.16. Blood supply to the flexor compartment is mainly from the perforating branches of the profunda femoris, with a small contribution from the inferior gluteal artery (Fig. 7.12).

The nerve supply to the flexor compartment is from the sciatic nerve (Fig. 7.13).

Adductor compartment of the thigh

The muscles of the adductor compartment are outlined in Figure 7.17. Blood supply to the adductor compartment is mainly from the perforating branches of the profunda femoris, with a small contribution from the inferior gluteal artery (Fig. 7.12). All of the muscles are innervated by the obturator nerve, except for the hamstring part of the adductor magnus muscle, which is supplied by the tibial nerve, a branch of the sciatic nerve (Fig. 7.13).

Femoral vein

The femoral vein lies posterior to the artery in the adductor canal. Below the inguinal ligament the vein lies medial to the artery in the femoral sheath. It passes posterior to the inguinal ligament to become the external iliac vein. It receives the venae comitantes of the profunda femoris artery and the great saphenous vein (whose tributaries are the venae comitantes of the femoral artery).

CLINICAL NOTE

Clinical examination

During lower limb examination the femoral, popliteal, dorsalis pedis and tibialis posterior pulses are assessed. The femoral pulse is palpable at the mid-inguinal point, midway between the anterior superior iliac spine and the pubic symphysis. The popliteal pulse is palpable posterior to the knee (the popliteal pulse lies deep within the fossa and so is difficult to feel), with the knee partially flexed. The posterior tibial pulse can be palpated approximately 2 cm inferior and posterior to the medial malleolus. The dorsalis pedis pulse is palpable on the dorsum of the foot, lateral to the tendon of extensor hallucis longus tendon and distal to the navicular bone.

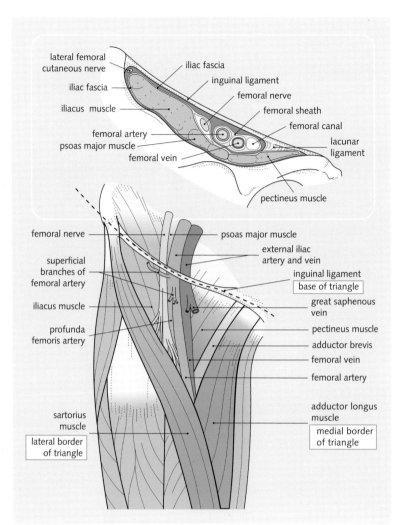

Fig. 7.14 Right femoral triangle and its contents. Inset shows the femoral canal from below.

Fig. 7.15 Muscles of the flexor compartment of the thigh.

Name of muscle (nerve supply)	Origin	Insertion	Action
Biceps femoris: Long head (tibial division of sciatic nerve) **Short head** (common peroneal division of the sciatic nerve)	Ischial tuberosity	Head of fibula	Flexes leg at knee joint and extends thigh at hip joint
Semitendinosus (tibial division of the sciatic nerve)	Ischial tuberosity	Proximal tibia (medial to tibial tuberosity)	Flexes leg at knee joint and extends thigh at hip joint
Semimembranosus (tibial division of sciatic)	Ischial tuberosity	Medial condyle of the tibia, forms the oblique popliteal ligament	Flexes leg at knee joint and extends thigh at hip joint

Fig. 7.16 Muscles of the posterior aspect of the right thigh.

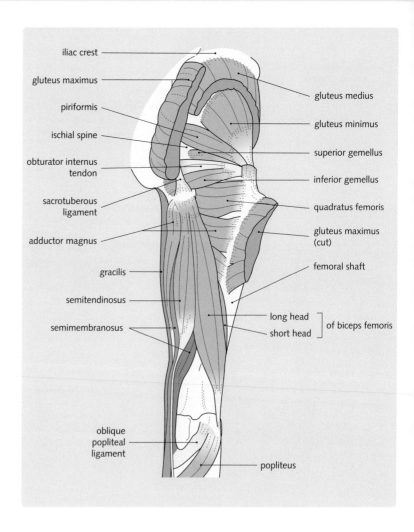

iliac crest
gluteus maximus
piriformis
ischial spine
obturator internus tendon
sacrotuberous ligament
adductor magnus
gracilis
semitendinosus
semimembranosus
oblique popliteal ligament

gluteus medius
gluteus minimus
superior gemellus
inferior gemellus
quadratus femoris
gluteus maximus (cut)
femoral shaft
long head
short head
} of biceps femoris
popliteus

Fig. 7.17 Muscles of the adductor compartment of the thigh.

Name of muscle (nerve supply)	Origin	Insertion	Action
Gracilis (obturator nerve)	Ischiopubic ramus	Proximal medial surface of tibia	Adducts thigh at hip joint Flexes leg at knee joint and medially rotates leg when knee is flexed
Adductor longus (obturator nerve)	Body of pubis	Linea aspera of femur	Adducts and flexes thigh at hip joint
Adductor brevis (obturator nerve)	Inferior ramus of pubis	Linea aspera of femur	Adducts and flexes thigh at hip joint
Adductor magnus (adductor part – obturator nerve; hamstring part – sciatic nerve)	Adductor part – ischiopubic ramus Hamstring part – ischial tuberosity	Adductor part – posterior surface of femur Hamstring part – adductor tubercle of femur	Adductor part – adducts and flexes thigh at hip joint Hamstring part – extends thigh at hip joint
Obturator externus (obturator nerve)	Outer surface of obturator membrane	Greater trochanter of femur	Lateral rotation of thigh at hip joint

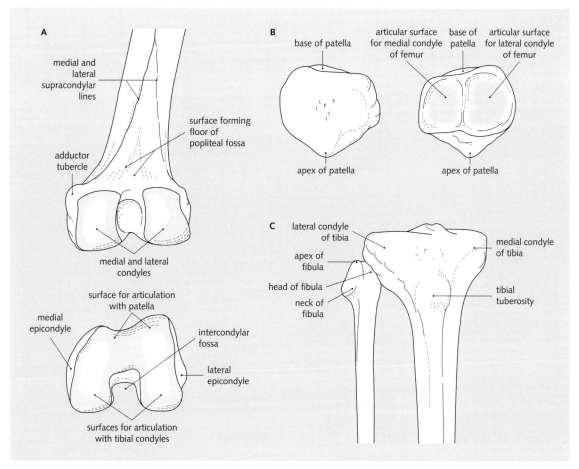

Fig. 7.18 Skeleton of the knee. A, Posterior and inferior aspects of the lower end of the right femur. B, Anterior and posterior aspects of the patella. C, Anterior aspect of the upper end of the right tibia and fibula.

THE KNEE AND POPLITEAL FOSSA

Popliteal fossa

The diamond-shaped popliteal fossa lies posterior to the knee joint. It is bordered by the biceps femoris muscle (superolaterally), semitendinosus and semi-membranosus muscles (superomedially) and by the medial and lateral heads of gastrocnemius muscle inferiorly (Fig. 7.19). Its roof is formed by skin, superficial fascia and deep fascia which is pierced by the small saphenous vein and three cutaneous nerves. The floor is formed by the femur, the oblique popliteal ligament, capsule of the knee joint and the popliteus muscle.

CLINICAL NOTE

Orthopaedics

A fracture of the femoral neck causes the affected limb to become shortened and externally (laterally) rotated. This is due to the unopposed action of gluteus maximus, piriformis, obturator internus and gemelli muscles which laterally rotate the hip. It is important to determine whether the fracture is within the joint capsule (intracapsular) or outside (extracapsular). Intracapsular fractures may interrupt the blood supply to the femoral head causing avascular necrosis. A dislocated hip causes the affected limb to become shortened and medially rotated.

Fig. 7.19 Right popliteal fossa and its contents.

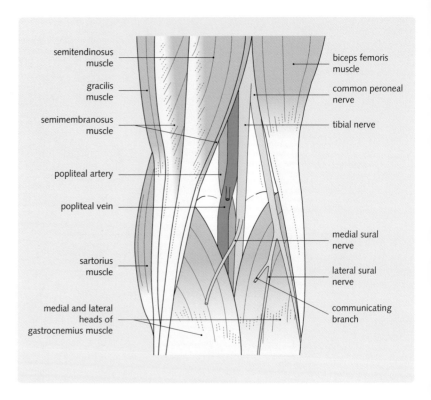

semitendinosus muscle

gracilis muscle

semimembranosus muscle

popliteal artery

popliteal vein

sartorius muscle

medial and lateral heads of gastrocnemius muscle

biceps femoris muscle

common peroneal nerve

tibial nerve

medial sural nerve

lateral sural nerve

communicating branch

Contents of the popliteal fossa

From deep to superficial include the following:

Popliteus muscle

The popliteus muscle is attached proximally to the lateral condyle of the femur, the fibula and the lateral meniscus. It inserts onto the popliteal surface of the tibia. It is supplied by the tibial nerve. It medially rotates the tibia and 'unlocks' the knee from a fully extended position (i.e. it initiates flexion of the knee).

Popliteal artery

This is the continuation of the femoral artery as it passes through the adductor hiatus. It lies deep in the fossa, in direct contact with the popliteal surface of the femur and the capsule of the knee joint. It terminates at the lower border of popliteus muscle, where it divides into the anterior and posterior tibial arteries. The popliteal artery gives off muscular branches, branches to the knee joint (superior, middle and inferior genicular arteries) and cutaneous branches. The genicular arteries form an intricate anastomosis with descending branches of the profunda femoris and femoral arteries, and ascending branches of the tibial arteries. This forms a collateral supply if the main vessels become occluded.

Popliteal vein

This passes superiorly in the popliteal fossa, medial to and then superficial to the artery before entering the adductor hiatus. It receives the small saphenous vein together with the venae comitantes of the popliteal artery.

Common peroneal nerve

This nerve is closely related to the tendon of biceps femoris in the popliteal fossa. It exits the fossa by passing superficial to the lateral head to the gastrocnemius muscle. It crosses the posterior aspect of the head of the fibula and then winds around the neck of the fibula. Branches in the popliteal fossa include:

- The lateral sural nerve, which supplies the skin of the calf
- A communicating branch with the medial sural nerve
- Branches to the knee joint.

Tibial nerve

This is a branch of the sciatic nerve. It lies superficially in the fossa, immediately deep to the popliteal fascia. It travels inferiorly through the centre of the fossa, giving off several branches:

- Articular branches to the knee joint
- Muscular branches to all of the muscles of the posterior leg (soleus, gastrocnemius, plantaris and popliteus)
- The medial sural cutaneous nerve, which joins the communicating branch of the lateral sural cutaneous nerve to form the sural nerve. The sural nerve supplies the skin over the lateral side of the calf and heel.

Short saphenous vein

In the popliteal fossa this normally penetrates the deep fascia to drain into the popliteal vein.

Popliteal lymph nodes

The majority of the popliteal nodes drain into the deep inguinal nodes.

Knee joint

The knee joint consists of two articulations between the femoral and tibial condyles, and between the patella and the femur (Fig. 7.18). It is a synovial hinge joint which allows some rotation. The articular surfaces, i.e. the femoral condyles, the patella and the superior surface of the tibial condyles, are covered by hyaline cartilage.

Menisci

Between the femoral and tibial condyles lie the lateral and medial menisci (Fig. 7.20). Menisci are formed from fibrocartilage. They help to transmit load, increase the area of contact between the femur and the tibia, contribute to joint stability, and assist in proprioception.

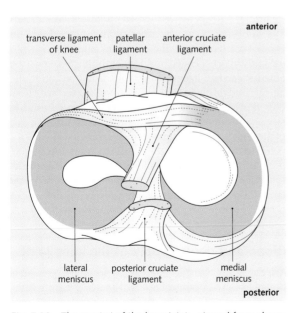

Fig. 7.20 The menisci of the knee joint - viewed from above.

Both menisci are attached to the intercondylar fossa of the tibia. At the periphery they are loosely attached via the coronary ligament to the capsule. The medial meniscus is also attached to the medial collateral ligament and the joint capsule. The menisci are commonly injured as a result of a sudden twisting of the knee, with the medial meniscus being more commonly injured than the lateral.

Capsule

The joint capsule encloses the articular surfaces posteriorly. It is incomplete:

- Anterosuperiorly to allow communication between the joint cavity and the suprapatellar bursa
- Posteroinferiorly to allow passage of the popliteus tendon.

Anteriorly it is replaced by the articular surface of the patella where the capsule blends with and it strengthened by the patellar retinacula, which are expansions of the tendons of the vastus medialis and lateralis.

Synovial membrane

Synovial membrane lines the joint capsule (Fig. 7.21). Superiorly it becomes continuous with the suprapatellar bursa. The cruciate ligaments and popliteus tendon lie outside the synovial cavity.

Bursae around the knee joint

The bursae around the knee joint include:

- The suprapatellar bursa (lies between the infero-anterior surface of the femur and the deep surface of the quadriceps femoris)
- The prepatellar bursa (lies between the patella and the skin)
- The superficial and deep infrapatellar bursae (lie between the patellar ligament and skin and the upper part of the tibia and the patellar ligament).

Ligaments

Several ligaments help to stabilize the knee joint (Fig. 7.21):

- The anterior and posterior cruciate ligaments (ACL and PCL respectively) cross over each other, forming an X. They help to keep the articular surfaces of the knee joint apposed, and prevent displacement of the femur on the tibia (or vice versa). The ACL runs between the medial surface of the lateral femoral condyle and the anterior intercondylar region of the tibia. It prevents anterior displacement of the tibia on the femur (or posterior displacement of the femur on the tibia), as well as limiting extension of the lateral femoral condyle. In knee joint extension the ACL becomes taut; this prevents hyperextension of the knee. The PCL runs between the lateral surface of the medial femoral condyle and the posterior

Fig. 7.21 Synovial membrane and the ligaments of the knee.

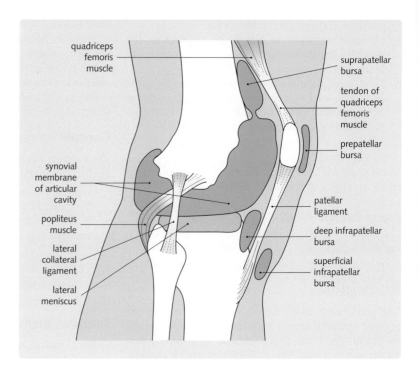

quadriceps femoris muscle

suprapatellar bursa

tendon of quadriceps femoris muscle

prepatellar bursa

synovial membrane of articular cavity

popliteus muscle

lateral collateral ligament

lateral meniscus

patellar ligament

deep infrapatellar bursa

superficial infrapatellar bursa

intercondylar region of the tibia. The PCL prevents anterior displacement of the femur on the tibia (or posterior displacement of the tibia on the femur).

- The patellar ligament is a continuation of the quadriceps tendon. It attaches from the apex of the patella to the tibial tuberosity. Its tension is controlled by the quadriceps muscle, which stabilizes the knee joint through its full range of movement.
- The medial (tibial) and lateral (fibular) collateral ligaments stabilize the knee during flexion and extension. The lateral collateral ligament attaches from the lateral femoral epicondyle to the lateral aspect of the head of the fibula. It prevents adduction of the knee. The medial collateral ligament attaches from the medial femoral epicondyle to the medial tibial condyle. It is also attached to the medial meniscus. It prevents abduction of the knee.
- The oblique popliteal ligament is an expansion of the semimembranosus tendon, which reinforces the knee joint capsule posteriorly.

CLINICAL NOTE

Orthopaedics

Around the knee there are several bursae (pouches filled with synovial fluid). Pressure or friction in the area of a bursa can result in inflammation (bursitis) and localized swelling (increased synovial fluid), e.g.

housemaid's knee (prepatellar bursitis) or clergyman's knee (infrapatellar bursitis). Treatment includes rest, use of ice packs, anti-inflammatory medications and aspiration of the synovial fluid, with injection of steroid medication.

Movements at the knee joint

The movements at the knee joint are outlined in Figure 7.22. 'Locking of the knee joint' puts the knee into a slightly hyperextended position. As the knee extends, the anterior cruciate ligament becomes taut, preventing the lateral condyle of the femur from extending further. However, due to the larger surface area of the medial condyle (Fig. 7.18) extension continues medially around the axis of the anterior cruciate ligament. This produces medial rotation of the femur upon the tibia and causes the oblique, popliteal, medial collateral and lateral collateral ligaments to tighten. At the end of this movement the knee becomes locked. The knee joint must be unlocked before flexion can occur. This is performed by the popliteus muscle, which laterally rotates the femur and loosens the ligaments.

Blood and nerve supply of the knee joint

Arterial supply to the knee arises from the genicular branches of the popliteal artery. The nerve supply comprises articular branches of the sciatic, femoral and obturator nerves.

Fig. 7.22 Movements at the knee joint.

Movement	Muscle
Flexion	Initiated by popliteus hamstrings, gastrocnemius, gracilis, sartorius
Extension	Quadriceps femoris
Medial rotation	Semitendinosus and semimembranosus (when knee is flexed), popliteus (when knee is extended)
Lateral rotation	Biceps femoris (when knee is flexed)
Unlocking of knee	Popliteus
Locking of knee – a passive rotation of the femur upon the tibia	Is caused at the end of extension by the anterior cruciate ligament becoming taut and the femoral medial condyle moving round this ligament

THE LEG AND DORSUM OF FOOT

Osteology of the leg

The skeleton of the leg is illustrated in Figure 7.23.

The interosseous membrane is a tough band of tissue connected to the interosseous borders of the tibia and fibula. It is pierced superiorly by the anterior tibial artery and inferiorly by branches of the peroneal (fibular) artery.

Superior tibiofibular joint

This is an articulation between the head of the fibula and the lateral condyle of the tibia. It is a synovial joint, stabilized by the anterosuperior and posterosuperior tibiofibular ligaments. Small sliding movements occur at this joint.

Inferior tibiofibular joint

This is an articulation between the distal ends of the tibia and fibula. It is a fibrous joint stabilized by an interosseous ligament, along with the anteroinferior and posteroinferior tibiofibular ligaments. There is very little movement at this joint. It contributes to the stability of the ankle joint by ensuring that the lateral malleolus remains closely apposed to the lateral surface of the talus.

Compartments of the leg

The leg is divided into extensor (anterior), flexor (posterior), and peroneal (lateral) compartments (Fig. 7.24) by anterior and posterior intermuscular septa. The muscles of the posterior compartment are divided into

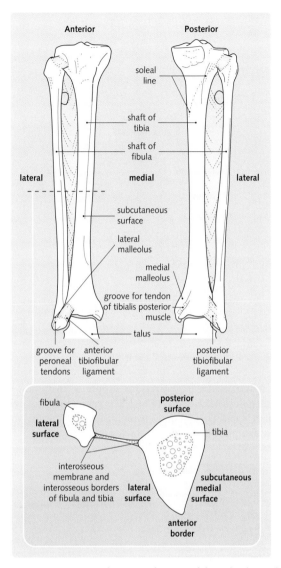

Fig. 7.23 Anterior and posterior features of the right tibia and fibula, and the cross section of the two bones showing the interosseous membrane.

superficial and deep groups by the deep transverse fascia of the leg.

Extensor compartment of the leg

Muscles of the extensor compartment of the leg are illustrated in Figures 7.25 and 7.26. The arterial supply to the compartment is provided by the anterior tibial artery (Figs 7.27 and 7.28). It is a terminal branch of the popliteal artery.

The common peroneal nerve exits the popliteal fossa and winds around the neck of the fibula, dividing into the superficial and deep peroneal nerves (Fig. 7.29). The deep nerve passes around the neck of the fibula to enter the extensor compartment of the leg, which it supplies.

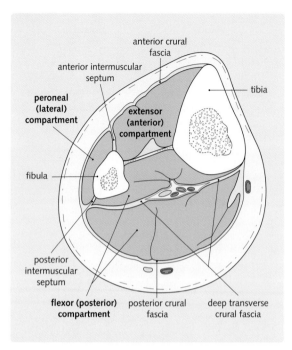

Fig. 7.24 Compartments of the left leg.

It terminates as the cutaneous supply to the skin between the first and second toes. The superficial peroneal nerve supplies the lateral compartment of the leg and the skin on the dorsum of the foot.

CLINICAL NOTE

Compartment syndrome

The intramuscular septa of the upper and lower limbs do not stretch. Trauma, fractures or haemorrhage can lead to swelling in any compartment of a limb, although this most commonly occurs in the lower leg and forearm.

Swelling increases the pressure within the compartment, which can result in compression of veins arteries nerves and muscles (in that order). This is known as compartment syndrome and is characterized by 6 P's: pain (severe and constant), pulselessness (arterial compression results in an impalpable dorsalis pedis pulse), paralysis, paraesthesia (due to nerve compression), perishingly cold (due to reduced perfusion) and pallor (due to reduced perfusion).

Treatment involves surgery to relieve pressure within the affected compartment. The wound is left open and closed at a later stage. Delayed treatment may result in permanent limb damage or amputation.

Dorsum of the foot

The structures from the extensor compartment of the leg pass into the dorsum of the foot. The tendons of extensor digitorum longus pass to the lateral four digits of the foot and join an extensor expansion. These expansions have the same arrangement as those found in the medial four digits of the hand. Over the proximal phalanx each expansion splits into a central slip, which inserts into the middle phalanx and two lateral slips, which insert into the distal phalanx. The interossei and lumbrical muscles attach to the expansions.

The extensor digitorum brevis and extensor hallucis brevis muscles are the only muscles intrinsic to the dorsum of the foot. Arising from the calcaneum, the three tendons of extensor digitorum brevis join the lateral sides of the extensor digitorum longus tendons of the middle three toes over the metatarsophalangeal joint. From a similar origin, the extensor hallucis brevis tendon inserts into the proximal phalanx of the great toe (hallux). The nerve supply is via the deep peroneal nerve and the muscle extends the digits (toes).

Name of muscle (nerve supply)	Origin	Insertion	Action
Extensor digitorum longus (deep peroneal nerve)	Fibula and interosseous membrane	Phalanges of lateral four digits	Extends toes and dorsiflexes foot at ankle joint
Extensor hallucis longus (deep peroneal nerve)	Fibula and interosseous membrane	Base of distal phalanx of great toe	Extends great toe, and dorsiflexes foot at ankle joint
Peroneus tertius (deep peroneal nerve)	Fibula and interosseous membrane	Base of 5th metatarsal bone	Dorsiflexes at ankle joint and everts foot
Tibialis anterior (deep peroneal nerve)	Tibia and interosseous membrane	Medial cuneiform and base of 1st metatarsal bone	Dorsiflexes and inverts foot

Fig. 7.25 Muscles of the extensor compartment of the leg.

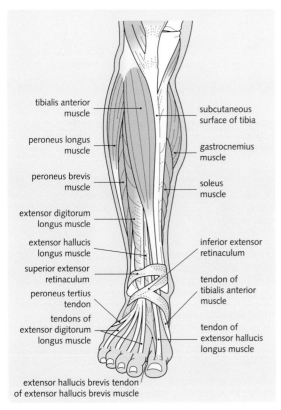

tibialis anterior muscle
subcutaneous surface of tibia
peroneus longus muscle
gastrocnemius muscle
peroneus brevis muscle
soleus muscle
extensor digitorum longus muscle
extensor hallucis longus muscle
inferior extensor retinaculum
superior extensor retinaculum
peroneus tertius tendon
tendon of tibialis anterior muscle
tendons of extensor digitorum longus muscle
tendon of extensor hallucis longus muscle
extensor hallucis brevis tendon of extensor hallucis brevis muscle

Fig. 7.26   Muscles of the extensor compartment of the right leg.

Extensor retinacula

The superior and inferior extensor retinacula keep the extensor tendons firmly bound down to the dorsum of the foot (Fig. 7.30). The retinacula are derived from the deep fascia of the leg.

The superior band passes from the anterior border of the tibia to the anterior border of the fibula. The inferior band is Y-shaped, and it runs from the calcaneus to the medial malleolus and plantar fascia.

Nerves and vessels of the dorsum of the foot

The deep peroneal nerve and anterior tibial artery enter the foot beneath the extensor retinaculum. The anterior tibial artery continues as the dorsalis pedis artery (see Fig. 7.28). It can be palpated between the tendons of extensor hallucis longus and extensor digitorum longus.

Cutaneous innervation of the dorsum of the foot is via the superficial peroneal, deep peroneal, sural and saphenous nerves.

Peroneal compartment of the leg

The peroneal compartment of the leg is illustrated in Figure 7.31. The muscles and their functions are outlined in Figure 7.32. The arterial supply to the peroneal compartment is via the anterior and posterior tibial arteries. The nerve supply is via the superficial peroneal nerve, which lies superficially and is vulnerable to damage. Damage to the nerve will result in foot drop.

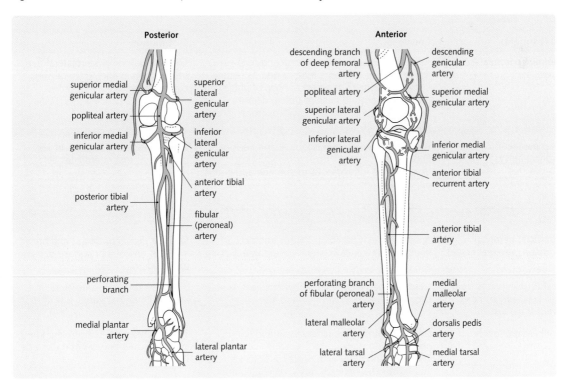

Posterior

superior medial genicular artery
popliteal artery
inferior medial genicular artery
posterior tibial artery
superior lateral genicular artery
inferior lateral genicular artery
anterior tibial artery
fibular (peroneal) artery
perforating branch
medial plantar artery
lateral plantar artery

Anterior

descending branch of deep femoral artery
descending genicular artery
popliteal artery
superior lateral genicular artery
superior medial genicular artery
inferior lateral genicular artery
inferior medial genicular artery
anterior tibial recurrent artery
anterior tibial artery
perforating branch of fibular (peroneal) artery
medial malleolar artery
lateral malleolar artery
dorsalis pedis artery
lateral tarsal artery
medial tarsal artery

Fig. 7.27   Arterial supply to the flexor and extensor compartments of the right leg.

Fig. 7.28 Arterial supply to the leg.

Artery (origin)	Course	Distribution
Popliteal (continuation of femoral artery at adductor hiatus)	Passes through popliteal fossa to enter the leg; ends at lower border of popliteus muscle dividing into anterior and posterior tibial arteries	Superior, middle, and inferior genicular arteries to both lateral and medial aspects of knee
Anterior tibial (popliteal artery)	Passes into anterior compartment through gap in superior part of interosseous membrane then descends on the surface of the membrane	Extensor compartment of leg
Dorsalis pedis (continuation of anterior tibial artery distal to extensor retinaculum)	Runs over the dorsum of the foot. Gives tarsal, arcuate and first dorsal metatarsal arteries before descending into the first interosseous space to join plantar arch	Muscles on dorsum of foot; pierces first dorsal interosseous muscle to contribute to formation of plantar arch
Posterior tibial (popliteal artery)	Passes through flexor compartment of leg and terminates distal to flexor retinaculum by dividing into medial and lateral plantar arteries	Flexor and lateral compartments of leg. Nutrient artery passes to tibia, contributes to anastomoses around the knee
Peroneal (posterior tibial artery)	Descends in flexor compartment adjacent to posterior intermuscular septum	Flexor compartment of leg. Perforating branches supply lateral compartment of leg

Fig. 7.29 Nerves of the leg.

Nerve (origin)	Course	Distribution
Common peroneal (sciatic nerve)	Arises at apex of popliteal fossa and follows medial border of biceps femoris and its tendon. Passes over posterior aspect of head of fibula and then winds around neck of fibula, deep to peroneus longus, where it divides into deep and superficial peroneal nerves	Supplies skin on posterolateral part of leg via its branch – lateral sural cutaneous nerve
Deep peroneal (common peroneal nerve)	Arises between peroneus longus and neck of fibula. Descends on interosseous membrane and enters dorsum of foot	Supplies extensor muscles of leg, and skin of first interdigital cleft
Saphenous (femoral nerve)	Descends with femoral vessels and the great saphenous vein	Supplies skin on medial side of leg and foot
Superficial peroneal (common peroneal nerve)	Arises between peroneus longus and neck of fibula and descends in lateral compartment of leg	Supplies peroneus longus and brevis and skin on anterior surface of leg and dorsum of foot
Sural (usually arises from both tibial and common peroneal nerves)	Descends between heads of gastrocnemius and becomes superficial at middle of leg	Supplies skin on posterolateral aspects of leg and lateral side of foot
Tibial (sciatic nerve)	Descends through popliteal fossa and lies on popliteus. Then runs inferiorly with posterior tibial vessels and terminates beneath flexor retinaculum by dividing into medial and lateral plantar nerves	Supplies flexor muscles of leg, knee joint, skin, and muscles of the sole of the foot

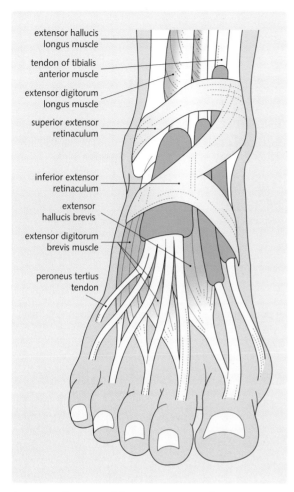

Fig. 7.30 Structure of the extensor retinacula.

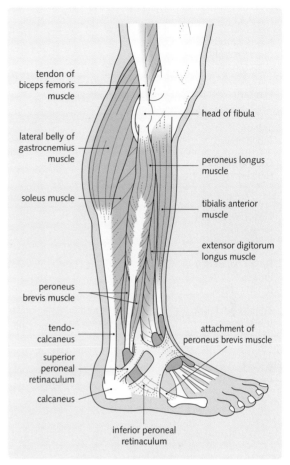

Fig. 7.31 Peroneal compartment of the leg.

Flexor compartment of the leg

Figure 7.33 outlines the muscles of the flexor compartment. Soleus is an antigravity muscle, which contracts alternately with the extensor muscles of the leg whilst standing, to help maintain balance. It is a slow plantar flexor of the ankle joint, unlike gastrocnemius which causes rapid flexion. Contraction of soleus helps to initiate walking by overcoming the inertia of the body's weight. Contraction of gastrocnemius increases the speed of movement (e.g. jumping).

The return of blood to the heart from the lower limb occurs against gravity. Contraction of soleus and gastrocnemius creates pressure within the veins of the lower limb, and aids venous return of blood to the heart. This mechanism is known as the calf muscle pump.

Flexor retinaculum

The flexor retinaculum runs from the medial malleolus to the calcaneus and plantar fascia (Fig. 7.34). The deep flexor tendons pass beneath the retinaculum, surrounded by synovial sheaths, together with the tibial nerve and the posterior tibial artery.

Fig. 7.32 Muscles of the peroneal compartment of the leg.

Name of muscle (nerve supply)	Origin	Insertion	Action
Peroneus longus (superficial peroneal nerve)	Fibula	1st metatarsal and medial cuneiform	Plantarflexes and everts the foot
Peroneus brevis (superficial peroneal nerve)	Fibula	5th metatarsal bone	Plantarflexes and everts the foot

Fig. 7.33 Muscles of the flexor compartment of the leg.

Name of muscle (nerve supply)	Origin	Insertion	Action
		Superficial group	
Plantaris (tibial nerve)	Lateral supracondylar ridge of femur	Via tendocalcaneus (Achilles tendon) into calcaneus	These muscles plantarflex the foot at the ankle joint
Soleus (tibial nerve)	Tibia and fibula		
Gastrocnemius (tibial nerve)	Medial and lateral condyles of femur		
		Deep group	
Flexor digitorum longus (tibial nerve)	Tibia	Distal phalanges of lateral four toes	Flexes lateral four toes Plantarflexes foot
Flexor hallucis longus (tibial nerve)	Fibula	Distal phalanx of great toe	Flexes hallux Plantarflexes foot
Tibialis posterior (tibial nerve)	Tibia and fibula and interosseous membrane	Navicular bone and surrounding bones	Plantarflexes and inverts foot

Fig. 7.34 Medial view of the foot showing the flexor retinaculum.

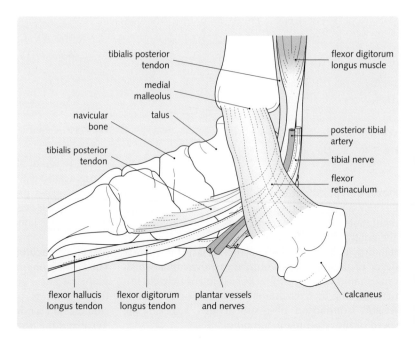

ANKLE AND FOOT

Osteology of the ankle and foot

Ankle joint

The ankle joint is a synovial hinge joint between the medial and lateral malleoli of the tibia and fibula, and the trochlea of the talus. Plantarflexion and dorsiflexion can occur at this joint. Dorsiflexion involves tibialis anterior, extensor digitorum longus and extensor hallucis longus. Plantarflexion involves gastrocnemius, soleus, flexor digitorum longus, flexor hallucis longus and tibialis posterior.

The joint is surrounded by a capsule that is lax anteroposteriorly and reinforced by strong medial and lateral ligaments. The medial (deltoid) ligament runs from the medial malleolus to the tuberosity of the navicular bone, the sustentaculum tali and the medial tubercle of the talus. The lateral ligaments (anterior talofibular ligament, calcaneofibular ligament and posterior talofibular ligament) are commonly damaged in ankle sprains. The articular surface of the talus is wider anteriorly. Therefore, when the ankle is dorsiflexed the joint is at its most stable, with the talus firmly wedged between the malleoli.

The blood supply to the ankle is via branches of the peroneal artery along with the anterior and posterior tibial arteries. Nerve supply arises from the tibial nerve and the deep peroneal nerve.

Foot

The skeleton of the foot consists of the hindfoot, midfoot and forefoot. The hindfoot is composed of the talus and the calcaneus (Fig. 7.35). The midfoot is composed

of five of the seven tarsal bones, the navicular, cuboid and three cuneiform bones, arranged in two rows. There are five tarsometatarsal joints between the midfoot and forefoot. There are also multiple joints within the midfoot itself. The forefoot comprises the five metatarsal bones, along with the phalanges. The metatarsal bones are composed of a base proximally, a body and a head distally. The great toe (the hallux) has two phalanges; the other digits have three (proximal, middle and distal).

Body weight is transferred from the tibia and fibula to the talus and calcaneus, then across the remaining tarsal and metatarsal bones. The weight is transferred to the ground via the calcaneus and the heads of the metatarsals.

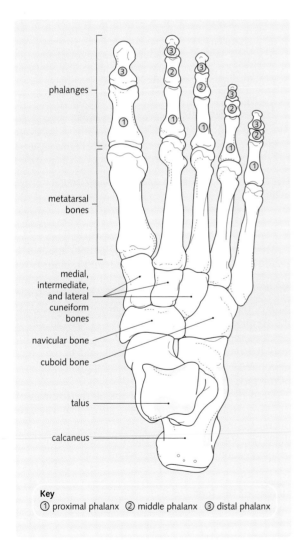

phalanges

metatarsal bones

medial, intermediate, and lateral cuneiform bones

navicular bone

cuboid bone

talus

calcaneus

Key
① proximal phalanx ② middle phalanx ③ distal phalanx

Fig. 7.35 Skeleton of the foot.

> **HINTS AND TIPS**
>
> For the structures passing behind the medial malleolus remember the mnemonic: Tom, Dick And Very Naughty Harry (tibialis posterior, flexor digitorum longus, artery, vein, nerve, flexor hallucis longus).

> **CLINICAL NOTE**
>
> **Orthopaedics**
>
> Ankle sprains occur when the ankle is turned in any direction that results in overstretching of the ligaments. The lateral ligament, consisting of three bands is weaker than the medial ligament, and is more prone to injury. The anterior talofibular ligament, part of the lateral ligament complex, is the most frequently damaged. There are three grades of sprain: (i) stretching of ligament with microscopic damage, but no instability, (ii) partial tear with some instability, and (iii) complete tear, with significant damage and instability. Damage to ligaments can result in an unstable ankle that is prone to invert involuntarily.

Intertarsal joints of the foot

The intertarsal joints of the foot are formed by the articulating tarsal bones. All are synovial joints except the cuboideonavicular joint, which is a fibrous joint. The important intertarsal joints are described below:

- The subtalar (talocalcaneal) joint is a synovial joint and is an articulation between the talus and the calcaneus. It is strengthened by the medial, lateral and posterior talocalcaneal ligaments. Inversion and eversion occur at this joint.
- The midtarsal joint (transverse tarsal joint) is formed by the talocalcaneonavicular (TCN) joint and the calcaneocuboidal joint.

- The talocalcaneonavicular (TCN) joint is a ball-and-socket joint formed between the head of the talus and the calcaneus and navicular bones. It is supported by the spring (plantar calcaneonavicular) ligament. Inversion and eversion occur at this joint, and it is also involved with pronation and supination.
- The calcaneocuboid joint is part of the transverse tarsal joint and resembles a saddle joint between the calcaneus and the cuboid bones. It is supported by the short plantar (plantar calcaneocuboid), long plantar and bifurcate ligaments, and by the tendon of the peroneus longus muscle.

Other tarsal joints

The cuneonavicular, cuboideonavicular, intercuneiform and cuneocuboidal joints are strengthened by dorsal, plantar and interosseous ligaments. There is very little movement between these joints.

Arches of the foot

The foot has three arches which support the weight of the body and act as shock absorbers during standing, and when walking over uneven ground. They are the medial longitudinal arch, the lateral longitudinal arch and the transverse arch (each foot contributing half of the transverse arch). They are maintained by the shape of the bones, muscles and ligaments.

The medial longitudinal arch is higher than the lateral arch, and consists of the calcaneus, talus, navicular, three cuneiform bones and the medial three metatarsals. The talus acts as a keystone in the centre of the arch. The arch is supported by the plantar aponeurosis, the plantar calcaneonavicular (spring), deltoid ligament, long and short plantar ligaments, and strong dorsal ligaments. The plantar aponeurosis, flexor hallucis longus and flexor digitorum longus muscles, the tibialis muscles, and the tendon of peroneus longus also support the arch.

The lateral arch consists of the calcaneus, the cuboid and the lateral two metatarsals. This is maintained by the long and short (calcaneocuboidal) plantar ligaments, the plantar aponeurosis, flexor digitorum longus, and the peroneus longus and brevis tendons.

Each foot contains half of the transverse arch. Each half consists of the metatarsal bases, cuboid, and the three cuneiforms. It is maintained by the wedge-shaped cuneiform bones and metatarsal bases, the long and short plantar ligaments, the deep transverse ligaments and the peroneus longus tendon.

Sole of the foot

The sole bears the weight of the body. The skin is thick and hairless. Fibrous septa divide the subcutaneous fat into small loculi, and they anchor the skin to the deep fascia or plantar aponeurosis (Fig. 7.36). This makes subcutaneous injections difficult.

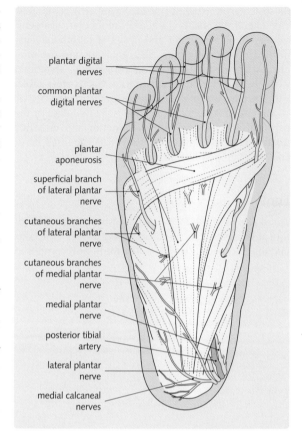

Fig. 7.36 Plantar fascia and cutaneous innervation of the sole of the foot.

The plantar aponeurosis (like the palmar aponeurosis of the hand) lies deep to the skin and extends from the calcaneal tuberosity and divides into five bifurcating slips which insert into the flexor fibrous sheaths at the base of the toes. The bifurcations allow the passage of the flexor tendons. The aponeurosis is very strong; it supports the longitudinal arch like a tie beam and protects the underlying muscles, vessels and nerves. It is perforated by the cutaneous nerves supplying the sole of the foot.

Deep to the plantar aponeurosis lie the muscles of the foot, arranged in four layers (Fig. 7.37). The axis of abduction and adduction passes through the second digit. Therefore, digits either move towards (adduction) or away (abduction) from the second digit.

Nerves of the foot

The nerves of the foot are described in Figures 7.38 and 7.39.

Fig. 7.37   Intrinsic plantar muscles of the foot.

Muscle (nerve supply)	Origin	Insertion	Action
	First layer		
Abductor hallucis (medial plantar nerve)	Calcaneus, flexor retinaculum, plantar aponeurosis	Proximal phalanx of hallux	abducts great toe
Flexor digitorum brevis (medial plantar nerve)	Calcaneus, plantar aponeurosis	Each tendon bifurcates and inserts into the middle phalanx of the lateral four digits	Flexes lateral four digits
Abductor digiti minimi (lateral plantar nerve)	Calcaneus, plantar aponeurosis	Proximal phalanx of digitus minimus	Abducts digitus minimus (little toe)
	Second layer		
Flexor accessorius or **Quadratus plantae** (lateral plantar nerve)	Calcaneus	Tendon of flexor digitorum longus	Pulls on the tendon of flexor digitorum longus and takes up the slack of this tendon when the ankle is plantarflexed. This allows the digits to be flexed in this position
Lumbricals (first medial lumbrical – medial plantar nerve; lateral three lumbricals – lateral plantar nerve)	Tendons of flexor digitorum longus	Extensor expansions of lateral four digits	Maintains extension of the digits at DIP and PIP joints while flexor digitorum longus tendons are flexing the lateral four digits at the MTP
	Third layer		
Flexor hallucis brevis (medial plantar nerve)	Cuboid and three cuneiforms	Proximal phalanx of hallux	Flexes hallux (great toe)
Adductor hallucis (lateral plantar nerve) Oblique head Transverse head	2nd to 4th metatarsal bases and plantar ligament Deep transverse ligament	Both heads insert into the proximal phalanx of the hallux	Adducts hallux towards second toe
Flexor digiti minimi brevis (lateral plantar nerve)	5th metatarsal	Proximal phalanx of digitus minimus	Flexes digitus minimus (little toe)
	Fourth layer		
Plantar interossei (lateral plantar nerve)	3rd, 4th, 5th metatarsals	Proximal phalanx of digits and their extensor expansions	Adduct digits towards second digit
Dorsal interossei (lateral plantar nerve)	1st and 2nd; 2nd and 3rd; 3rd and 4th; 4th and 5th metatarsals	Proximal phalanx of digits and their extensor expansions	Abduct digits away from second digit. With plantar interossei and lumbricals they extend the DIP, PIP joints and flex the MTP joint

IP, interphalangeal joint; PIP, proximal interphalangeal joint; DIP, distal interphalangeal joint; MTP, metatarsophalangeal joint.

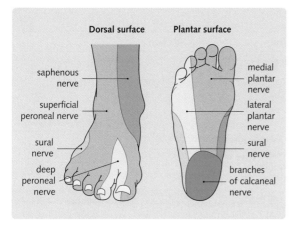

Dorsal surface   Plantar surface

saphenous nerve
superficial peroneal nerve
sural nerve
deep peroneal nerve

medial plantar nerve
lateral plantar nerve
sural nerve
branches of calcaneal nerve

Fig. 7.38 Distribution of nerves of the foot.

Fig. 7.39 Nerves of the foot.

Nerve (origin)	Distribution
Saphenous (femoral nerve)	Supplies skin on medial side of foot as far anteriorly as head of 1st metatarsal
Superficial peroneal (common peroneal nerve)	Supplies skin on dorsum of foot and all digits, except adjoining sides of first and second digits
Deep peroneal (common peroneal nerve)	Supplies extensor digitorum brevis, extensor hallucis brevis and skin on contiguous sides of first and second digits
Medial plantar (larger terminal branch of the tibial nerve)	Supplies skin of medial side of sole of foot and plantar surfaces of first three-and-one-half digits Also supplies abductor hallucis, flexor digitorum brevis, flexor hallucis brevis and first lumbrical
Lateral plantar (smaller terminal branch of tibial nerve)	Supplies quadratus plantae, abductor digiti minimi and flexor digiti minimi brevis Deep branch supplies plantar and dorsal interossei, lateral three lumbricals, and adductor hallucis Supplies skin on sole lateral to a line splitting fourth digit
Sural (tibial and common peroneal nerves)	Lateral aspect of foot
Calcaneal nerves (tibial and sural nerves)	Skin of heel

Blood supply to the foot

The posterior tibial artery terminates by dividing into the medial and lateral plantar arteries under the flexor retinaculum (Fig. 7.40).

The medial plantar artery passes forward with the medial plantar nerve, along the medial aspect of the sole of the foot. It gives off muscular branches and terminates as digital branches (which join with the plantar metatarsal branches of the plantar arch) supplying the toes.

The lateral plantar artery passes obliquely across the sole of the foot, giving off muscular and cutaneous branches. At the level of the base of the 5th metatarsal the artery passes medially and anastomoses with the dorsalis pedis artery to form the plantar arch, which gives rise to metatarsal arteries. These in turn give rise to the plantar digital arteries which contribute to the supply of the toes (see above).

Fibrous flexor and flexor synovial sheaths

Fibrous flexor sheaths in the foot are similar to those of the hand. They run from the head of the metatarsal bone to the base of the distal phalanx and surround the synovial sheaths. The sheath has anular fibres over the bones and cruciate fibres over the joints (to allow movement).

> **HINTS AND TIPS**
>
> Note that the lateral plantar nerve in the foot has a similar distribution to the ulnar nerve in the hand (both have a superficial and a deep branch) and that the medial plantar nerve in the foot has a similar distribution to the median nerve in the hand.

The synovial sheaths covering the flexor digitorum longus tendons surround them from just above the flexor retinaculum to the navicular bone. The tendon of flexor hallucis longus is covered by a synovial sheath from above the retinaculum to the base of the 1st metatarsal. As the tendons described above enter their fibrous flexor sheath, they are again covered by a synovial sheath. The synovial sheath for tibialis posterior extends from the flexor retinaculum to the insertion of the tendon onto the navicular bone.

Functions of the feet

The feet serve to:

- Support the body weight
- Maintain balance and allow movement on uneven surfaces
- Act as propulsive levers, e.g. in walking and running.

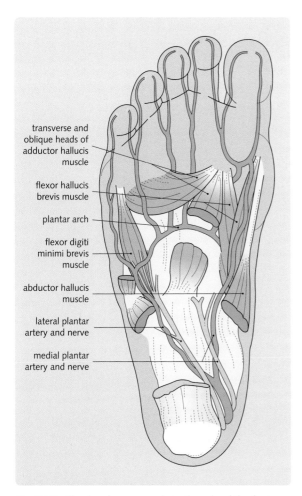

transverse and oblique heads of adductor hallucis muscle

flexor hallucis brevis muscle

plantar arch

flexor digiti minimi brevis muscle

abductor hallucis muscle

lateral plantar artery and nerve

medial plantar artery and nerve

Fig. 7.40 Blood and nerve supply to the sole of the foot.

RADIOLOGICAL ANATOMY

Imaging of the bones and joints

When there are symptoms and/or signs of joint problems or a fracture, an X-ray is the first imaging investigation to be performed. Two images are taken at 90° to each other and, in some cases, include the joint above and below the injury, especially if the lower leg (or the forearm) is involved.

Normal radiographic anatomy

Figures 7.41, 7.42 and 7.43 show the normal articulations of the hip, knee and foot. The osteology of the lower limb is demonstrated.

CLINICAL NOTE

Osteoarthritis

X-rays of the joints of the limbs, particularly of the knee and hip, are commonly requested in order to confirm a suspected diagnosis of osteoarthritis. The typical changes of osteoarthritis found on an X-ray are: loss of joint space, subchondral sclerosis (bone appears whiter under joint hyaline cartilage), osteophytes (smooth spur-like bony growths) and subchondral cysts (seen as darkened areas within the bone adjacent to a joint).

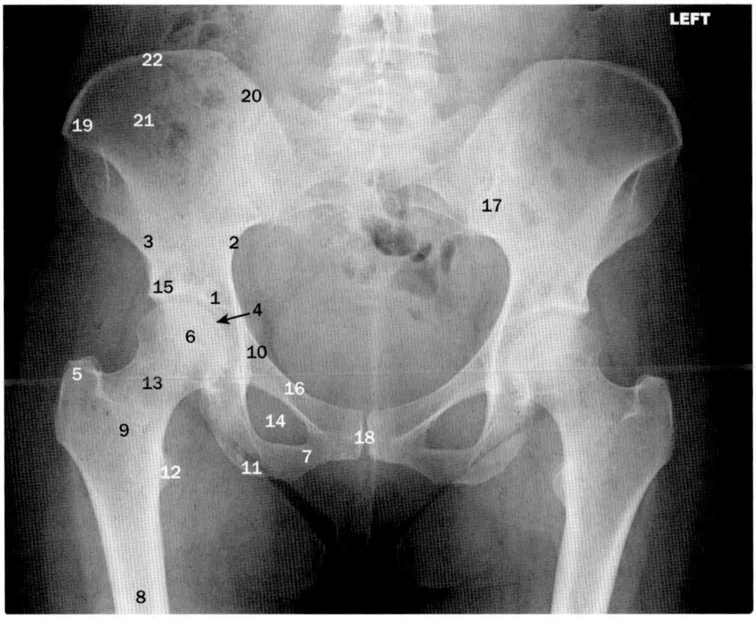

LEFT

1. Acetabulum
2. Arcuate line
3. Ilium
4. Fovea
5. Greater trochanter of femur
6. Head of femur
7. Inferior ramus of pubis
8. Shaft of the femur
9. Intertrochanteric line
10. Ischial spine
11. Ischial tuberosity
12. Lesser trochanter
13. Neck of femur
14. Obturator foramen
15. Rim of the acetabulum
16. Superior ramus of pubis
17. Sacro-iliac joint
18. Pubic symphysis
19. Anterior superior iliac spine
20. Posterior superior iliac spine
21. Ala of ilium
22. Iliac crest

Fig. 7.41 An anteroposterior X-ray of the right hip and pelvis.

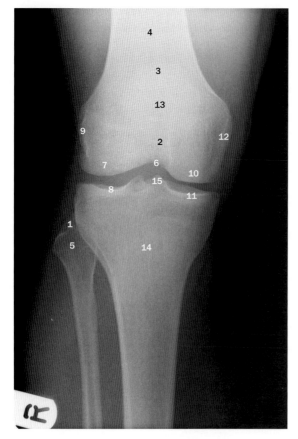

Fig. 7.42 An anteroposterior X-ray of the knee.

1. Apex (styloid process) of fibula
2. Apex of the patella
3. Base of the patella
4. Femur
5. Head of fibula
6. Intercondylar fossa
7. Lateral condyle of femur
8. Lateral condyle of tibia
9. Lateral epicondyle of femur
10. Medial condyle of femur
11. Medial condyle tibia
12. Medial epicondyle of femur
13. Patella
14. Tibia
15. Tubercles of intercondylar eminence

How to examine an X-ray methodically

See Chapter 3 for a description of how to examine an X-ray of the bones, as the explanation provided can be applied to the lower limb as well as the upper limb.

> **HINTS AND TIPS**
>
> On a normal hip X-ray a smooth curved line can be traced with your finger, starting at the shaft of the femur medially, trace proximally across the femoral neck (medially) to the superior pubic ramus (anterior border). This is known as Shenton's line and any disruption to its smooth convex course suggests a femoral neck fracture.

Angiography of the lower limb

In Figures 7.44, 7.45 and 7.46 arteriography highlights the arterial supply to the hip, thigh, knee, leg and foot.

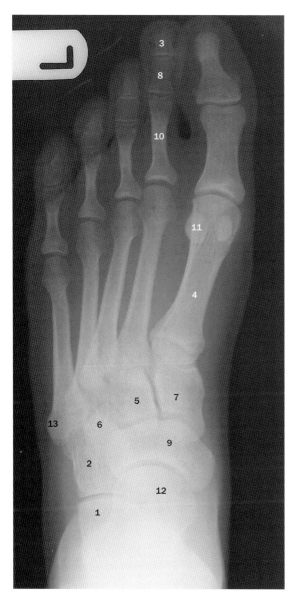

1. Calcaneus
2. Cuboid
3. Distal phalanx of second toe
4. First metatarsal
5. Intermediate cuneiform
6. Lateral cuneiform
7. Medial cuneiform
8. Middle phalanx of second toe
9. Navicular
10. Proximal phalanx of second toe
11. Sesamoid bones in flexor hallucis brevis muscle
12. Talus
13. Tuberosity of base of 5th metatarsal

Fig. 7.43   An X-ray of the foot.

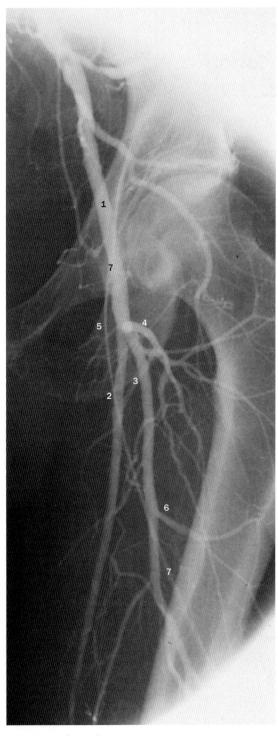

1. Profunda femoris artery
2. Common femoral artery
3. Superficial femoral artery
4. Lateral circumflex artery
5. Medial circumflex artery
6. Perforating artery
7. Catheter introduced into distal
   abdominal aorta via femoral artery

Fig. 7.44   A femoral arteriogram.

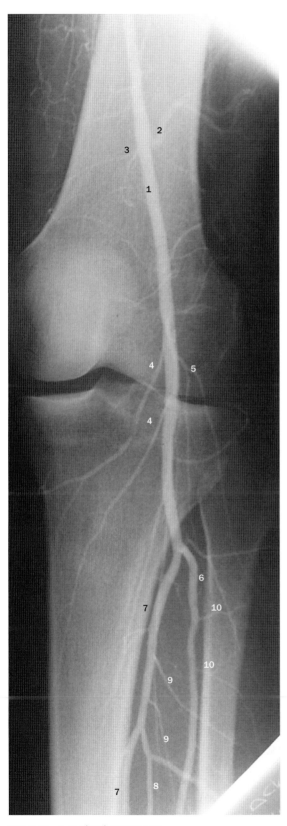

1. Popliteal artery
2. Superior lateral genicular artery
3. Superior medial genicular artery
4. Inferior medial genicular artery
5. Inferior lateral genicular artery
6. Anterior tibial artery
7. Posterior tibial artery
8. Peroneal artery
9. Muscular branches of posterior tibial artery
10. Muscular branches of anterior tibial artery

Fig. 7.45 A popliteal arteriogram.

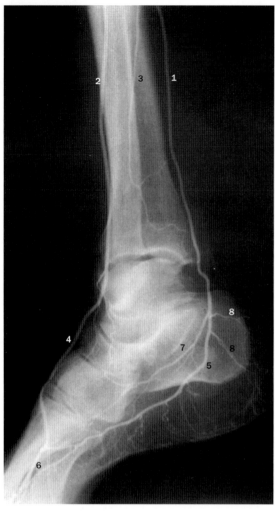

1. Posterior tibial artery
2. Anterior tibial artery
3. Peroneal artery
4. Dorsalis pedis artery
5. Lateral plantar artery
6. Plantar arch
7. Medial plantar artery
8. Medial calcaneal artery

Fig. 7.46 A foot arteriogram.

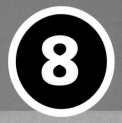
Objectives

In this chapter you will learn to:
* List the individual bones of which the skull is composed and name their foraminae.
* Describe the blood supply, venous drainage and innervation of the face and scalp.
* Describe the arrangement of the dura mater and its reflections, including the dural venous sinuses.
* Describe the blood supply to the brain and explain the function of the circulus arteriosus (circle of Willis).
* List the cranial nerves and their functions.
* Discuss the contents of the orbit, including the intraocular muscles, their actions and their innervation.
* Describe the anatomy of the parotid gland and the structures passing through it.
* List the branches of the trigeminal and facial nerves, as well as their motor and sensory branches.
* Describe the fascial columns of the neck and their contents.
* Understand the muscular structures of the pharynx, tongue and palate, their innervation and blood supply.
* Describe the structure of the larynx, including its cartilages, membranes, muscles and innervation.
* Review an x-ray of the skull, recognizing the major features.

REGIONS AND COMPONENTS OF THE HEAD AND NECK

Skull

The skull is composed of a number of bones, joined at sutures (Figs 8.1–8.5). The skull consists of:

* The cranium (composed of outer and inner tables of bone, separated by diploë – Fig. 8.7)
* The facial skeleton.

The cranium is subdivided into an upper part – the vault, and a lower part – the base of the skull.

Foramina of the skull

There are numerous foramina in the skull which transmit nerves, arteries and veins (Figs 8.5, 8.6 and 8.13). Some foramina are clinically important.

Fetal skull

The fetal skull differs from the adult skull in the following ways:

* The facial skeleton is proportionately smaller
* Alveolar and mastoid processes are undeveloped
* There is a midline suture between the frontal bones: the metopic suture, which usually disappears by 6 years of age

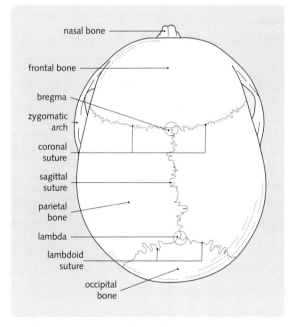

Fig. 8.1 Superior view of the skull.

* There are two fibrous defects between the skull bones known as fontanelles. The two frontal and parietal bones meet at the anterior fontanelle, which closes by 18–24 months of age, to form the bregma. The two parietal bones and the occipital bone meet at

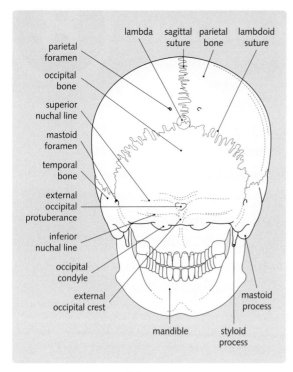

Fig. 8.2 Posterior view of the skull.

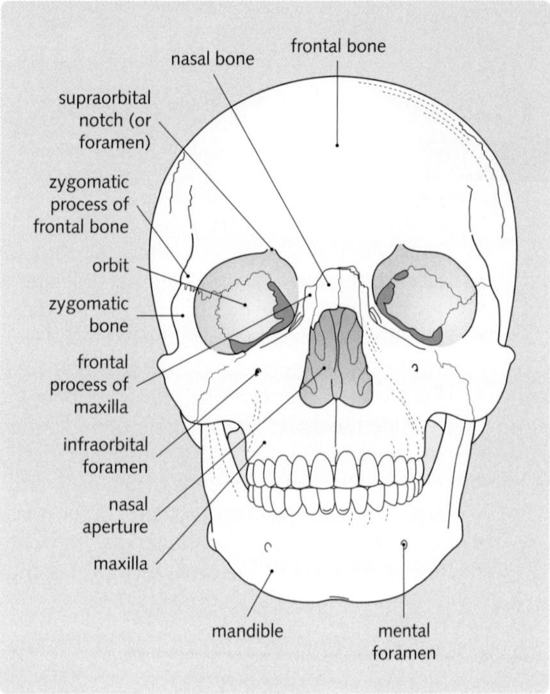

Fig. 8.3 Anterior view of the skull.

Fig. 8.4 Lateral view of the skull.

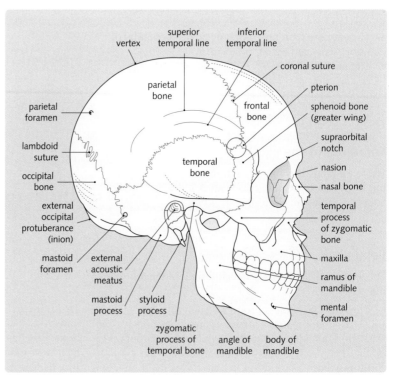

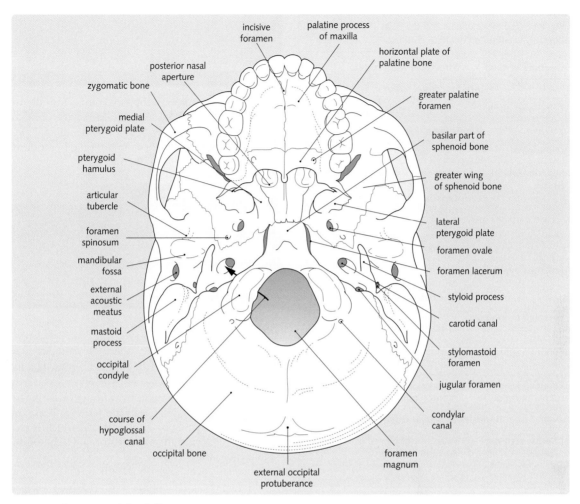

Fig. 8.5 Inferior view of the skull.

the posterior fontanelle, which closes by approximately 5 months of age to form the lambda.

Joints of the head and neck

There are seven cervical vertebrae forming the skeleton of the neck. The atlanto-occipital joint lies between the C1 vertebra and the occipital condyles. The atlanto-axial joint lies between the axis and atlas (Fig. 2.3B).

THE FACE AND SCALP

Scalp

The scalp consists of five layers (Fig. 8.7). It has a rich blood supply (Fig. 8.8). The veins of the scalp closely mirror the arterial supply and connect with the diploic veins in the skull bones and the intracranial venous sinuses via valveless emissary veins. Infections of the scalp are therefore potentially very serious, as they may spread intracranially.

> **HINTS AND TIPS**
>
> The layers of the scalp from superficial to deep are:
> **S** Skin
> **C** Connective tissue
> **A** Aponeurosis
> **L** Loose connective tissue
> **P** Pericranium (periostium).

Sensory nerve supply to the scalp is shown in Figure 8.8. The muscles of the scalp and external ear are supplied by the facial nerve.

Fig. 8.6 The major openings in the base of the skull and the structures transmitted through them

Opening in skull	Structures transmitted
Anterior cranial fossa	
Cribriform plate	Olfactory nerves
Middle cranial fossa	
Optic canal	Optic nerve, ophthalmic artery
Superior orbital fissure	Lacrimal, frontal and nasociliary branches of V_1 (ophthalmic branch of trigeminal nerve); oculomotor, abducent, and trochlear nerves; superior ophthalmic vein
Foramen ovale	V_3 (mandibular division of trigeminal nerve), lesser petrosal nerve
Foramen rotundum	V_2 (maxillary division of trigeminal nerve)
Foramen spinosum	Middle meningeal artery and vein
Foramen lacerum (upper part only)	Internal carotid artery, greater petrosal nerve
Posterior cranial fossa	
Internal acoustic meatus	Facial, vestibulocochlear nerves; labyrinthine artery
Jugular foramen	Glossopharyngeal, vagus, accessory nerves; sigmoid sinus becomes internal jugular vein
Hypoglossal canal	Hypoglossal nerve
Foramen magnum	Medulla oblongata, spinal part of accessory nerve, upper cervical nerves; right and left vertebral arteries

Face

The skin of the face is connected to the facial bones by loose connective tissue, in which the muscles of facial expression lie. There is no deep fascia. Like the scalp, the skin of the face is very vascular and highly sensitive.

CLINICAL NOTE

Scalp laceration

The scalp has a rich blood supply, and bleeds profusely because blood vessels are anchored to connective tissue, which holds them open. A wound which passes transversely through the aponeurotic layer will gape, but one which runs longitudinally or is superficial will not.

Sensory innervation of the face comes from the trigeminal nerve (V). It has three divisions: the ophthalmic (V_1), the maxillary (V_2), and the mandibular (V_3) nerves which supply the upper, middle and lower thirds of the face respectively (Fig. 8.9).

CLINICAL NOTE

Subaponeurotic haematoma

Bleeding deep to the aponeurosis of occipitofrontalis, e.g. from a blow to the back of the head or a scalp laceration, can track forward into the eyelids and the root of the nose, resulting in black eyes.

Muscles of the face

Most of the muscles of facial expression are attached to the overlying skin (Fig. 8.10). They are supplied by the facial nerve (VII). The major muscles are:

- Occipitofrontalis: formed by a frontal belly anteriorly, and an occipital belly posteriorly. These are joined by a flat, aponeurotic tendon which is part of the scalp (epicranial aponeurosis). Occipitofrontalis raises the eyebrows.
- Orbicularis oculi: consists of orbital (closes the eye) and palpebral (blinking of the eyelids) parts – connected to bone via the medial palpebral ligament at the medial angle of the eye
- Buccinator: lies in the cheek. It forces food out of the vestibule of the mouth and into the oral cavity
- Orbicularis oris: lies around the mouth and closes/purses the lips.

Motor nerve supply to the face

The facial nerve (VII), exits the skull through the stylomastoid foramen, to lie between the ramus of the mandible and the mastoid process. It enters the parotid gland and divides into its five terminal branches supplying the muscles of facial expression (Fig. 8.9).

Before entering the parotid gland the facial nerve gives off the posterior auricular nerve and a muscular branch, which supplies the occipital belly of occipitofrontalis, stylohyoid and the posterior belly of digastric.

Vessels of the face

The face has a very rich blood supply, largely from the facial and superficial temporal arteries. Both are branches of the external carotid artery (Fig. 8.11). The facial artery

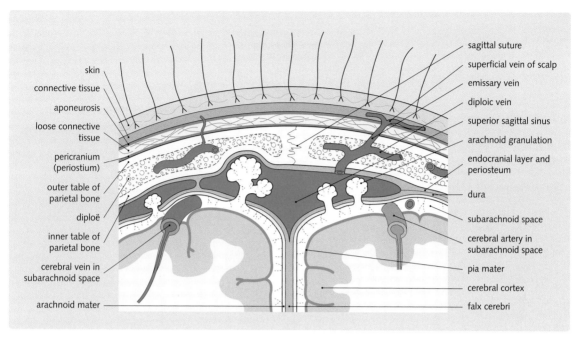

Fig. 8.7 Layers of the scalp.

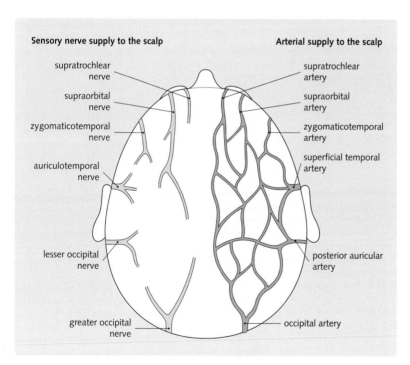

Fig. 8.8 Nerve and arterial supply to the scalp.

arises from the anterior side of the external carotid artery. It ascends medial to the mandible, then winds around its inferior border, and enters the face. It gives off inferior labial, superior labial and lateral nasal branches and terminates as the angular artery at the medial canthus of the eye.

The superficial temporal artery commences in the parotid gland, and ascends superficial to the zygomatic process of the temporal bone. It then divides into frontal and parietal branches. Its pulse is palpable anterior to the tragus. The superficial temporal artery anastomoses with

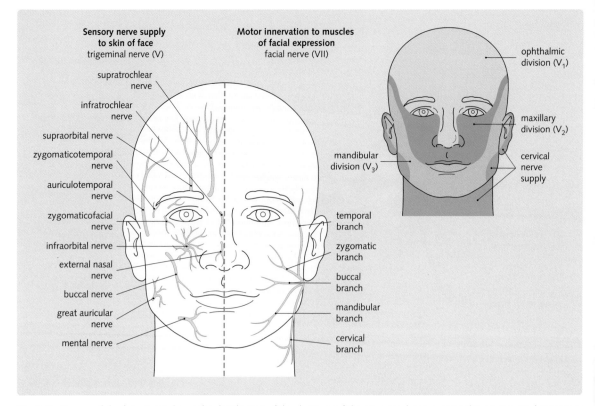

Sensory nerve supply to skin of face
trigeminal nerve (V)

Motor innervation to muscles of facial expression
facial nerve (VII)

supratrochlear nerve

infratrochlear nerve

supraorbital nerve

zygomaticotemporal nerve

auriculotemporal nerve

zygomaticofacial nerve

infraorbital nerve

external nasal nerve

buccal nerve

great auricular nerve

mental nerve

ophthalmic division (V₁)

maxillary division (V₂)

mandibular division (V₃)

cervical nerve supply

temporal branch

zygomatic branch

buccal branch

mandibular branch

cervical branch

Fig. 8.9 Nerves of the face. Inset shows the distribution of the divisions of the trigeminal nerve. Note the great auricular nerve is not part of the trigeminal nerve.

Fig. 8.10 Major muscles of the face.

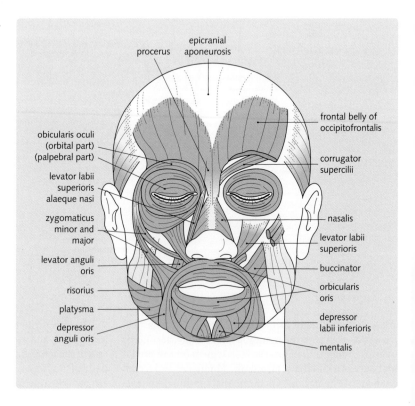

procerus

epicranial aponeurosis

frontal belly of occipitofrontalis

obicularis oculi (orbital part) (palpebral part)

levator labii superioris alaeque nasi

zygomaticus minor and major

levator anguli oris

risorius

platysma

depressor anguli oris

corrugator supercilii

nasalis

levator labii superioris

buccinator

orbicularis oris

depressor labii inferioris

mentalis

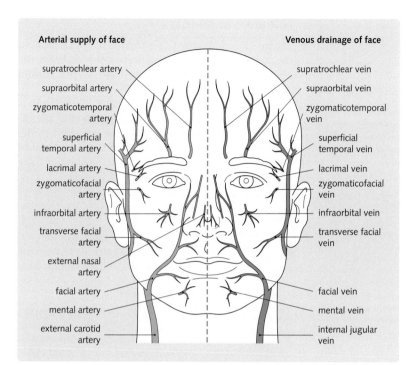

Fig. 8.11 Arterial supply and venous drainage of the face.

Arterial supply of face

- supratrochlear artery
- supraorbital artery
- zygomaticotemporal artery
- superficial temporal artery
- lacrimal artery
- zygomaticofacial artery
- infraorbital artery
- transverse facial artery
- external nasal artery
- facial artery
- mental artery
- external carotid artery

Venous drainage of face

- supratrochlear vein
- supraorbital vein
- zygomaticotemporal vein
- superficial temporal vein
- lacrimal vein
- zygomaticofacial vein
- infraorbital vein
- transverse facial vein
- facial vein
- mental vein
- internal jugular vein

(among others) the supraorbital artery of the internal carotid artery.

The supraorbital and supratrochlear arteries are terminal branches of the ophthalmic artery – a branch of the internal carotid artery.

> **HINTS AND TIPS**
>
> The terminal branches of the facial nerve can be remembered by the following mnemonic: **T**en **Z**ebras **B**ought **M**y **C**ar (**t**emporal, **z**ygomatic, **b**uccal, **m**andibular, **c**ervical).

Veins draining the face follow a similar course to the arteries (Fig. 8.11):

- The supraorbital and supratrochlear veins unite to form the facial vein, which descends in the face, receiving tributaries corresponding to the branches of the facial artery.
- The superficial temporal and maxillary veins form the retromandibular vein in the parotid gland.
- The posterior auricular and posterior division of the retromandibular veins form the external jugular vein.
- Occipital veins drain into the suboccipital venous complex.
- The facial vein and the anterior division of the retromandibular vein drain into the internal jugular vein.

Lymphatic drainage of the face

Lymph nodes of the face drain to the deep cervical nodes (Fig. 8.12).

THE CRANIAL CAVITY AND MENINGES

The cranium protects the brain and its surrounding meninges. The cranium is covered by periosteum: pericranium on the outer surface and endocranium on the inner surface, which are continuous with each other at the sutures of the skull.

The cranial bones consist of outer and inner tables of compact bone, separated by cancellous bone (the diploë) containing red marrow throughout life (see Fig. 8.7).

The internal surface of the base of the skull is divided into anterior, middle and posterior cranial fossae (Fig. 8.13). The foramina of the cranial fossae and the structures passing through each are outlined in Figure 8.6.

Cranial fossae

Anterior cranial fossa

The anterior cranial fossa contains the frontal lobes of the brain and the olfactory bulbs. The ethmoid bone of the fossa contains the cribriform plate (perforated by the olfactory nerves).

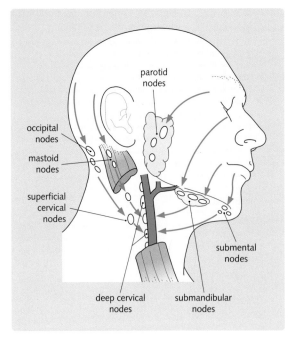

Fig. 8.12 Lymphatic drainage of the face.

Middle cranial fossa

The middle cranial fossa contains the temporal lobes of the cerebral hemispheres, the floor of the forebrain, the optic chiasma, the termination of the internal carotid arteries and the pituitary gland. A shallow depression (trigeminal impression) near the apex of the petrous temporal bone houses the sensory ganglion of the trigeminal nerve. The optic chiasma lies superior to the optic groove. The optic canals lie at the lateral end of the groove. The pituitary gland lies in the pituitary fossa or sella turcica, inferior to the optic chiasma.

Posterior cranial fossa

The posterior cranial fossa is roofed by the tentorium cerebelli, a shelf-like fold in the dura mater. It contains the pons, the medulla, the cerebellum and the midbrain.

CLINICAL NOTE

Pituitary tumour

A tumour of the pituitary gland may compress the optic chiasma. As this carries fibres from the temporal visual fields, the patient will complain of 'tunnel vision' (bitemporal hemianopia).

Fig. 8.13 Internal surface of the base of the skull, showing the cranial fossae.

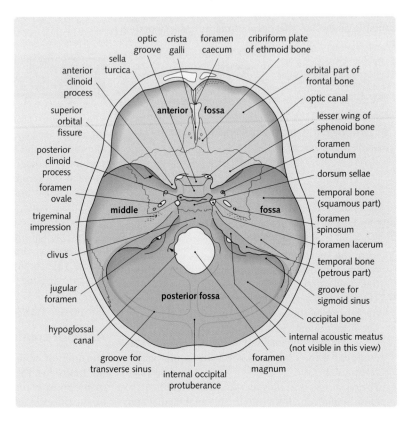

Meninges

There are three meningeal layers surrounding the brain and spinal cord (Fig. 8.7).

Dura mater

The dura mater is composed of two layers. The outer layer is known as the endosteal layer (and serves as the periosteum covering the inside of the skull). The inner layer is the meningeal layer – a dense fibrous layer covering the brain. The two layers of dura are firmly adherent to each other throughout most of the skull, separating at intervals to form dural venous sinuses (described below). These sinuses drain cerebrospinal fluid and blood from the brain, which drains into the internal jugular veins.

The dura is continuous with the dura mater of the spinal cord through the foramen magnum. Sleeves of dura surround the cranial nerves, which fuse with the epineurium of the nerves outside the skull. The dura gives rise to the following septae which support the brain and restrict its movement:

- Falx cerebri: a sickle-shaped fold of dura which lies between the two cerebral hemispheres. It attaches anteriorly to the crista galli, and blends posteriorly with the tentorium cerebelli. The superior sagittal sinus runs in its superior margin (attached to the endocranium on the vault of the skull). The inferior sagittal sinus runs in its free inferior margin. The straight sinus runs along its attachment to the tentorium cerebelli (Figs 8.14A & 8.14B).
- Tentorium cerebelli: a crescent-shaped fold of dura mater which roofs the posterior cranial fossa. It covers the cerebellum and supports the occipital lobes of the cerebral hemispheres. The tentorium is attached to either side of the posterior clinoid process, passes back along the petrous temporal bone and curves around the inner aspect of the occipital bone. Posteriorly the falx cerebri and falx cerebelli are attached to its upper and lower surfaces. Its free margin is anchored to the anterior clinoids, forming the tentorial notch through which the midbrain passes. The superior petrosal and transverse venous sinuses run along its attachment to the petrous and occipital bones, respectively (Figs 8.14A and 8.14B).
- Falx cerebelli: projects anteriorly between the two cerebellar hemispheres, and is attached to the internal occipital crest. Its posterior margin contains the occipital sinus (Figs 8.14A & 8.14B).
- Diaphragma sellae: a small circular fold of dura forming the roof of the pituitary fossa (Fig. 8.14B).

Arachnoid mater

The arachnoid mater lies deep to the dura. It is separated from the pia mater by the subarachnoid space, containing cerebrospinal fluid. Where the arachnoid passes over the contours of the brain, the subarachnoid and pia mater are not closely apposed; the spaces formed in this way contain CSF. Some spaces are large and are known as subarachnoid cisterns.

Pia mater

The pia mater closely invests the brain surface. It continues as a sheath around the small vessels entering the brain substance.

Blood and nerve supply of the meninges

The meninges are supplied by the middle meningeal artery and branches of the internal carotid, maxillary, ascending pharyngeal, occipital and vertebral arteries. Dura mater in the anterior and middle cranial fossae is innervated by the trigeminal nerve. The dura of the posterior fossa is supplied by the upper three cervical nerves, with meningeal branches of the vagal and hypoglossal nerves.

Dural venous sinuses

The dural venous sinuses lie between the two layers of the dura, are lined by endothelium and have no valves. Veins draining the brain, the diploë, the scalp, the orbit and the inner ear drain into the sinuses as described below and illustrated in Figure 8.14A:

- Superior sagittal sinus: this runs in the upper border of the falx cerebri. It commences at the foramen caecum and passes posteriorly, grooving the vault of the skull. At the internal occipital protuberance, it forms the confluence of the sinuses, and continues as a transverse sinus (usually the right). It receives numerous cerebral veins. CSF drains into the sinus via arachnoid granulations (Fig. 8.7).
- Inferior sagittal sinus: this lies in the free margin of the falx cerebri. It joins with the great cerebral vein to form the straight sinus. It drains cerebral veins from the medial side of the cerebral hemispheres.
- Straight sinus: this lies between the falx cerebri and tentorium cerebelli and is formed by the junction of the inferior sagittal sinus and the great cerebral vein. It terminates by turning to form (usually the left) transverse sinus.
- Transverse sinuses: these commence at the internal occipital protuberance and run in the attachment of the tentorium cerebelli. They end by turning inferiorly to form the sigmoid sinuses. They receive the superior petrosal sinuses and the inferior cerebral, cerebellar and diploic veins.
- Sigmoid sinuses: these turn inferiorly and medially to groove the mastoid process. It then turns downward through the posterior part of the jugular

Fig. 8.14 A, The positions of the cranial venous sinuses. B, The falx cerebri, falx cerebelli, diaphragma sellae and tentorium cerebelli.

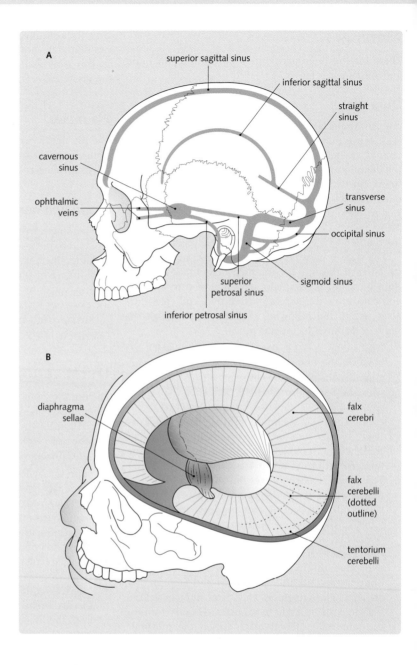

foramen to become continuous with the internal jugular vein.

- Occipital sinus: this lies in the attached margin of the falx cerebelli. It drains into the bases of the sigmoid sinuses.
- Cavernous sinuses: the cavernous sinuses lie on either side of the body of the sphenoid, and they extend from the superior orbital fissure anteriorly to the apex of the petrous temporal bone posteriorly. They receive:

- The superior and inferior ophthalmic veins
- The cerebral veins
- The sphenoparietal sinus
- The central vein of the retina.

The cavernous sinuses drain posteriorly into the superior and inferior petrosal sinuses and inferiorly into the pterygoid venous plexus. The two sinuses communicate via anterior and posterior intercavernous sinuses.

The internal carotid artery, its sympathetic nerve plexus and the abducens nerve run through the sinus

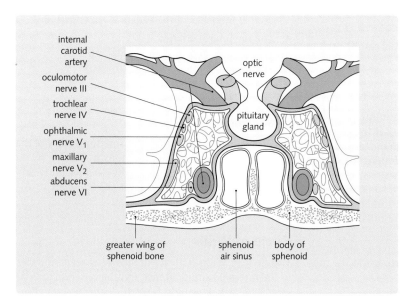

Fig. 8.15 A coronal section of the cavernous sinus showing its relations.

internal carotid artery

oculomotor nerve III

trochlear nerve IV

ophthalmic nerve V$_1$

maxillary nerve V$_2$

abducens nerve VI

optic nerve

pituitary gland

greater wing of sphenoid bone

sphenoid air sinus

body of sphenoid

(Fig. 8.15). The oculomotor and trochlear nerves and the ophthalmic and maxillary divisions of the trigeminal nerves lie in the lateral wall of the sinus, between the endothelium and the dura:

- Superior and inferior petrosal sinuses: the superior and inferior petrosal sinuses emerge from the cavernous sinus, and lie at the superior and inferior borders of the petrous temporal bone respectively. The superior sinus drains into the transverse sinus and the inferior into the internal jugular vein.

CLINICAL NOTE

Intracranial haemorrhages

- Extradural (epidural) – due to bleeding from the branches of the middle meningeal artery (e.g. due to a fracture of the pterion) into the space between the periosteum and dura. A history of head trauma with brief unconsciousness is common. This is followed by a lucid interval of several hours. Headache, nausea/vomiting and focal neurological signs, e.g. weakness, then develop (due to raised intracranial pressure).

- Subdural – sudden movement or trauma may shear the veins leading from the brain to the dural venous sinuses. This results in bleeding between the dura and arachnoid mater. They generally develop more slowly than extradural haemmorhages since the site of bleeding is venous (extradural haemorrhages are arterial).

- Subarachnoid – an artery in the subarachnoid space (e.g. part of the circle of Willis) ruptures, bleeding into the CSF. This results in severe headache, loss of consciousness and in some cases, death.

CLINICAL NOTE

Spread of infection from the face

The facial vein connects with the cavernous sinus in the skull via the superior ophthalmic vein. This provides a path for spread of infection from the face, e.g. a boil or spot, to the cavernous sinus. This gives rise to the 'danger area of the face' – a triangular region with its base at the top lip and its apex at the bridge of the nose from which infection may spread. Infection may lead to cavernous sinus thrombosis, resulting in meningitis, sepsis and cranial nerve palsy. Venous drainage from the orbit may also become obstructed, causing oedema and papilloedema and loss of vision.

Arteries of the cranial cavity

The brain is supplied by the two internal carotid arteries and the two vertebral arteries.

Internal carotid artery

The internal carotid artery (ICA) is a terminal branch of the common carotid artery (Fig. 8.16). It travels in the carotid sheath, enters the skull through the carotid canal and enters the middle cranial fossa through the foramen lacerum in the floor of the cavernous sinus. The artery runs forward in the cavernous sinus, turning superiorly to pierce the roof at the anterior end. It then enters the subarachnoid space and gives off the ophthalmic artery. Inferior to the anterior perforated substance of the brain, the ICA gives off the anterior cerebral and posterior communicating arteries then continues as the middle cerebral artery.

Vertebral artery

The vertebral artery arises from the first part of the subclavian artery. It ascends in the foramina transversaria of the C6–C1 vertebrae and enters the skull through the foramen magnum. It ascends superiorly on the surface of the medulla oblongata (Fig. 8.16), and joins the vertebral artery from the opposite side to form the basilar artery.

Cranial branches of the vertebral artery include:

- The meningeal arteries
- The anterior and posterior spinal arteries
- The posterior inferior cerebellar artery
- The medullary arteries.

Basilar artery

The basilar artery ascends on the anterior surface of the pons (Fig. 8.16) supplying the pons as it does so. At the upper border of the pons, it divides into the posterior cerebral arteries. It also gives off branches to the cerebellum and internal ear.

Circle of Willis

The circle of Willis is an anastomosis between branches of the internal carotid arteries and the vertebral arteries (Fig. 8.16), allowing blood entering either artery to flow to any part of either cerebral hemisphere. It lies in the interpeduncular fossa beneath the forebrain. An anterior communicating artery connects the two anterior cerebral arteries and posterior communicating arteries connect the internal carotid to the posterior cerebral artery.

Cranial nerves

The cranial nerves are summarized in Figure 8.17.

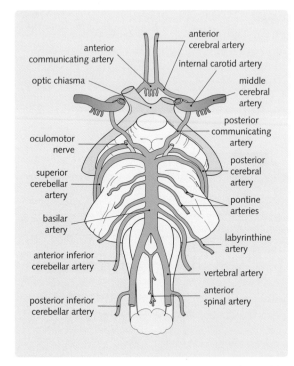

Fig. 8.16 Internal carotid and vertebral arteries on base of the brain.

labels:
- anterior communicating artery
- optic chiasma
- oculomotor nerve
- superior cerebellar artery
- basilar artery
- anterior inferior cerebellar artery
- posterior inferior cerebellar artery
- anterior cerebral artery
- internal carotid artery
- middle cerebral artery
- posterior communicating artery
- posterior cerebral artery
- pontine arteries
- labyrinthine artery
- vertebral artery
- anterior spinal artery

> **CLINICAL NOTE**
>
> **Stroke (cerebrovascular accident – CVA)**
>
> A stroke is loss of function of part(s) of the brain secondary to a disturbance in blood supply to the brain. Strokes can be classified as ischaemic (approximately 87% of all strokes) and haemmorhagic (approximately 13% of all strokes). Ischaemic strokes occur due to thrombosis, emboli or hypoperfusion. Haemmorhagic strokes occur secondary to an aneurysm or arteriovenous malformation. The symptoms and signs of stroke depend on which part of the brain is affected. Patients commonly present with sudden onset unilateral limb weakness, unilateral facial droop or speech or visual disturbance. Symptoms occur rapidly, over minutes to hours. A transient ischaemic attack (TIA) produces symptoms often identical to that of stroke, however the symptoms resolve in less than 24 hours, and often last only for a few minutes. In these patients the risk of a stroke is high, and they must undergo further investigation and receive prophylactic treatment.

Fig. 8.17   Summary of cranial nerves

Nerve	Distribution and functions
Olfactory (I)	Smell from nasal mucosa of roof of each nasal cavity
Optic (II)	Vision from retina
Oculomotor (III)	Motor to superior, medial and inferior oblique; parasympathetic innervation to sphincter pupillae and ciliary muscle (constricts pupil and accommodates lens of eye) carries sympathetic nerve fibres (from carotid plexus) to smooth muscle part of levator palpebrae superioris
Trochlear (IV)	Motor to superior oblique
Trigeminal (V) – ophthalmic division (V_1)	Sensation from upper third of face, including cornea, scalp, eyelids, external nose and paranasal sinuses
Trigeminal (V) – maxillary division (V_2)	Sensation from the middle third of face, including upper lip, maxillary teeth, mucosa of nose, maxillary sinuses, and palate; supplies dura mater anteriorly
Trigeminal (V) – mandibular division (V_3)	Motor to muscles of mastication, mylohyoid, anterior belly of digastric, tensor veli palatini and tensor tympani; sensation from lower third of face, including temporomandibular joint, and mucosa of mouth and anterior two-thirds of tongue, supplies dura mater anteriorly
Abducent (VI)	Motor to lateral rectus
Facial (VII)	Motor to muscles of facial expression and scalp, stapedius, stylohyoid, and posterior belly of digastric; taste from anterior two-thirds of tongue, floor of mouth, and palate; sensation from skin of external acoustic meatus; parasympathetic innervation to submandibular and sublingual salivary glands, lacrimal gland, and glands of nose and palate
Vestibulocochlear (VIII)	Vestibular sensation from semicircular ducts, utricle, and saccule; hearing from the organ of Corti
Glossopharyngeal (IX)	Motor to stylopharyngeus, parasympathetic innervation to parotid gland; visceral sensation from parotid gland, carotid body and sinus, pharynx, and middle ear; taste and general sensation from posterior third of tongue
Vagus (X)	Motor to constrictor muscles of pharynx, intrinsic muscles of larynx, and muscles of palate (except tensor veli palatini) and superior two-thirds of oesophagus; parasympathetic innervation to smooth muscle of trachea, bronchi, digestive tract and cardiac muscle of heart; visceral sensation from pharynx, larynx, trachea, bronchi, heart, to the splenic flexure oesophagus, stomach, and intestine; taste from epiglottis and palate; sensation from auricle, external acoustic meatus and dura mater of posterior cranial fossa
Accessory (XI) cranial root Spinal root	Motor to striated muscles of soft palate, pharynx, and larynx via fibres that join X in jugular foramen Motor to sternocleidomastoid and trapezius
Hypoglossal (XII)	Sensory to dura mater, posteriorly; motor to intrinsic and extrinsic muscles of tongue (except palatoglossus)

CLINICAL NOTE

Subclavian steal syndrome

Where the two vertebral arteries join to form the basilar artery there is potential for anastomosis. For example, if the first part of the right subclavian artery becomes blocked, blood from the left vertebral artery will pass down the right vertebral artery to supply the right upper limb. This causes cerebral or brainstem ischaemia, and hence blackouts when using the affected arm.

THE ORBIT

The eyeball and its associated structures are protected by the bony orbital cavity. The eyelids protect the eyes anteriorly.

Eyelids

The superficial surface of the lids is covered by skin; the deep surface is covered by mucosa – the conjunctiva, which reflects at the superior and inferior fornices onto the anterior surface of the eyeball; the space between eyeball and eyelid is called the conjunctival sac (Fig. 8.18). The opening between the eyelids is the palpebral fissure. The fibrous framework of the eyelids is formed by the orbital septum (Figs 8.18 and 8.19). The septum is thickened at the lid margins to form the tarsal plates, which medially and laterally form the medial and lateral palpebral ligaments. The tarsal plates contain tarsal glands which empty at the margins of the eyelids. Levator palpebrae superioris muscle is attached to the superior tarsal plate. Sebaceous and ciliary glands also empty onto the eyelid.

The lacrimal gland, composed of an orbital and a palpebral part, lies at the superolateral aspect of the orbit, wrapped around the tendon of levator palpebrae superioris. Its ducts open into the conjunctival sac. The nerve supply to the lacrimal gland is parasympathetic

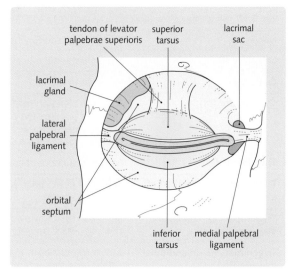

Fig. 8.19 Orbital septum, tarsi and palpebral ligaments.

secretomotor, originating in the lacrimal nucleus. Parasympathetic fibres travel initially with the facial nerve and eventually with the greater petrosal nerve, to synapse in the pterygopalatine ganglion. The postganglionic fibres then join the maxillary nerve, pass into the zygomaticotemporal nerve and the lacrimal nerve to supply the lacrimal gland.

Tears produced by the lacrimal gland are spread medially over the conjunctiva and cornea by blinking, preventing dehydration of the conjunctiva. They gather in the lacrimal lake and drain into the lacrimal punctum (Fig. 8.20), to enter the lacrimal canaliculi, which drain into the lacrimal sac (Fig. 8.20). The sac is the superior end of the nasolacrimal duct, which opens into the inferior meatus of the nose.

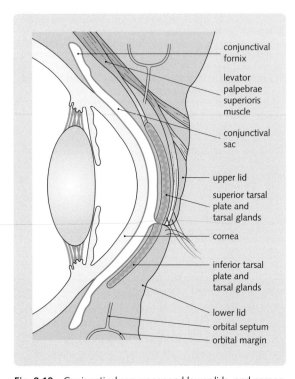

Fig. 8.18 Conjunctival sac, upper and lower lids, and cornea.

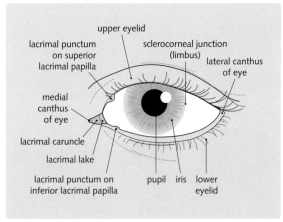

Fig. 8.20 Eyelids, palpebral fissure and eyeball.

Osteology of the orbit

The orbital cavity is composed of the following bones (Fig 8.21):

- Superiorly (roof) – frontal (orbital part), lesser wing of sphenoid
- Medial wall – maxilla, lacrimal, ethmoid, body of sphenoid
- Inferiorly (floor) – maxillary, zygomatic, palatine
- Lateral wall – zygomatic (frontal process), greater wing of sphenoid.

Figure 8.22 lists the openings within the orbit and the structures passing through each.

Muscles of the orbit

The muscles of the orbit are outlined in Figure 8.23 and illustrated in Figure 8.24.

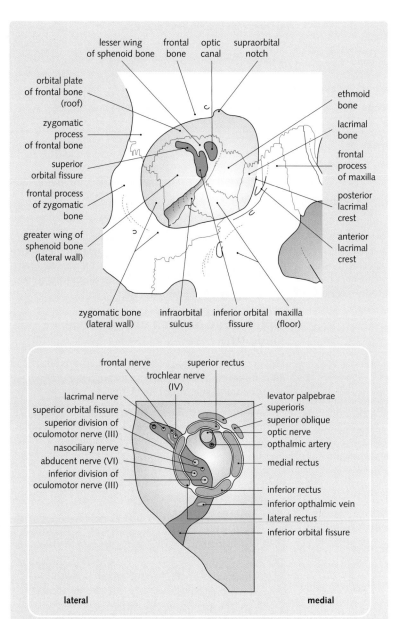

Fig. 8.21 Bones of the orbit and structures in the back of the orbit.

lesser wing of sphenoid bone — frontal bone — optic canal — supraorbital notch

orbital plate of frontal bone (roof)

zygomatic process of frontal bone

superior orbital fissure

frontal process of zygomatic bone

greater wing of sphenoid bone (lateral wall)

ethmoid bone

lacrimal bone

frontal process of maxilla

posterior lacrimal crest

anterior lacrimal crest

zygomatic bone (lateral wall) — infraorbital sulcus — inferior orbital fissure — maxilla (floor)

frontal nerve — superior rectus

trochlear nerve (IV)

lacrimal nerve

superior orbital fissure

superior division of oculomotor nerve (III)

nasociliary nerve

abducent nerve (VI)

inferior division of oculomotor nerve (III)

levator palpebrae superioris

superior oblique

optic nerve

opthalmic artery

medial rectus

inferior rectus

inferior opthalmic vein

lateral rectus

inferior orbital fissure

lateral

medial

Openings	Bones	Contents
Supraorbital notch (foramen)	Orbital plate of the frontal bone	Supraorbital nerve and vessels
Infraorbital groove and canal	Orbital plate of the maxilla	Infraorbital nerve and vessels
Inferior orbital fissure	Maxilla and greater wing of the sphenoid bone	Communicates with the pterygopalatine fossa and transmits the maxillary nerve and its zygomatic branch, the inferior ophthalmic vein and sympathetic nerves
Superior orbital fissure	Greater and lesser wing of the sphenoid bone	Lacrimal, frontal, trochlear, oculomotor, abducens and nasociliary nerves, and superior ophthalmic vein
Optic canal	Lesser wing of the sphenoid bone	Optic nerve and ophthalmic artery
Zygomaticotemporal and zygomaticofacial foramina	Zygomatic bone	Zygomaticotemporal and zygomaticofacial nerves
Anterior and posterior ethmoidal foramina	Ethmoid bone	Anterior and posterior ethmoidal nerves and vessels

Fig. 8.22 Openings within the orbit and the structures transmitted through them

Vessels of the orbit

The ophthalmic artery supplies the orbit. Initially it lies within the subarachnoid space of the optic nerve and pierces its dural sheath (Fig. 8.25). The superior ophthalmic vein communicates anteriorly with the facial vein and posteriorly, it drains to the cavernous sinus. The inferior ophthalmic vein communicates via the inferior orbital fissure with the pterygoid venous plexus (a route for transmission of infection).

Nerves of the orbit

Optic nerve (II)

The optic nerve is surrounded by meninges as it enters the orbit. It passes forward and laterally within the cone of rectus muscles and pierces the sclera. The meningeal layer fuses with the sclera here. The nerve carries afferent fibres from the retina to the visual cortex.

Oculomotor nerve (III)

The oculomotor nerve is divided into superior and inferior divisions:

- The superior division supplies superior rectus and levator palpebrae superioris.
- The inferior division supplies inferior rectus, medial rectus and inferior oblique.
- The nerve to inferior oblique sends a branch to the ciliary ganglion. This carries parasympathetic fibres to the sphincter pupillae (constricts the pupil) and the ciliary muscle.

Trochlear nerve (IV)

The trochlear nerve leaves the lateral wall of the cavernous sinus to enter the orbit. It runs forward and medially, across the origin of levator palpebrae superioris to supply the superior oblique muscle.

Ophthalmic division of trigeminal nerve (VI)

This runs in the lateral wall of the cavernous sinus and gives three branches which pass through the superior orbital fissure to the orbit (Fig. 8.21):

- **Lacrimal nerve**: passes along the upper part of the lateral rectus muscle to supply the skin and conjunctiva of the upper lid laterally. It is joined by a branch of the zygomaticotemporal nerve carrying parasympathetic fibres to the lacrimal gland.

CLINICAL NOTE

Oculomotor nerve palsy

This results in ptosis (loss of innervation of levator palpabrae superioris), a dilated pupil (loss of parasympathetic innervation) and an eye which is deviated downwards and outwards (unopposed lateral rectus and superior oblique).

Fig. 8.23 Muscles of the eyeballs and eyelids

Name of muscle (nerve supply)	Origin	Insertion	Action
Extrinsic muscles of eyeball (striated skeletal muscle)			
Superior rectus (III nerve)	Common tendinous ring on posterior wall of orbital cavity	Superior surface of eyeball just posterior to corneoscleral junction	Moves eye upward and medially
Inferior rectus (III nerve)	Common tendinous ring on posterior wall of orbital cavity	Inferior surface of eyeball just posterior to corneoscleral junction	Moves eye downward and medially
Medial rectus (III nerve)	Common tendinous ring on posterior wall of orbital cavity	Medial surface of eyeball just posterior to corneoscleral junction	Moves eye medially
Lateral rectus (VI nerve)	Common tendinous ring on posterior wall of orbital cavity	Lateral surface of eyeball just posterior to corneoscleral junction	Moves eye laterally
Superior oblique (IV nerve)	Body of sphenoid bone	Passes through trochlea and is attached to superior surface of eyeball beneath superior rectus, behind the equator	Moves eye downward and laterally
Inferior oblique (III nerve)	Floor of orbital cavity, anteriorly and medially	Lateral surface of eyeball deep to lateral rectus	Moves eye upward and laterally
Intrinsic muscles of eyeball (smooth muscle)			
Sphincter pupillae of iris (parasympathetic via III nerve)	Ring of smooth muscle passing circumferentially around pupil	–	Constricts pupil
Dilator pupillae of iris (sympathetic)	Ciliary body	Sphincter pupillae	Dilates pupil
Ciliary muscle (parasympathetic via III nerve)	Corneoscleral junction	Ciliary body	Controls shape of lens; in accommodation, makes lens more globular
Muscles of eyelids			
Orbicularis oculi (VII nerve)	Medial palpebral ligament, lacrimal bone	Skin around orbit, tarsal plates	Closes eyelids (helps spread tears across conjunctiva)
Levator palpebrae superioris (striated muscle: III nerve; smooth muscle: sympathetic)	Lesser wing of sphenoid bone	Superior tarsal plate	Raises upper lid

HINTS AND TIPS

Motor innervation of the extraocular muscles is from the 3rd cranial nerve (oculomotor), except for superior oblique – innervated by the trochlear nerve (4th cranial nerve – SO4) and lateral rectus – innervated by the abducens nerve (6th cranial nerve - LR6).

HINTS AND TIPS

Note that the pterygopalatine ganglion, NOT the ciliary ganglion, supplies the lacrimal gland.

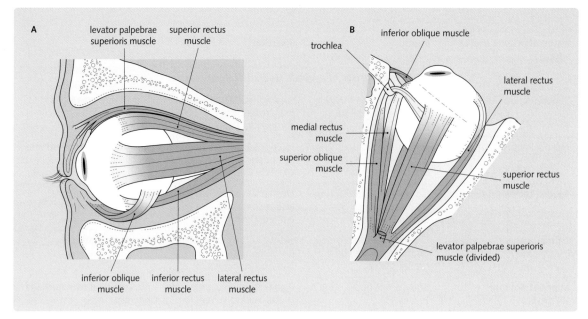

Fig. 8.24 Muscles of the orbit via branches of the ophthalmic artery.

Fig. 8.25 Arterial supply to the orbit via branches of the ophthalmic artery.

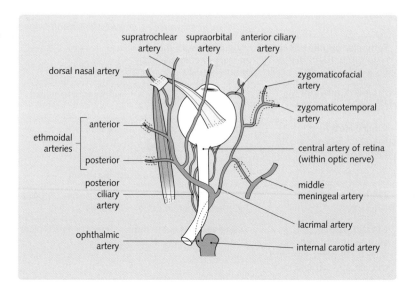

- **Frontal nerve**: passes forward on the superior surface of levator palpebrae superioris. Before it reaches the orbital margin it divides into supraorbital and supratrochlear nerves, which supply the skin of the forehead and scalp, and the frontal sinus.
- **Nasociliary nerve**: enters the orbit, crossing above the optic nerve to reach the medial wall of the orbit. It runs anteriorly on the superior margin of medial

rectus, gives off the posterior ethmoidal branch and ends by dividing into anterior ethmoidal and infratrochlear nerves (Fig. 8.26).

Abducent nerve (VI)

The abducent nerve enters the orbit and supplies the lateral rectus muscle.

Fig. 8.26 Branches of the nasociliary nerve

Branch	Action
Communicating branch	Communicates with the ciliary ganglion – general sensory fibres from the eyeball pass to the ciliary ganglion via the short ciliary nerves and then to the nasociliary nerve via the communicating branch
Long ciliary nerve	2–3 branches containing sympathetic fibres for the dilator pupillae – runs with the short ciliary nerves and pierces the sclera to reach the iris
Posterior ethmoidal nerve	Exits through the posterior ethmoidal foramen to supply the ethmoidal and sphenoidal air sinuses
Infratrochlear nerve	Passes below the trochlea to supply the skin over the upper eyelid
Anterior ethmoidal nerve	Exits via the anterior ethmoidal foramen and enters the anterior cranial fossa on the cribriform plate of the ethmoid; then enters the nasal cavity via an opening opposite the crista galli to supply the mucosa of the nose; then supplies the skin of the nose as the external nasal nerve

Ciliary ganglion

The ciliary ganglion is one of four parasympathetic ganglia found in the head (the others are the otic, pterygopalatine and submandibular ganglia). They all share a common structure, consisting of:

- Preganglionic parasympathetic fibres, which synapse within the ganglion (from cranial nerves III, VII, IX, X)
- Postganglionic sympathetic fibres, which travel to the ganglion on adjacent blood vessels (all are vasoconstrictor)
- Sensory fibres travelling through the ganglion are always one of the branches of the 5th cranial nerve.

The ciliary ganglion is situated posteriorly in the orbit, lateral to the optic nerve. Preganglionic parasympathetic fibres from the Edinger–Westphal nucleus travel with the oculomotor nerve and synapse in the ganglion.

> **CLINICAL NOTE**
>
> **Abducent nerve palsy**
>
> The long intracranial course of the abducent nerve (supplying lateral rectus muscle) makes it particularly vulnerable to compression if raised intracranial pressure occurs. The affected eye is unable to abduct when eye movements are tested. The eye may also appear adducted when the patient is asked to look straight ahead (as medial rectus is unopposed).

Postganglionic parasympathetic fibres pass to the back of the eye via the short ciliary nerves to supply the constrictor pupillae and ciliary muscle. Sympathetic fibres (from the internal carotid plexus) pass through the ganglion to enter the long ciliary nerves to supply the dilator pupillae. General sensory fibres enter the ganglion via the nasociliary nerve. The long ciliary nerve also carries sympathetic (vasoconstrictor) and sensory fibres to the eyeball.

THE PAROTID REGION

Parotid gland

The parotid gland is the largest salivary gland. It lies between the ramus of the mandible and the sternocleidomastoid muscle (Fig. 8.27). The gland is surrounded by a capsule derived from the investing layer of deep cervical fascia. The free edge of the deep fascial layer forms the stylomandibular ligament, passing from the angle of the mandible to the styloid process, and separating parotid and submandibular glands.

The parotid duct emerges from the anterior border of the gland. It passes over the masseter muscle and at its anterior border, it turns medially to pierce the buccal fat pad and buccinator muscle, to open into the oral cavity opposite the upper second molar tooth.

Structures within the parotid gland

The structures of the parotid gland from superficial to deep are as follows (Fig. 8.28):

- Facial nerve (VII): this divides into its five terminal branches in the parotid gland
- Retromandibular vein: this is formed in the gland by the union of the superficial temporal and maxillary veins. It divides into anterior and posterior divisions, which exit the lower border of the gland. The anterior division joins the facial vein to drain into the internal jugular vein; the posterior division joins with the posterior auricular vein to form the external jugular vein
- External carotid artery: this divides into its two terminal branches at the neck of the mandible – the maxillary and superficial temporal arteries.

Fig. 8.27 Parotid gland and its relations. (Adapted from Snell RS, 1992, *Clinical Anatomy for Medical Students,* 4th edn, Little Brown & Co. Reproduced with the permission of Lippincott Williams & Wilkins. http://lww.com.)

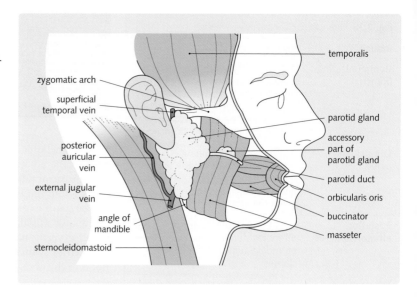

Fig. 8.28 Transverse section, showing structures within the parotid gland. (Adapted from Snell RS, 1992, *Clinical Anatomy for Medical Students,* 4th edn, Little Brown & Co. Reproduced with the permission of Lippincott Williams & Wilkins. http://lww.com.)

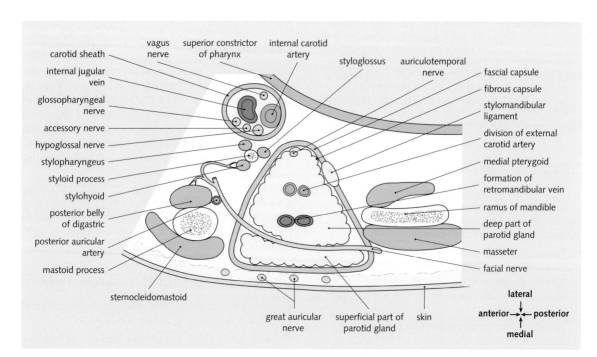

CLINICAL NOTE

Parotid duct stone

A stone in the parotid duct causes intense pain on salivation (i.e. during eating). Treatment is surgical.

Blood supply, innervation and lymphatic drainage of the parotid gland

Blood supply is from the external carotid artery and its terminal branches.

Parasympathetic secretomotor fibres from the glossopharyngeal nerve (IX) pass to the otic ganglion via the tympanic branch of the glossopharyngeal nerve and the lesser petrosal nerve (page 198). Postganglionic fibres pass to the parotid via the auriculotemporal nerve (a branch of the trigeminal nerve (V_3)). The great auricular nerve supplies sensory fibres to the gland capsule. The auriculotemporal nerve supplies sensory fibres to the gland itself. Parotid lymph nodes drain the gland to the deep cervical nodes.

CLINICAL NOTE

Bell's palsy

The term Bell's palsy is reserved for any acute onset lower motor neuron facial paralysis, for which there is no other identifiable cause (although viral infection is thought to be associated with the condition). The facial nerve is thought to swell within the facial canal leading to damage to the nerve or impaired blood flow to the nerve. Bell's palsy produces an ipsilateral weakness of the facial muscles. The corner of the mouth and eye droop – a patient cannot blow out their cheeks, raise their eyebrow or close their eye.

THE TEMPORAL AND INFRATEMPORAL FOSSAE

Temporal fossa

The temporal fossa lies on the lateral aspect of the skull. It is bounded by the superior temporal line of the temporal bone superiorly, by the frontal process of the zygomatic bone anteriorly and by the zygomatic arch inferiorly. The contents of the temporal fossa are:

- The temporalis muscle
- Temporal fascia – the temporal fascia attaches inferiorly to the zygomatic arch and superiorly to the superior temporal line, covering temporalis in this region
- The deep temporal nerves and vessels – from the mandibular nerve (V_3) and the maxillary artery respectively, emerge from the border of lateral pterygoid to supply temporalis
- The auriculotemporal nerve – from the mandibular nerve (V_3), supplies the skin of the auricle, the external auditory meatus and the scalp over the temporal region
- The superficial temporal artery – emerges from behind the temporomandibular joint, crosses the zygomatic arch and ascends to the scalp.

Infratemporal fossa

The infratemporal fossa lies beneath the base of the skull between the pharynx and the ramus of the mandible (Fig. 8.29). It communicates with the temporal region deep to the zygomatic arch.

The infratemporal fossa (Fig. 8.30) contains the medial and lateral pterygoid muscles, branches of the mandibular nerve, the otic ganglion, the chorda tympani, the maxillary artery and the pterygoid venous plexus – detailed below.

Muscles of mastication

There are four muscles of mastication (Fig. 8.31), all supplied by the trigeminal nerve (V_3).

CLINICAL NOTE

Neurological examination

The muscles of mastication can be clinically tested by asking the patient to:
- Clench the teeth (masseter and temporalis muscles)
- Move the chin from side to side in a chewing motion (lateral and medial pterygoid muscles).

Mandible

Major features of the mandible are shown in Figure 8.32. The two halves of the mandible unite at the midline symphysis menti.

Temporomandibular joint

The temporomandibular joint (TMJ) is the articulation between the condylar head of the mandible and the mandibular fossa of the temporal bone (Figs 8.33 & 8.34). It is a synovial joint; the joint space is divided into upper and lower compartments by a fibrocartilaginous articular

Fig. 8.29	Boundaries of the infratemporal fossa
Boundary	**Components**
Anterior	Posterior surface of the maxilla
Posterior	Styloid process
Superior	Infratemporal surface of the greater wing of the sphenoid bone
Medial	Lateral pterygoid plate
Lateral	Ramus of the mandible

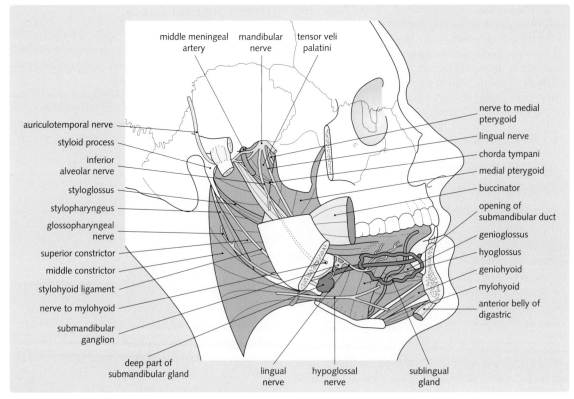

Fig. 8.30 Infratemporal fossa and its relations (the ramus, condyloid and coronoid processes, and most of the body of the mandible have been removed).

Fig. 8.31 Muscles of mastication			
Muscle (nerve supply)	**Origin**	**Insertion**	**Action**
Temporalis (V_3 nerve)	Temporal fossa floor up to inferior temporal line	Coronoid process	Elevates mandible; posterior fibres retract a protruded mandible
Masseter (V_3 nerve)	Lower border and deep surface of zygomatic arch	Lateral surface of ramus of mandible	Elevates and protrudes mandible
Lateral pterygoid (V_3 nerve)			
Superior head	Infratemporal surface of sphenoid bone	Neck of the mandible	Acting together they protrude the mandible and pull the articular disc anteriorly; acting alone on one side produces deviation of mandible to contralateral side
Inferior head	Lateral surface of lateral pterygoid plate	Articular disc	
Medial pterygoid (V_3 nerve)			
Superficial head	Tuberosity of maxilla	Medial surface of ramus and angle of the mandible	Acting together they elevate the mandible; acting alone on one side produces deviation of mandible to contralateral side
Deep head	Medial surface of lateral pterygoid plate		

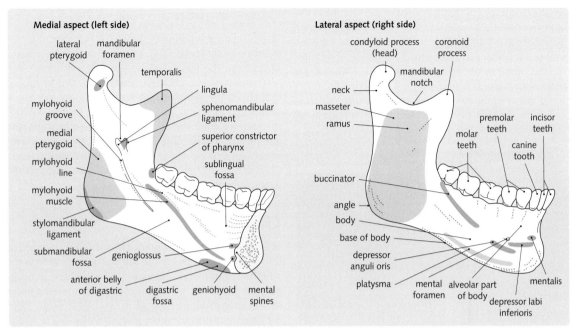

Fig. 8.32 Features of the mandible.

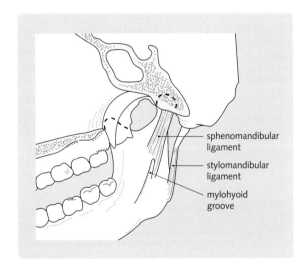

Fig. 8.33 Ligaments of the temporomandibular joint (medial view).

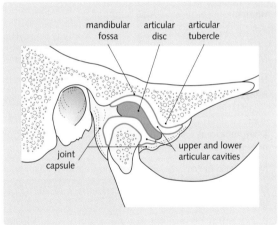

Fig. 8.34 Temporomandibular joint (lateral view).

disc, attached to the lateral pterygoid muscle anteriorly and to the joint capsule.

The capsule surrounds the joint, and is attached to the margins of the mandibular fossa and the neck of the mandible. It is strengthened by the lateral (temporomandibular) ligament. The sphenomandibular and stylomandibular ligaments are also functionally associated with the joint.

Hinge-like movements (elevation and depression) take place in the lower joint space (between the condyle and the articular disc). When the mouth is opened widely, a gliding movement occurs in the upper joint space as the head and disc are pulled forward (protracted) by the medial pterygoid.

Mandibular nerve

This is the third division of the trigeminal nerve (V_3). It is composed of a motor and a sensory root, both of which exit the skull through the foramen ovale to enter the infratemporal fossa. At this point they immediately join the motor root of the trigeminal nerve. Inferior to the foramen ovale, the nerve is separated from the pharynx by the tensor veli palatini muscle and lies deep to the superior head of the lateral pterygoid muscle. It divides into anterior and posterior divisions. The anterior division of the mandibular nerve is concerned with supplying the muscles of mastication, except for its buccal branch which is sensory to the skin of the cheek, mucosa and gingivae (Fig. 8.35).

CLINICAL NOTE

Dislocation of the **TMJ**

When yawning, if the lateral pterygoid muscle contracts too much the mandibular head may pass anteriorly over the articular tubercle and dislocate the TMJ. An affected individual is unable to close his or her mouth. Dislocation is reduced by pressing on the molar teeth with the thumbs in the mouth while pulling up the chin.

Otic ganglion

This is a parasympathetic ganglion lying inferior to the foramen ovale (page 195). Preganglionic secretomotor fibres from the inferior salivary nucleus of the glossopharyngeal nerve (IX) are carried in the tympanic branch to the tympanic plexus and tympanic membrane, and then from here are carried in the lesser petrosal nerve to enter the otic ganglion. The fibres synapse and postganglionic fibres hitchhike on the auriculotemporal nerve to enter the parotid gland. Postganglionic sympathetic and sensory fibres also pass through the ganglion without synapsing.

Chorda tympani

The chorda tympani is a branch of the facial nerve in the temporal bone. It enters the infratemporal fossa via the petrotympanic fissure and joins the lingual nerve. It transmits preganglionic parasympathetic secretomotor fibres to the submandibular ganglion, and taste fibres from the anterior two-thirds of the tongue via the lingual nerve.

Fig. 8.35 Branches of the mandibular nerve and the areas they supply.

Branch	Area supplied
Main trunk	
Meningeal branch	Re-enters cranial cavity via foramen spinosum
Nerve to medial pterygoid	Medial pterygoid and a branch that passes through otic ganglion to supply tensor tympani and tensor veli palatini
Anterior division (motor except the buccal nerve)	
Deep temporal nerves	Two or three nerves emerge from the upper border of lateral pterygoid – enter and supply temporalis
Masseteric nerve	Passes through mandibular notch to supply masseter muscle
Nerve to lateral pterygoid	Enters deep surface of lateral pterygoid and supplies it
Buccal nerve	Passes anteriorly between heads of lateral pterygoid to appear at anterior border of masseter; is sensory to skin of cheek and underlying buccal mucosa and gingiva
Posterior division (mainly sensory)	
Lingual nerve	Appears at lower border of lateral pterygoid and runs over superior surface of medial pterygoid to lie just beneath mucosa lining inner aspect of mandible adjacent to 3rd molar tooth (its subsequent course is described with the mouth); deep to lateral pterygoid, the nerve receives the chorda tympani
Inferior alveolar nerve	Runs parallel with lingual nerve over medial pterygoid; enters mandibular foramen and supplies teeth of lower jaw; at mental foramen, a branch of the nerve, the mental nerve, exits mandible to supply lower lip and chin region; mylohyoid nerve arises from inferior alveolar nerve just above mandibular foramen to supply mylohyoid and anterior belly of digastric
Auriculotemporal nerve	Emerges from behind the temporomandibular joint, crosses the root of the zygomatic arch behind the superficial temporal artery; supplies the skin of the auricle, the external auditory meatus and scalp over the temporal region

Maxillary artery

The maxillary artery is the large terminal branch of the external carotid artery in the parotid gland. It passes anteriorly, medial to the neck of the mandible, reaching the lower border of lateral pterygoid and entering the infratemporal fossa. It then passes between the heads of lateral pterygoid and enters the pterygopalatine fossa through the pterygomaxillary fissure. Figure 8.36 lists the branches of the maxillary artery.

Pterygoid venous plexus

The pterygoid venous plexus lies around the muscles of mastication, in the infratemporal fossa. It drains veins from the orbit, oral cavity and nasal cavity. It communicates with the cavernous sinus and with the facial vein.

HINTS AND TIPS

The pterygoid venous plexus is devoid of valves (as are all veins of the head and neck). It communicates with the cavernous sinus, and so infections of the face may spread into the cavernous sinus. This results in headaches, loss of vision and paralysis of cranial nerves which pass through the cavernous sinus.

THE EAR AND VESTIBULAR APPARATUS

The ear is the organ of hearing and balance. It may be divided into the external ear, the middle ear and the internal ear.

External ear

The external ear is composed of the auricle and the external auditory meatus.

Auricle

The auricle is composed of skin and cartilage. It captures sound and conducts it to the tympanic membrane.

External auditory (acoustic) meatus

The meatus extends from the auricle to the tympanic membrane (Fig. 8.37). The lateral third is cartilaginous and the medial two-thirds are bony. It is lined by a layer of thin skin and contains ceruminous and sebaceous glands which produce cerumen (earwax).

Tympanic membrane

The tympanic membrane is a thin membrane separating the external ear and middle ear (tympanic cavity) (Fig. 8.37). It is covered by skin externally and by mucous membrane internally. The tympanic membrane is outwardly concave, with a central depression – the umbo.

The membrane moves in response to air vibration. Movements of the membrane are transmitted across the middle ear to the internal ear by three small bones. The auriculotemporal nerve and a small auricular branch of the vagus nerve supply the external surface of the tympanic membrane. The glossopharyngeal nerve supplies the internal surface.

Middle ear

The middle ear lies in the petrous temporal bone. It consists of the tympanic cavity and the epitympanic recess, which lies superior to the tympanic cavity. It is connected

---

Fig. 8.36 Branches of the maxillary artery

Branch	Site of origin	Area supplied
Middle meningeal artery	Infratemporal fossa	Enters cranial cavity via foramen spinosum to supply meninges
Inferior alveolar artery	Infratemporal fossa	Follows inferior alveolar nerve into mandibular canal and supplies lower jaw and teeth, and surrounding mucosa
Deep temporal arteries Masseteric artery Pterygoid branches	Infratemporal fossa	Muscles of mastication
Posterior superior alveolar artery	Pterygopalatine fossa	Enters posterior aspect of maxilla to supply molar and premolar teeth of maxilla
Anterior superior alveolar artery	Infraorbital canal	Incisor and canine teeth

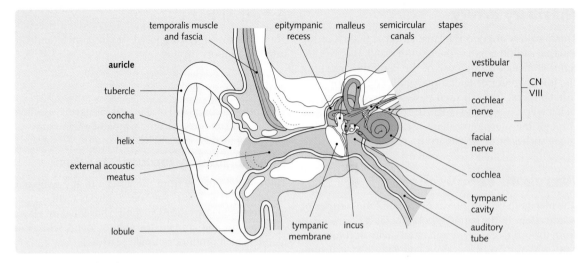

Fig. 8.37   External auditory meatus.

to the nasopharynx via the auditory tube (Eustachian tube) and to the mastoid air cells and antrum via the aditus. The mucosa of the tympanic cavity is continuous with that of the auditory tube, mastoid cells and the mastoid antrum.

The middle ear contains:

- The ossicles (malleus, incus and stapes)
- Stapedius and tensor tympani muscles
- The chorda tympani
- The tympanic plexus of nerves.

Figure 8.38 describes the walls of the middle ear.

Fig. 8.38   Walls of the middle ear

Wall	Components
Roof (tegmental wall)	Tegmen tympani (thin plate of bone): separates cavity from dura in floor of middle cranial fossa
Floor (jugular wall)	A layer of bone separates tympanic cavity from superior bulb of internal jugular vein
Lateral wall (membranous)	Tympanic membrane with epitympanic recess superiorly
Medial wall (labyrinthine)	Separates tympanic cavity from inner ear
Anterior wall (carotid)	Separates tympanic cavity from carotid canal; superiorly lies opening of auditory tube and canal for tensor tympani
Posterior wall	Connected by aditus to mastoid antrum and air cells

Mastoid antrum

The aditus connects the mastoid antrum to the epitympanic recess of the tympanic cavity. The tegmen tympani separates the antrum from the middle cranial fossa. The floor of the antrum communicates with the mastoid air cells via several openings. Anteroinferiorly the antrum is related to the bony canal in which the facial nerve lies.

Auditory tube

The auditory tube connects the tympanic cavity to the nasopharynx. The posterior third is bony and the remainder is cartilaginous. The mucosa is continuous with that of the tympanic cavity and nasopharynx. The tube allows pressure in the middle ear to equalize with atmospheric pressure, allowing free movement of the tympanic membrane. Pressure changes, e.g. during flying, can be equalized by swallowing or chewing or performing the Valsalva manoeuvre – these movements open the auditory tubes. Its nerve supply arises from the tympanic plexus (mainly the tympanic branch of CN IX).

Ossicles

The ossicles are the malleus, incus and stapes. The malleus is attached to the tympanic membrane. The incus connects the malleus to the stapes, which is attached to the oval window (Fig. 8.39). The ossicles transmit vibration from the tympanic membrane to the oval window.

There are two muscles associated with the ossicles: tensor tympani (medial pterygoid nerve – V_3) dampens vibration of the tympanic membrane, and stapedius (VII) dampens vibration of the stapes, thus limiting the impact of loud noise.

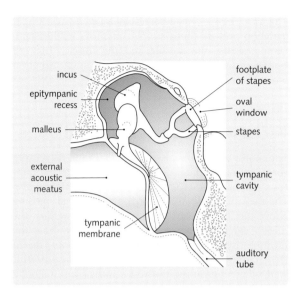

Fig. 8.39 Coronal section of the tympanic cavity showing the ossicles in situ.

Internal ear

This is the site of amplification and transformation of mechanical energy to electrical energy. The internal ear is contained within the petrous temporal bone (Fig. 8.40). It consists of the bony labyrinth which contains the membranous labyrinth. These are separated by a space containing fluid called perilymph, which is similar in composition to cerebrospinal fluid.

Bony labyrinth

Vestibule

The central vestibule contains the utricle and saccule, components of the balance system. It is continuous with the cochlea anteriorly, with the semicircular canals posteriorly, and with the posterior cranial fossa via the aqueduct of the vestibule. The aqueduct extends to the posterior surface of the petrous temporal bone to open into the internal auditory meatus. It contains the endolymphatic ducts and blood vessels.

CLINICAL NOTE

Eustachian (auditory tube) and infection

The Eustachian tube provides a passage for infection to spread from the nasopharynx to the tympanic cavity (middle ear). Infections occur more commonly in children as the tube is shorter, more horizontal and so drainage of fluid from the middle ear is more difficult, resulting in otitis media (infection of the middle ear).

Cochlea

The cochlea contains the cochlear duct, and is concerned with hearing. It makes 2.5 turns around a bony core – the modiolus. The large basal turn of the cochlea (the promontory) protrudes into the medial wall of the tympanic cavity.

Fig. 8.40 Internal ear.

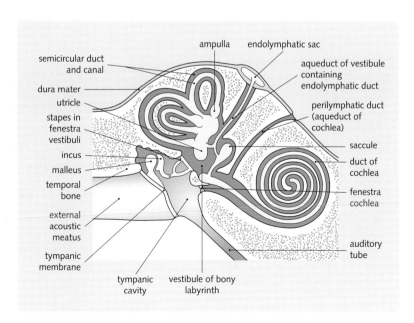

Semicircular canals

These three lie perpendicular to one other. At one end of each canal is a swelling – the ampulla. The semicircular ducts lie in the canals.

Membranous labyrinth

This is a series of ducts and sacs which are contained in the bony labyrinth and contain endolymph.

Saccule and utricle

These contain receptors which respond to vertical and horizontal linear acceleration respectively, as well as the static pull of gravity.

Cochlear duct

This lies within the bony cochlea, separating the interior of the cochlea into three parts. The scala vestibuli lies superior to the duct and the scala tympani lies inferior to it. Both are filled with perilymph, and communicate with each other at the tip of the cochlea. The duct contains the organ of Corti, which contains the receptors of the auditory apparatus.

Semicircular ducts

These contain receptors which respond to rotational acceleration in three different planes.

Endolymphatic duct

This duct opens into the endolymphatic sac. Endolymph has a composition similar to that of intracellular fluid.

Vestibulocochlear nerve (VIII)

Near the lateral end of the internal auditory meatus this nerve divides into an anterior cochlear nerve (hearing) and a posterior vestibular nerve (balance) (Fig. 8.41).

The vestibular nerve enlarges to form the vestibular ganglion and its fibres supply receptors in the semicircular ducts, the saccule and the utricle. The cell bodies of the cochlear nerve form the spiral ganglion which innervates the organ of Corti.

Facial nerve in the temporal bone

The motor part of the facial nerve (VII) and its sensory root – the nervus intermedius – enter the internal auditory meatus together with the vestibulocochlear nerve. The two roots fuse and enter the facial canal, passing above the internal ear to reach the medial wall of the middle ear. The nerve then turns posteriorly above the promontory (the geniculate ganglion (sensory) lies at this sharp bend) and passes posteriorly to the posterior wall, where it turns inferiorly to exit the temporal bone through the stylomastoid foramen.

Branches in the temporal bone

Branches in the temporal bone comprise:

- The greater petrosal nerve – branches off at the geniculate ganglion and enters the middle cranial fossa. It is joined by the deep petrosal nerve (sympathetic) to form the nerve of the pterygoid canal
- The nerve to stapedius
- The chorda tympani. This arises superior to the the stylomastoid foramen. It passes to the lateral wall of the middle ear, crosses the deep surface of the tympanic membrane, and enters a canal leading to the petrotympanic fissure. It joins the lingual nerve in the infratemporal fossa.

Fig. 8.41   Vestibulocochlear nerve.

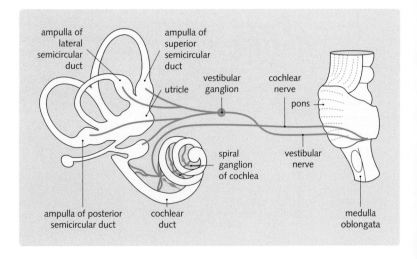

ampulla of lateral semicircular duct

ampulla of superior semicircular duct

vestibular ganglion

cochlear nerve

utricle

pons

spiral ganglion of cochlea

vestibular nerve

ampulla of posterior semicircular duct

cochlear duct

medulla oblongata

Damage to the facial nerve

The course of the facial nerve is complex. It is composed of a motor and sensory root (known as the nervus intermedius, which also carries parasympathetic fibres). The nerve exits the cranial cavity and travels with the the vestibulocochlear nerve (CN VIII) along the internal acoustic meatus. It then travels alone along the facial canal within the petrous temporal bone. Within the petrous temporal bone it gives off the following branches:

• The greater petrosal nerve, carrying parasympathetic fibres which synapse in the ptergyopalatine ganglion, to supply glands in the nasal cavity, palate and lacrimal gland
• Motor branch to stapedius
• Chorda tympani which carries parasympathetic fibres, which are secretomotor, to the submandibular ganglion and also sensory fibres for taste from the anterior two-thirds of the tongue.

It then passes through the stylomastoid foramen, passing close to the middle ear cavity. At the exit from stylomastoid foramen, it gives branches to the posterior belly of digastric and stylohyoid muscles. It terminates within the substance of the parotid gland giving the five motor branches to the muscles of facial expression (temporal, zygomatic, buccal mandibular and cervical).

Damage to the facial nerve proximally, within the petrous temporal bone, at the internal acoustic foramen would result in facial paralysis, hyperacusis (due to paralysis of stapedius), loss of taste and some salivation (due to damage to chorda tympani). At this level it may also affect vestibulocochlear nerve (loss of hearing and balance). Damage to the nerve at or distal to the stylomastoid foramen will result in paralysis of facial muscles only.

THE NECK

The neck is the region between the head and the thorax.

Soft tissues of the neck

Fascial layers of the neck

The fascial layers of the neck are illustrated in Figure 8.42. They are described below:

Superficial fascia

The superficial fascia is a thin layer which encloses the platysma muscle. Cutaneous nerves, superficial vessels and superficial lymph nodes lie in the fascia.

Deep fascia

This lies beneath the superficial fascia. It condenses to form the following:

• Investing layer of deep cervical fascia: this completely encircles the neck, splitting to enclose the sternocleidomastoid and trapezius muscles. Posteriorly it is attached to the ligamentum nuchae. Superiorly, it is attached to the lower border of the mandible, the zygomatic arch and the base of the skull. It splits to enclose the parotid and submandibular glands and attaches to the hyoid. Inferiorly the fascia is attached to the acromion, clavicle and sternum. It attaches to the anterior and posterior borders of the manubrium to form the suprasternal space, containing the jugular arch, which connects the anterior jugular veins.
• Pretracheal fascia: this fascia is attached superiorly to the thyroid and cricoid cartilages. Inferiorly, it enters the thorax to blend with the fibrous pericardium. Laterally, it blends with the carotid sheath. It encloses the thyroid and parathyroid glands, and lies deep to the infrahyoid muscles.
• Prevertebral fascia: this fascia covers the vertebral column and its associated muscles (Fig. 8.42), attaching posteriorly to the ligamentum nuchae. It forms the axillary sheath around the axillary artery and brachial plexus. Superiorly, it is attached to the base of the skull, and inferiorly it enters the thorax to blend with the anterior longitudinal ligament of the vertebral column. The retropharyngeal space lies between the prevertebral fascia and the pharynx, extending down into the thorax.
• Carotid sheath: this is a condensation of the fascia surrounding the common and internal carotid arteries, the internal jugular vein, the deep cervical chain of nodes, and the vagus nerve. It extends from the base of the skull to the root of the neck.

Posterior triangle of the neck

The inferior belly of omohyoid divides the posterior triangle into a large occipital triangle and a small supraclavicular triangle (Fig. 8.43).

The margins and contents of the posterior triangle are detailed in Figures 8.44 and 8.45 respectively.

Figure 8.46 outlines the muscles on the lateral aspect of the neck.

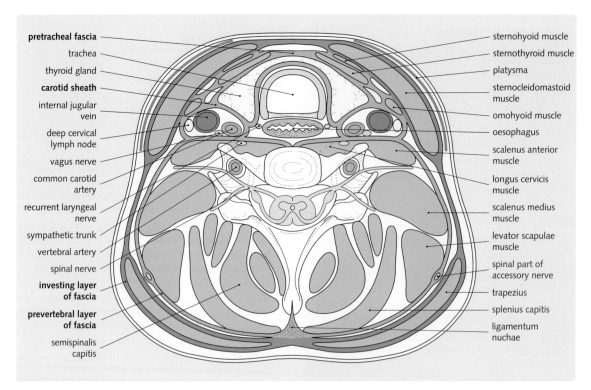

pretracheal fascia
trachea
thyroid gland
carotid sheath
internal jugular vein
deep cervical lymph node
vagus nerve
common carotid artery
recurrent laryngeal nerve
sympathetic trunk
vertebral artery
spinal nerve
investing layer of fascia
prevertebral layer of fascia
semispinalis capitis

sternohyoid muscle
sternothyroid muscle
platysma
sternocleidomastoid muscle
omohyoid muscle
oesophagus
scalenus anterior muscle
longus cervicis muscle
scalenus medius muscle
levator scapulae muscle
spinal part of accessory nerve
trapezius
splenius capitis
ligamentum nuchae

Fig. 8.42 Fascial layers of the neck.

Fig. 8.43 Posterior triangle of the neck.

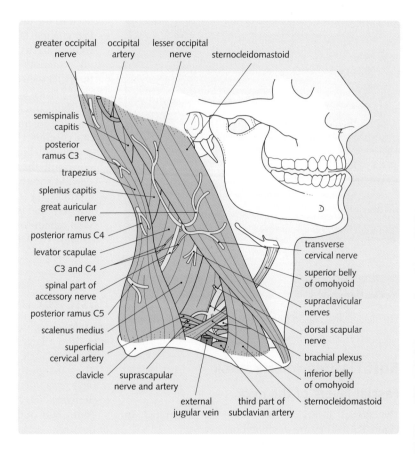

greater occipital nerve
occipital artery
lesser occipital nerve
sternocleidomastoid
semispinalis capitis
posterior ramus C3
trapezius
splenius capitis
great auricular nerve
posterior ramus C4
levator scapulae
C3 and C4
spinal part of accessory nerve
posterior ramus C5
scalenus medius
superficial cervical artery
clavicle
suprascapular nerve and artery
external jugular vein
third part of subclavian artery
transverse cervical nerve
superior belly of omohyoid
supraclavicular nerves
dorsal scapular nerve
brachial plexus
inferior belly of omohyoid
sternocleidomastoid

Fig. 8.44 Margins of the posterior triangle

Margin	Components
Anterior	Posterior border of sternocleidomastoid
Posterior	Anterior border of trapezius
Inferior	Middle third of clavicle
Roof	Skin, superficial fascia, platysma, investing layer of deep fascia
Floor	Prevertebral fascia over prevertebral muscle

Fig. 8.45 Contents of the posterior triangle

Structure	Origin
3rd part of subclavian artery	Enters anterior inferior angle of triangle
Superficial cervical artery	Branch of thyrocervical trunk of subclavian artery
Suprascapular artery	Branch of thyrocervical trunk
Brachial plexus	Roots of plexus enter posterior triangle by emerging between scalenus anterior and medius; trunks and divisions also lie in posterior triangle before entering the axilla
Accessory nerve	Spinal part of accessory nerve enters posterior triangle by emerging from deep to posterior border of sternocleidomastoid
Cervical plexus	The four cutaneous branches emerge from posterior border of sternocleidomastoid

CLINICAL NOTE

Infection in fascial planes of the neck

Abscess formation behind the prevertebral fascia can extend laterally in the neck, forming a swelling posterior to the sternocleidomastoid muscle. If it perforates the fascia anteriorly it enters the retropharyngeal space and can narrow the pharynx, causing difficulties in swallowing (dysphagia) and speaking (dysarthria) before spreading into the superior mediastinum, anterior to the pericardium.

Cervical plexus

The cervical plexus (Fig. 8.47) is formed by the anterior rami of C1–C4 spinal nerves in the substance of the prevertebral muscles. It is covered by the prevertebral fascia and is related to the internal jugular vein in the carotid sheath.

External jugular vein

The external jugular vein is formed by the posterior auricular vein and the posterior division of the retromandibular vein behind the angle of the mandible. It crosses sternocleidomastoid and pierces the deep fascia just above the clavicle in the posterior triangle to enter the subclavian vein.

Anterior triangle of the neck

The anterior triangle is formed by the anterior border of sternocleidomastoid muscle, the midline of the neck and the inferior border of the mandible. It is subdivided by the anterior and posterior bellies of digastric and the superior belly of omohyoid into the digastric (submandibular), carotid and muscular triangles (Figs 8.48, 8.49 & 8.50).

Vessels of the anterior triangle

Common carotid artery

The left common carotid artery arises from the aortic arch, the right from the brachiocephalic trunk. Both ascend in the neck deep to sternocleidomastoid. At the upper border of the thyroid cartilage (level of C3) the arteries divide into the external and internal carotids (Fig. 8.51).

At the terminal part of the common carotid artery (the origin of the internal carotid artery) there is a dilatation, the carotid sinus. This contains baroreceptors which respond to changes in arterial blood pressure. The carotid body lies in the tunica adventitia of the artery. It contains chemoreceptors which monitor blood carbon dioxide levels.

Both the carotid sinus and the carotid body are innervated by the carotid sinus branch of the glossopharyngeal nerve.

HINTS AND TIPS

The carotid pulse is palpable at the superior border of the thyroid cartilage, anterior to the sternocleidomastoid muscle.

Fig. 8.46 Major muscles of the lateral aspect of the neck

Name of muscle (nerve supply)	Origin	Insertion	Action
Platysma (VII nerve)	Inferior border of mandible; skin and subcutaneous tissues of lower part of the face	Fascia covering superior parts of pectoralis major and deltoid muscles	Used to express sadness and fright by pulling angles of mouth down
Sternocleidomastoid [XI nerve (spinal part), C2, C3]	Anterior surface of manubrium of sternum; medial third of clavicle	Mastoid process of temporal bone and superior nuchal line	Individually each muscle laterally flexes neck and rotates it so face is turned upwards toward opposite side; both muscles act together to flex neck
Trapezius [XI nerve (spinal part), C2, C3]	Superior nuchal line; external occipital protuberance; ligamentum nuchae; spinous processes of C7–T12 vertebrae	Lateral third of clavicle; acromion; spine of scapula	Elevates, retracts, and rotates scapula laterally so that the glenoid 'looks upwards'

Fig. 8.47 Branches of the cervical plexus.

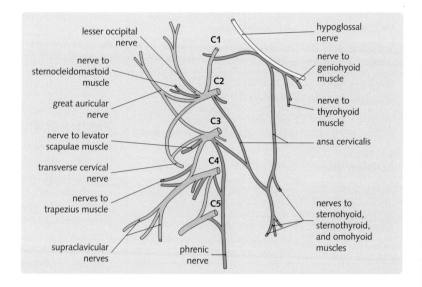

External carotid artery

This commences at the superior border of the thyroid cartilage and ascends to enter the parotid gland. Its branches are:

- Ascending pharyngeal (to the pharynx)
- Superior thyroid (to the superior pole of the thyroid)
- Lingual (passes to the tongue)
- Facial (loops over the submandibular gland and mandible to supply the face)
- Occipital
- Posterior auricular
- Superficial temporal
- Maxillary

Internal carotid artery

This artery commences at the upper border of the thyroid cartilage and ascends in the carotid sheath, to pass through the carotid canal in the base of the skull. It supplies the cerebral hemispheres and the orbital contents. It gives off no branches in the neck.

Internal jugular vein

This vein commences at the end of the sigmoid sinus and exits the cranial cavity through the jugular foramen. It descends through the neck in the carotid sheath, at first posterior, then lateral to the carotid artery. It unites

Fig. 8.48	Contents of the anterior triangle of the neck
Triangle	**Main contents**
Carotid	External carotid artery; larynx and pharynx, and internal and external laryngeal nerves
Muscular	Sternothyroid and sternohyoid muscles, superior belly of omohyoid; thyroid gland, trachea, and oesophagus
Digastric (submandibular)	Submandibular gland and lymph nodes; facial artery and vein; external carotid artery; internal carotid artery, internal jugular vein, glossopharyngeal (IX), vagus (X), and hypoglossal (XII) nerves
Submental	Submental lymph nodes

with the subclavian vein to form the brachiocephalic vein posterior to the sternoclavicular joint.

The vein has dilatations at its upper and lower ends – the superior and inferior bulbs.

Tributaries include the inferior petrosal sinus and the facial, pharyngeal, lingual and superior and middle thyroid veins.

Deep cervical nodes

These nodes form a chain along the internal jugular vein in the carotid sheath. They drain the entire head and neck. Efferent vessels join to form the jugular lymph trunk, which in turn drains into the thoracic duct, right lymph duct or subclavian trunk (Fig. 8.12).

> **CLINICAL NOTE**
>
> **Central venous catheter**
>
> A central venous catheter (CVC or 'central line') can be inserted into the internal jugular vein in order to allow the central venous pressure to be measured, to allow blood samples to be taken, to allow drugs to be administered or for feeding (total parenteral nutrition – TPN). The vein is normally located using ultrasound (veins can be seen to compress on ultrasound scan by gentle pressure with the ultrasound probe, arteries are more resistant to compression). A needle is introduced into the vein, a guidewire is inserted through the needle, and the catheter is then threaded over the guidewire and sutured in place.

Nerves of the triangles of the neck

All the following nerves (except the accessory nerve) are found in the anterior triangle (Fig. 8.51).

Glossopharyngeal nerve (IX)

This nerve emerges from the jugular foramen. It lies between the carotid arteries and passes lateral to stylopharyngeus, which it supplies. It gives a branch to the carotid body then passes between the superior and middle constrictors to supply sensory and taste fibres to the posterior third of the tongue and oropharynx.

Vagus nerve (X)

The vagus exits the skull through the jugular foramen, where its superior and inferior sensory ganglia lie. Inferior to the superior ganglion, the cranial part of the accessory nerve joins the vagus and together they form the pharyngeal and recurrent laryngeal nerves (Fig. 8.52). The vagus descends in the neck in the carotid sheath between the internal carotid artery and internal jugular vein. At the root of the neck it passes anterior to the first part of the subclavian artery to enter the thorax.

Accessory nerve (XI)

The spinal part of the accessory nerve arises from the upper five or six cervical segments and ascends to enter the skull via the foramen magnum. It joins the cranial root from the medulla oblongata and they exit the skull via the jugular foramen.

The cranial root joins the vagus nerve; the spinal root supplies sternocleidomastoid and trapezius.

> **HINTS AND TIPS**
>
> CN XI is the nerve of twos: it has two roots, passes through two foraminae and its spinal root supplies two muscles.

Hypoglossal nerve (XII)

This emerges from the hypoglossal canal and descends in the neck between the internal carotid artery and internal jugular vein. At the lower border of digastric, the nerve loops around the occipital artery passing lateral to internal and external carotid arteries to enter the submandibular region. It provides a motor supply to the muscles of the tongue.

The nerve is joined by fibres of C1. Some of these are given off in the superior root of the ansa cervicalis, others pass directly to thyrohyoid and geniohyoid.

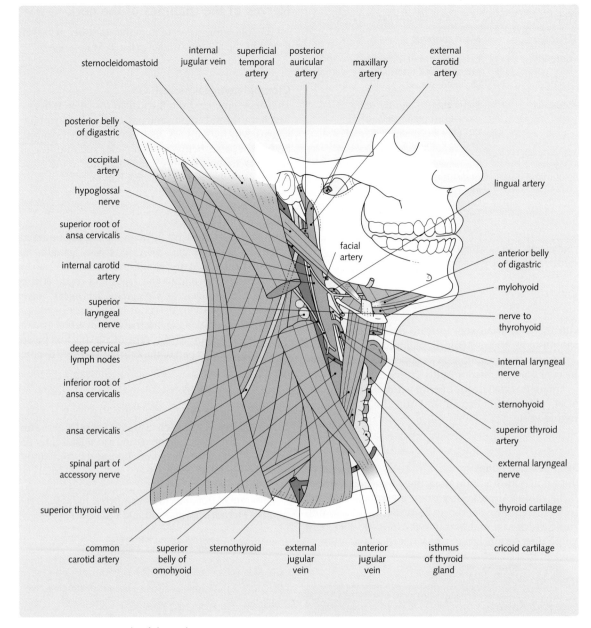

Fig. 8.49 Anterior triangle of the neck.

Ansa cervicalis

This nerve loop is formed from a superior root of C1 fibres travelling along the XII nerve and an inferior root from C2 and C3. It supplies omohyoid, sternohyoid and sternothyroid.

Sympathetic trunk

The trunk lies deep in the neck, between the carotid sheath and prevertebral fascia. It has superior, middle and inferior ganglia. The inferior ganglion usually fuses with the first thoracic ganglion to form the stellate ganglion. Postganglionic fibres form plexuses around the major arteries, to supply the structures of the head and neck. The trunks also give off cardiac branches.

> **HINTS AND TIPS**
>
> All sympathetic fibres to the head and neck are carried as plexuses on the surface of blood vessels.

Fig. 8.50 Suprahyoid and infrahyoid muscles.

Name of muscle (nerve supply)	Origin	Insertion	Action
Suprahyoid muscles			
Posterior belly of digastric (VII nerve)	Mastoid process	Intermediate tendon bound to hyoid bone	Depresses mandible and elevates hyoid bone
Anterior belly of digastric (inferior alveolar V_3 nerve)	Lower border of mandible near midline	Intermediate tendon bound to hyoid bone	Depresses mandible and elevates hyoid bone
Stylohyoid (VII nerve)	Styloid process of temporal bone	Body of hyoid bone	Elevates hyoid bone
Mylohyoid (inferior alveolar V_3 nerve)	Mylohyoid line on medial surface of mandible	Body of hyoid bone and mylohyoid raphe	Elevates floor of mouth and hyoid bone, and depresses mandible
Geniohyoid (C1 through XII nerve)	Inferior mental spine	Body of hyoid bone	Elevates hyoid bone and depresses mandible
Infrahyoid muscles			
Sternohyoid (ansa cervicalis C1–C3)	Manubrium sterni and clavicle	Body of hyoid bone	Depresses hyoid bone
Sternothyroid (ansa cervicalis C1–C3)	Manubrium sterni	Oblique line on lamina of thyroid cartilage	Depresses larynx
Thyrohyoid (C1 travelling with the XIIth nerve)	Oblique line on lamina of thyroid cartilage	Body of hyoid bone	Depresses hyoid bone and elevates larynx
Omohyoid–inferior belly (ansa cervicalis C1–C3)	Upper margin of scapula	Intermediate tendon bound to clavicle and first rib	Depresses hyoid bone
Omohyoid–superior belly (ansa cervicalis C1–C3)	Body of hyoid bone	Intermediate tendon bound to clavicle and first rib	Depresses hyoid bone

(Adapted from Hall-Craggs ECB (1995) *Anatomy as a Basis for Clinical Medicine.* Williams & Wilkins.)

MIDLINE STRUCTURES OF THE FACE AND NECK

Pharynx

The pharynx is a C-shaped fibromuscular tube lying posterior to the nasal cavity (nasopharynx), oral cavity (oropharynx) and larynx (laryngopharynx). It extends from the base of the skull to the inferior border of the cricoid cartilage (C6 vertebral level), where it is continuous with the oesophagus. There are three layers in the pharyngeal wall:

- The muscular layer is formed by the pharyngeal constrictors and longitudinal muscles (Figs 8.53 & 8.54). The constrictors sit inside each other like a series of stacking cups.
- The pharyngobasilar fascia separates the mucosa and the muscle layer. It blends with the periosteum of the base of the skull.
- The mucous membrane (Fig. 8.55).

CLINICAL NOTE

Horner's syndrome

A cervical sympathetic trunk lesion results in an ipsilateral partial ptosis (due to paralysis of the superior tarsal muscle, which is attached to levator palpebrae superioris muscle), miosis (pupillary constriction), and anhydrosis (lack of sweating). This is due to an interrupted sympathetic nerve supply, commonly secondary to an apical lung tumour, invading the sympathetic chain or the T1 ganglion (stellate ganglion) which lies on the neck of the first rib.

Nasopharynx

The nasopharynx lies posterior to the nasal cavity, above the soft palate. During swallowing, the soft palate

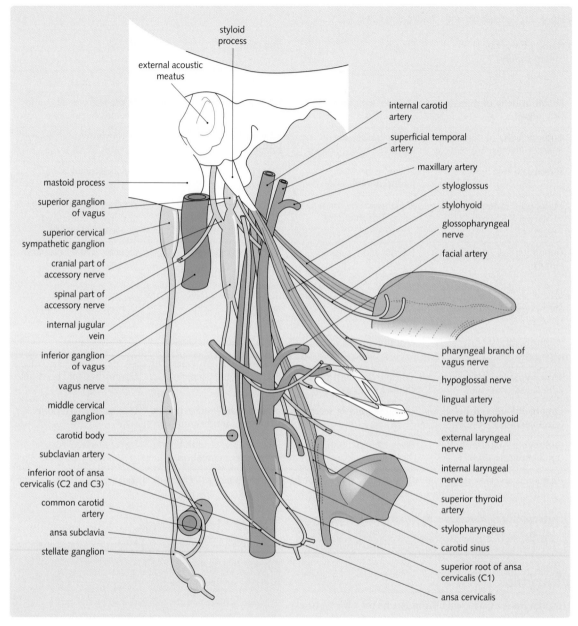

Fig. 8.51 The common carotid artery and the lower cranial nerves. (Adapted from Snell RS, 1992, *Clinical Anatomy for Medical Students*, 4th edn, Little Brown & Co. Reproduced with the permission of Lippincott Williams & Wilkins. http://lww.com.)

elevates and the pharyngeal wall is pulled forward to form a seal, preventing food entering the nasopharynx. The pharyngeal tonsil (adenoid) lies in the posterior wall. The auditory tube opens at the tubal elevation in the lateral wall – it also contains tonsillar tissue (the tubal tonsils). The tubal recess is a small depression in the lateral wall, posterior to the tubal elevation. Anteriorly, the nasopharynx is continuous with the nasal cavity through the choanae.

Fig. 8.52 Branches of the vagus nerve in neck and thorax

Branch	Course and distribution
Meningeal branch	Dura mater of posterior cranial fossa
Auricular branch	Medial surface of auricle, external auditory meatus, and adjacent tympanic membrane
Pharyngeal branch	Contains motor fibres from XI nerve (cranial part); combines with pharyngeal branches of IX nerve (sensory fibres) to form pharyngeal plexus, which supplies all pharyngeal muscles except stylopharyngeus (IX) and all soft-palate muscles except tensor veli palatini (V_3)
Superior laryngeal nerve-divides into internal and external laryngeal nerves	Internal laryngeal nerve is sensory to piriform fossa and mucosa of larynx above vocal folds; external laryngeal nerve is motor to cricothyroid muscle
Cardiac branches Pulmonary branches Oesophageal branches	Assist in forming cardiac plexus in thorax Assist in forming pulmonary plexus in thorax Assist in forming oesophageal plexus in thorax
Right recurrent laryngeal nerve	Arises from vagus nerve as it crosses subclavian artery; hooks backwards and upwards behind artery and ascends in a groove between trachea and oesophagus; supplies all laryngeal muscles (except cricothyroid) and laryngeal mucosa below vocal folds, trachea, and oesophagus
Left recurrent laryngeal nerve	Arises from X nerve as it crosses aortic arch; hooks beneath arch behind ligamentum arteriosum and passes into neck between trachea and oesophagus; has a similar distribution to right nerve

Fig. 8.53 Muscles of the pharynx

Name of muscle (nerve supply)	Origin	Insertion	Action
Superior constrictor (pharyngeal plexus)	Medial pterygoid plate, pterygoid hamulus, pterygomandibular raphe, mylohyoid line of mandible	Pharyngeal tubercle of occipital bone, midline pharyngeal raphe	Assists in separating oro- and nasopharynx and propels food bolus downward
Middle constrictor (pharyngeal plexus)	Stylohyoid ligament, lesser and greater cornua of hyoid bone	Pharyngeal raphe	Propels food bolus downward
Inferior constrictor (pharyngeal plexus)			
Thyropharyngeus	Lamina of thyroid cartilage	Pharyngeal raphe	Propels food bolus downward
Cricopharyngeus	Cricoid cartilage	Contralateral cricopharyngeus	Upper oesophageal sphincter
Palatopharyngeus (pharyngeal plexus)	Palatine aponeurosis Horizontal plate of palatine bone	Thyroid cartilage	Elevates pharyngeal wall and pulls palatopharyngeal folds medially
Salpingopharyngeus (pharyngeal plexus)	Auditory tube	Merges with palatopharyngeus	Elevates pharynx and larynx
Stylopharyngeus (IX)	Styloid process of temporal bone	Thyroid cartilage	Elevates larynx during swallowing

Fig. 8.54 Muscles of the pharynx.

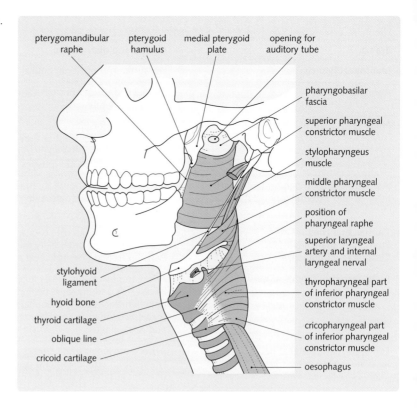

pterygomandibular raphe

pterygoid hamulus

medial pterygoid plate

opening for auditory tube

pharyngobasilar fascia

superior pharyngeal constrictor muscle

stylopharyngeus muscle

middle pharyngeal constrictor muscle

position of pharyngeal raphe

superior laryngeal artery and internal laryngeal nerval

thyropharyngeal part of inferior pharyngeal constrictor muscle

cricopharyngeal part of inferior pharyngeal constrictor muscle

oesophagus

stylohyoid ligament

hyoid bone

thyroid cartilage

oblique line

cricoid cartilage

CLINICAL NOTE

Pharyngeal pouch

Pharyngeal mucosa may bulge between the thyropharyngeus and cricopharyngeal muscles to form a pharyngeal pouch (Killian's dehiscence). As it enlarges, it pushes the oesophagus aside, resulting in severe dysphagia (difficulty swallowing) and the possibility of foodstuffs being aspirated into the lungs, causing infection. Treatment is surgical.

Oropharynx

The oropharynx lies between the soft palate and the upper border of the epiglottis, posterior to the oral cavity. The palatine tonsils lie in its lateral walls. The posterior third of the tongue forms the anterior wall of the oropharynx – it has an irregular surface owing to the presence of the underlying lingual tonsil.

The mucosa is reflected from the base of the tongue onto the epiglottis to form one median and two lateral glossoepiglottic folds, with two pouches – valleculae – lying between them.

Laryngopharynx

The laryngopharynx lies posterior to the laryngeal opening and the posterior surface of the larynx.

The piriform fossae are grooves on either side of the laryngeal inlet which direct food from the back of the tongue to the oesophagus, thus avoiding the airway.

Vessels of the pharynx

Blood supply is from branches of the ascending pharyngeal, ascending palatine, facial, maxillary and lingual arteries. Veins drain via the pharyngeal venous plexus to the internal jugular vein.

Lymphatics drain into the deep cervical nodes either directly or indirectly via the retropharyngeal or paratracheal nodes.

Nerve supply of the pharynx

The motor nerve supply of the pharynx is from the pharyngeal pleus, formed by branches of cranial nerves IX, and the cranial part of XI.

The sensory nerve supply is as follows:

- Nasopharynx – maxillary nerve (V_2)
- Oropharynx – IX nerve
- Laryngopharynx – internal laryngeal nerve (X).

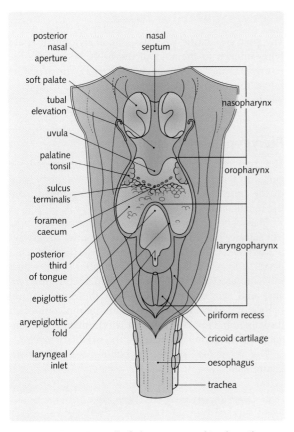

posterior nasal aperture
nasal septum
soft palate
tubal elevation
nasopharynx
uvula
palatine tonsil
oropharynx
sulcus terminalis
foramen caecum
laryngopharynx
posterior third of tongue
epiglottis
aryepiglottic fold
piriform recess
laryngeal inlet
cricoid cartilage
oesophagus
trachea

Fig. 8.55 Posterior wall of pharynx opened to show the mucous membrane and interior of the pharynx.

Nose

The nose consists of:

- The external nose – this has a bony (nasal bones and frontal process of the maxilla) and cartilaginous skeleton, separated by the nasal septum.
- The nasal cavities – these communicate with the exterior via the nares or nostrils and with the nasopharynx via the choanae.

Nasal cavity

The walls of the nasal cavity are listed in Figure 8.56. The openings in the lateral wall are listed in Figure 8.57. The nerve and blood supply of the lateral wall are illustrated in Figure 8.58.

Paranasal sinuses

The paranasal sinuses lie around the nasal cavity, in the bones of the face and skull:

- Maxillary – lying laterally within the maxilla
- Ethmoidal – lying medially within the ethmoid

Fig. 8.56	Walls of the nasal cavity
Surface	**Components**
Floor	Palatine process of maxilla, horizontal process of palatine bone, i.e. the hard palate
Roof	Nasal, frontal, sphenoid, and ethmoid bones; above lies the anterior cranial fossa and the sphenoidal sinus
Lateral wall	Maxillary, palatine, sphenoid, lacrimal, and ethmoid bones and the inferior concha; the superior and middle conchae are projections of the ethmoid bone; the superior, middle and inferior meatus lie beneath their respective conchae; sphenoethmoidal recess lies above the superior concha
Medial wall (nasal septum)	The perpendicular plate of the ethmoid, the vomer and the septal cartilage

Fig. 8.57	Openings in the lateral wall of the nose
Region of lateral wall	**Features and openings**
Sphenoethmoidal recess	Sphenoidal sinus
Superior meatus	Posterior ethmoidal air cells
Middle meatus	The hiatus semilunaris lies below the middle concha; the frontal sinus, anterior ethmoidal cells, and maxillary sinus open into the hiatus; the bulla ethmoidalis is formed by the underlying middle ethmoidal cells which open onto it
Inferior meatus	Nasolacrimal duct

- Frontal – lying directly behind the forehead in the frontal bone
- Sphenoidal – lying posterosuperiorly within the sphenoid. It is a direct relation of the pituitary gland and allows surgical access to it.

Mucous membrane of the nose

The vestibule lies just inside the anterior nares and is lined by hairy skin. The remainder of the nasal cavity is lined by ciliated columnar epithelium. There is a rich vascular plexus in the submucosa, together with numerous serous and mucous glands.

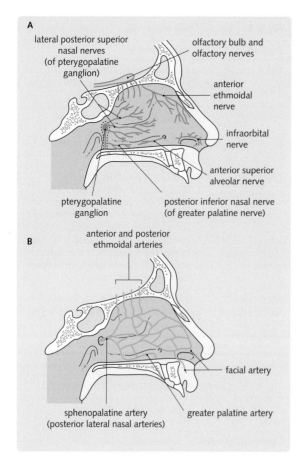

A

lateral posterior superior nasal nerves (of pterygopalatine ganglion)

olfactory bulb and olfactory nerves

anterior ethmoidal nerve

infraorbital nerve

anterior superior alveolar nerve

pterygopalatine ganglion

posterior inferior nasal nerve (of greater palatine nerve)

B

anterior and posterior ethmoidal arteries

facial artery

sphenopalatine artery (posterior lateral nasal arteries)

greater palatine artery

Fig. 8.58 Nerve (A) and blood (B) supplies of the lateral wall of the nose.

Dust from inspired air is removed by the nasal hairs and the mucus of the nasal cavity. The air is warmed by the vascular plexus and moistened before it enters the lower airway.

The roof and superior part of the lateral wall contain olfactory epithelium, which receives the distal processes of the olfactory nerve cells. These fibres play a role in both smell and taste sensations.

The sphenopalatine artery anastomoses with the septal branch of the superior labial artery around the vestibule of the nose.

CLINICAL NOTE

Nose bleed

The anastomosis around the vestibule of the nose (Little's area) is a very common site for nosebleeds. The anterior ethmoidal artery, posterior ethmoidal artery, sphenopalatine artery, greater palatine artery and superior labial artery anastomose at this site.

Pterygopalatine fossa

The pterygopalatine fossa is a small pyramidal space lying inferior to the apex of the orbit. It contains the terminal branches of the maxillary artery, the maxillary nerve, the nerve of the pterygoid canal and the pterygo-palatine ganglion (Fig. 8.59).

Pterygopalatine ganglion

The pterygopalatine ganglion is a parasympathetic ganglion lying in the pterygopalatine fossa, just lateral to the sphenopalatine foramen. It is suspended from the maxillary nerve (V_2).

Preganglionic parasympathetic fibres from the superior salivary nucleus of the facial nerve enter the greater petrosal nerve. This joins the deep petrosal (sympathetic) nerve to form the nerve of the pterygoid canal, which joins the ganglion. Here, the parasympathetic fibres synapse and sympathetic fibres (from the deep petrosal branch of the carotid plexus) pass uninterrupted through the ganglion. Fibres of common sensation enter the ganglion via ganglionic branches of the maxillary nerve.

The branches of the ganglion are shown in Figure 8.60.

HINTS AND TIPS

The pterygopalatine ganglion supplies the lacrimal gland, nasal cavity, nasopharynx, paranasal air sinuses and palate, so is known as 'The Ganglion of Hayfever'.

Branches of the maxillary nerve in the pterygopalatine fossa

- Infraorbital nerve – carries secretomotor fibres to the lacrimal gland
- Zygomatic nerve – divides into zygomaticotemporal and zygomaticofacial branches
- Posterior superior alveolar nerve.

Fig. 8.59	Communications of the pterygopalatine fossa
Surface	**Communicates with**
Lateral	Infratemporal fossa
Medial	Nasal cavity via the sphenopalatine foramen; hard palate via palatine canal
Anterior	Orbit via the inferior orbital fissure
Posterosuperior	Middle cranial fossa via the foramen rotundum and pterygoid canal
Posteromedial	Nasopharynx via palatovaginal canal

Fig. 8.60	Branches of the pterygopalatine ganglion
Branch	**Course and distribution**
Nasopalatine nerve	Passes through the sphenopalatine foramen to supply the nasal septum and incisive gum of the hard palate
Lateral posterior superior nasal nerve	Exits via the sphenopalatine foramen to supply the lateral wall of the nose
Greater palatine nerve	Passes through the greater palatine canal and foramen to supply the mucosa of the palate and the lateral wall of the nose
Lesser palatine nerve	Exits through the lesser palatine foramina to supply the soft palate and the mucosa over the palatine tonsil
Pharyngeal nerve	Passes via the palatovaginal canal to supply the nasopharynx
Lacrimal fibres	Parasympathetic fibres to the lacrimal gland join the zygomaticotemporal nerve of V_2 then the lacrimal nerve before supplying the gland

Oral cavity

The oral cavity is divided into two parts:

- The vestibule lies between the cheeks/lips and the teeth
- The oral cavity proper is bounded by the teeth and gums anteriorly and laterally. The palate forms the roof; the floor is formed by the anterior two-thirds of the tongue and the floor of the mouth. A midline fold of mucosa – the frenulum – lies beneath the tongue (Fig. 8.61).

The parotid, submandibular, sublingual and numerous minor salivary glands open into the oral cavity.

Its nerve supply is as follows:

- Roof – greater and lesser palatine and nasopalatine nerves
- Floor – lingual nerve
- Cheek – buccal nerve (from V_3).

Folds of mucosa over the palatoglossus and palatopharyngeus muscle posteriorly form the palatoglossal and palatopharyngeal arches.

Lips

The lips seal the oral cavity and assist in speech. They are covered by mucosa internally and by skin externally.

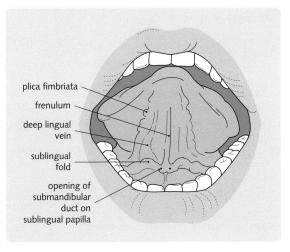

plica fimbriata
frenulum
deep lingual vein
sublingual fold
opening of submandibular duct on sublingual papilla

Fig. 8.61   Oral cavity.

The orbicularis oris muscle, the superior and inferior labial vessels and nerves, and numerous minor salivary glands lie in the substance of the lips.

Tongue

The tongue is a mobile muscular organ covered by mucous membrane. The anterior two-thirds lie in the mouth, the posterior third in the oropharynx (Fig. 8.62). A fibrous median septum runs from anterior to posterior. The intrinsic muscles of the tongue are listed in Figure 8.63.

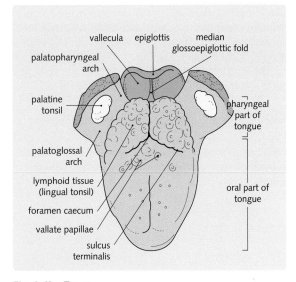

vallecula   epiglottis   median glossoepiglottic fold
palatopharyngeal arch
palatine tonsil
pharyngeal part of tongue
palatoglossal arch
lymphoid tissue (lingual tonsil)
foramen caecum
vallate papillae
sulcus terminalis
oral part of tongue

Fig. 8.62   Tongue.

Fig. 8.63 Muscles of the tongue

Name of muscle (nerve supply)	Origin	Insertion	Action
Intrinsic muscles			
Longitudinal (XII nerve)	Mucous membrane	Mucous membrane	Shortens tongue
Transverse (XII nerve)	Mucous membrane and median septum	Mucous membrane	Narrows tongue
Vertical (XII nerve)	Mucous membrane	Mucous membrane	Lowers tongue
Extrinsic muscles			
Palatoglossus (pharyngeal plexus)	Palatine aponeurosis	Lateral aspect of tongue	Pulls tongue upward and backward and narrows oropharyngeal isthmus
Genioglossus (XII nerve)	Superior mental spine (genial tubercle) of mandible	Merges with other tongue muscles	Draws tongue forward and pulls tip backward
Hyoglossus (XII nerve)	Body and greater cornu of hyoid bone	Merges with other tongue muscles	Depresses tongue
Styloglossus (XII nerve)	Styloid process of temporal bone	Merges with other tongue muscles	Draws tongue upward and backward

Mucous membrane of the tongue

The sulcus terminalis divides the tongue into the anterior two-thirds and the posterior third. It is V-shaped, with the foramen caecum lying at its apex, which it is the remnant of the upper end of the thyroglossal duct. Between 10 and 12 vallate papillae lie anterior to the sulcus.

The mucosa of the anterior two-thirds of the tongue is relatively smooth and it has numerous filiform and fungiform papillae on the dorsal surface. Lateral folds of mucosa, the plica fimbriata, are seen on the ventral surface of the tongue.

The irregular surface of the posterior third of the tongue is due to the underlying lingual tonsil.

Blood and nerve supply to the tongue

Vessels of the tongue comprise the lingual arteries and veins. Lymphatic drainage is to the deep cervical, the submandibular and the submental nodes. The nerve supply to the tongue is shown in Figure 8.64.

HINTS AND TIPS

Remember, the XII nerve is motor to all the muscles of the tongue except palatoglossus which is supplied by the pharyngeal plexus.

Fig. 8.64 Nerve supply to the tongue

	Posterior 1/3rd	Anterior 2/3rds
General sensory	Glossopharyngeal nerve (IX)	Lingual nerve (V$_3$)
Taste	Glossopharyngeal nerve (IX) (also vallate papillae)	Chorda tympani (VII) (via the lingual nerve)

CLINICAL NOTE

Tongue carcinoma

Carcinoma of the tongue may spread via the lymphatics to both sides of the neck (lymphatics cross the midline), dramatically worsening its prognosis.

Floor of the mouth and submandibular region

This region lies between the mandible and hyoid bone. It contains the following:

- Muscles – digastric, mylohyoid, hyoglossus, geniohyoid, genioglossus, and styloglossus
- Salivary glands – submandibular and sublingual

- Nerves – lingual, glossopharyngeal, and hypoglossal and the submandibular ganglion
- Blood vessels – facial and lingual
- Lymph nodes – submandibular.

Lingual nerve

From the third-molar region of the mandible, the lingual nerve crosses styloglossus to the lateral surface of hyoglossus and the submandibular duct. It gives branches to the mucosa of the tongue.

Hypoglossal nerve

The hypoglossal nerve runs forward below the deep part of the submandibular gland, the submandibular duct and the lingual nerve. It supplies all the muscles of the tongue except palatoglossus.

Submandibular gland

This consists of two parts – a large superficial part and a small deep part, which are continuous around the posterior border of mylohyoid. The deep part of the gland lies in the intramuscular cleft. Blood supply is from the facial and lingual arteries. Nerve supply is from the submandibular ganglion, a parasympathetic ganglion with the following connections:

- Sensory fibres from the lingual nerve (V3) pass through the ganglion (common sensation to anterior two-thirds of tongue)
- Sympathetic fibres from the superior cervical ganglion travelling on the facial artery pass through the ganglion (vasoconstrictor)

- Preganglionic parasympathetic fibres from the facial (VII) nerve pass to the ganglion via the nervus intermedius, the chorda tympani and the lingual nerve (secretomotor).

Postganglionic parasympathetic secretomotor fibres pass to the submandibular and sublingual glands via the lingual nerve or directly. The submandibular ducts open onto the sublingual papillae on either side of the frenulum of the tongue.

Sublingual gland

The sublingual gland lies superficially under the sublingual fold, extending back from the sublingual papilla under the tongue. Numerous short ducts open onto the fold. The lingual nerve and submandibular duct lie medially. It is supplied by the submandibular ganglion.

Palate and tonsils

The palate forms the roof of the mouth and the floor of the nose. It is divided into two components:

- The hard palate is composed of the palatine process of the maxilla and the horizontal process of the palatine bone. It is covered by mucous membrane.
- The soft palate is a mobile fibromuscular fold lying posteriorly. It is composed of muscles (Fig. 8.65) and the palatine aponeurosis – the expanded tendon of tensor veli palatini.

Blood supply to the palate is from the greater and lesser palatine arteries. Nerve supply is from the pterygopalatine ganglion.

Fig. 8.65 Muscles of the soft palate			
Name of muscle (nerve supply)	Origin	Insertion	Action
Tensor veli palatini (nerve to medial pterygoid V$_3$)	Spine of sphenoid, auditory tube, scaphoid fossa of pterygoid process	With muscle of other side, forms palatine aponeurosis	Tenses soft palate
Levator veli palatini (pharyngeal plexus)	Petrous part of temporal bone, auditory tube	Palatine aponeurosis	Elevates soft palate
Musculus uvulae (pharyngeal plexus)	Posterior border of hard palate	Mucous membrane of uvula	Elevates uvula
Palatopharyngeus (pharyngeal plexus)	Palatine aponeurosis horizontal plate of palatine bone	Posterior border of thyroid cartilage	Elevates pharyngeal wall and pulls palatopharyngeal folds medially and depresses soft palate
Palatoglossus (pharyngeal plexus)	Palatine aponeurosis	Lateral aspect of tongue	Pulls tongue upward and backward and narrows oropharyngeal isthmus and depresses soft palate

The palatine tonsils are masses of lymphoid tissue lying in the tonsillar fossae between the palatoglossal and palatopharyngeal arches, covered by mucous membrane. The surface is pitted by many openings that lead to the tonsillar crypts. Lymphatics drain to the deep cervical nodes.

Larynx

The larynx is continuous with the laryngopharynx superiorly and with the trachea inferiorly at the level of C6. It acts as a sphincter, separating the lower respiratory system from the alimentary system and is responsible for voice production.

The laryngeal cartilages are shown in Figure 8.66. The laryngeal membranes link these cartilages together, and join the larynx to the hyoid bone and the trachea (Fig. 8.67). The membranes thicken in places to form ligaments.

Mucous membrane of the larynx

The mucosa is tucked under the vestibular ligament to form the laryngeal ventricle between the vestibular ('false vocal') and vocal folds. Above the vocal fold the mucosa is supplied by the internal laryngeal nerve and the superior laryngeal artery. Below the vocal fold it is supplied by the recurrent laryngeal nerve and the inferior laryngeal artery (from the inferior thyroid artery).

Laryngeal cavity

The laryngeal inlet allows communication between the pharynx and the larynx. It is bounded by the epiglottis and the aryepiglottic and interarytenoid folds (Fig. 8.68).

The inlet leads to the vestibule, which extends to the vestibular folds. The laryngeal ventricle lies between the vestibular and vocal folds. The rima glottis is the space between the vocal folds. The infraglottic cavity lies below the vocal folds and is continuous with the trachea.

Intrinsic muscles of the larynx

The intrinsic muscles of the larynx are described in Figure 8.69. All intrinsic muscles are paired except the transverse arytenoid muscle. They can alter the tension and length of the vocal folds and the size and shape of the rima glottis (Fig. 8.70).

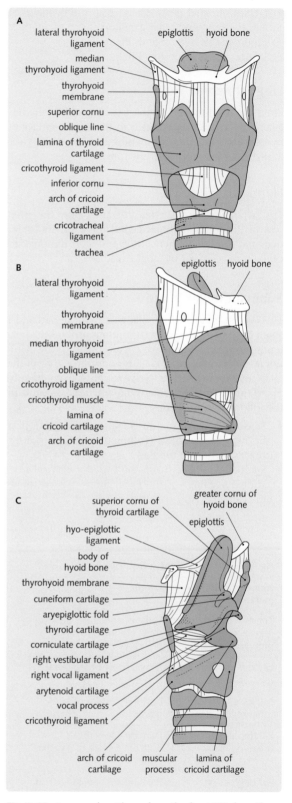

Fig. 8.66 Laryngeal cartilages from the front (A), from the right (B), and from the left without the left lamina of thyroid cartilage (C).

Fig. 8.67 Laryngeal membranes

Membrane	Attachments
Thyrohyoid	Runs between the thyroid cartilage and hyoid bone; has a midline thickening and two lateral thickenings, the median thyrohyoid ligament and lateral thyrohyoid ligaments, respectively
Quadrangular	Runs between the epiglottis and the arytenoid cartilage; its lower free border is the vestibular ligament
Cricothyroid	Joins the cricoid, thyroid, and arytenoid cartilages; its upper free border is the vocal ligament; there is also a midline thickening, the median cricothyroid ligament
Cricotracheal	Runs from the cricoid cartilage to the trachea

to tilt backward and forwards on the other. This alters the vocal fold tension and length.

The synovial cricoarytenoid joint has a lax capsule. This allows rotation and gliding movements of the arytenoid cartilages upon the cricoid cartilage. These movements widen or narrow a V-shaped rima glottis. Rotation of the arytenoids can open the rima glottis into a diamond shape or narrow it.

> **HINTS AND TIPS**
>
> All intrinsic muscles of the larynx are supplied by the recurrent laryngeal nerve, except for the cricothyroid muscle, which is supplied by the external laryngeal nerve.

> **CLINICAL NOTE**
>
> **Tracheostomy (tracheotomy) and cricothyroidotomy**
> During a tracheostomy the skin of the neck is incised and the strap muscles moved to one side, the thyroid isthmus is moved inferiorly or clamped and divided if necessary – an incision is then made though the 2nd to 4th tracheal cartilages and a tracheostomy tube inserted.
> A cricothyroidotomy (a short-term, emergency procedure) is performed by passing a needle through the cricothyroid membrane directly below the thyroid prominence. This is useful when there is a blockage at the rima glottidis, as the needle passes below this level.

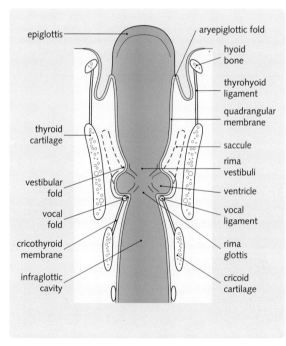

Fig. 8.68 Coronal section of the laryngeal cavity. (Adapted from Williams P (ed.) (1995) *Gray's Anatomy*, 38th edition. Churchill Livingstone.)

Joints of the larynx

The synovial cricothyroid joint is formed by the inferior cornu (horn) of the thyroid cartilage articulating with the facet of the cricoid cartilage, allowing one cartilage

Trachea

The trachea commences at the level of the C6 vertebra and is continuous with the larynx above. It ends at the sternal angle (T4 vertebral level) by dividing into the right and left main bronchi. Its walls are reinforced by C-shaped hyaline cartilages anteriorly.

Thyroid gland

The thyroid gland is an endocrine organ, lying between the trachea and infrahyoid strap muscles. It is covered by a capsule and pretracheal fascia. It has a narrow isthmus (overlying tracheal rings 2–4) connecting two lobes (which extend up to the middle of the thyroid cartilage) (Fig. 8.71). It produces the hormones thyroxine and calcitonin.

Fig. 8.69 Intrinsic muscles of the larynx

Muscle (nerve supply)	Origin	Insertion	Action
Cricothyroid (external laryngeal nerve)	Cricoid cartilage arch	Inferior border of thyroid cartilage and inferior cornu	Lengthens and tenses vocal cords by tilting cricoid and thus arytenoid cartilages
Posterior cricoarytenoid (recurrent laryngeal nerve)	Cricoid cartilage lamina	Muscular process of arytenoid cartilage	Abducts vocal cords by laterally rotating arytenoid cartilages on cricoid cartilage
Lateral cricoarytenoid (recurrent laryngeal nerve)	Cricoid cartilage arch	Muscular process of arytenoid cartilage	Adducts vocal cords by medially rotating arytenoid cartilages on cricoid cartilage
Thyroarytenoid (recurrent laryngeal nerve)	Posterior surface of thyroid cartilage	Muscular process of arytenoid cartilage	Shortens vocal cord
Transverse arytenoid (recurrent laryngeal nerve)	Body of arytenoid cartilage	Body of contralateral arytenoid cartilage	Closes rima glottis by adducting arytenoid cartilages
Oblique arytenoid (recurrent laryngeal nerve)	Muscular process of arytenoid cartilage	Apex of contralateral arytenoid cartilage	Closes rima glottis by drawing arytenoid cartilages together
Vocalis (recurrent laryngeal nerve)	Vocal process of arytenoid cartilage	Vocal ligament	Maintains/increases tension in anterior part of vocal ligament; relaxes posterior part of vocal ligament

Blood and nerve supply to the thyroid gland

The superior thyroid artery (the first branch of the external carotid artery) has the external laryngeal nerve running with it. The artery branches at the upper pole of the gland to supply it. The inferior thyroid artery (arising from the thyrocervical trunk of the subclavian artery) has the recurrent laryngeal nerve running with it. The four arteries (two each side) anastomose posteriorly.

The thyroid ima artery is present in only 3% of individuals, arising from either the brachiocephalic trunk or the aortic arch and entering the lower part of the isthmus.

The superior and middle thyroid veins join the internal jugular vein. The inferior thyroid veins join and empty into the left brachiocephalic vein.

Parathyroid glands

The parathyroid glands are four small glands (two on each side) embedded in the posterior border of the thyroid gland. They are important in the regulation of calcium metabolism and may be damaged during thyroid surgery.

Blood supply to the parathyroid glands

The upper and lower parathyroid glands are supplied by the inferior thyroid artery. Small veins join the thyroid veins.

CLINICAL NOTE

Thyroglossal cysts, goitre and thyroidectomy

The thyroid gland develops as a downgrowth from the back of the tongue – attached to it by the thyroglossal duct. This duct usually disappears; however, remnants may persist. A cyst may form in these remnants. These can be distinguished from a midline sebaceous cyst (or a goitre) by asking a patient to swallow or stick out the tongue, which will pull the thyroglossal cyst upwards. An enlargement of the thyroid is referred to as a goitre and may compress structures adjacent to the thyroid. A thyroidectomy (removal of the thyroid) may be total

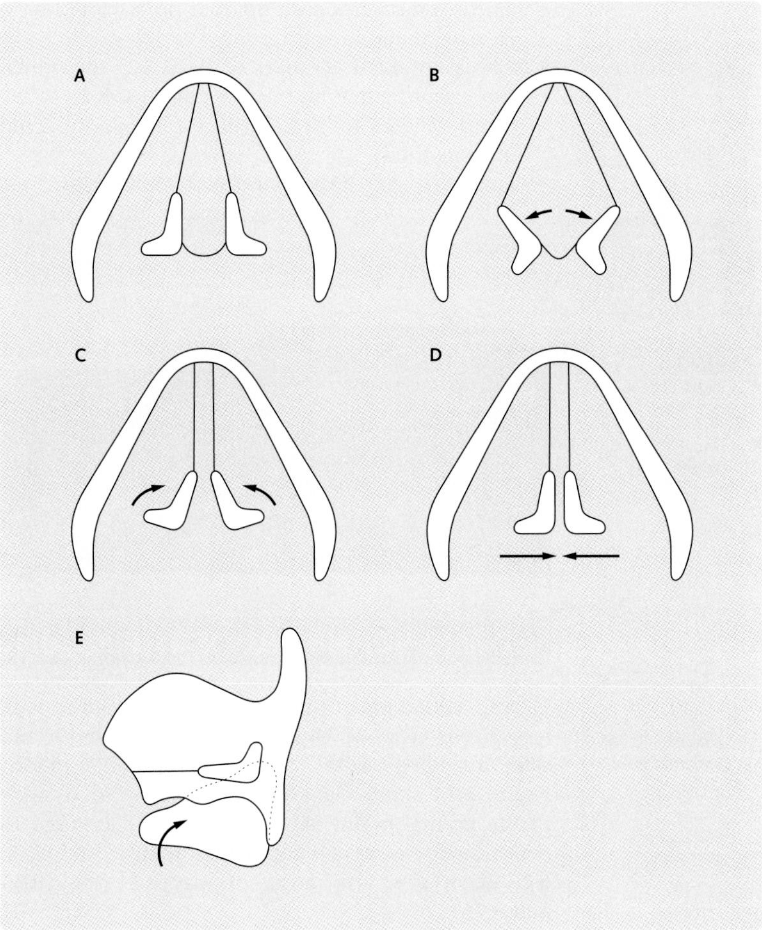

Fig. 8.70 Movements of the vocal folds, arytenoid and cricoid cartilages.

(e.g. for carcinoma) or subtotal (e.g. in the treatment of hyperthyroidism), where part of the gland is preserved. Due to the close relationship between the inferior thyroid arteries and the recurrent laryngeal nerve, these are tied rather than cut during a thyroidectomy – as damage to the nerve results in hoarseness.

RADIOLOGICAL ANATOMY

Imaging of the skull

X-rays of the cranium are used to evaluate the bones of the skull. Several different views are needed to assess and locate fractures as the bones become superimposed on x-ray images. The brain is imaged using CT and MRI scans.

Normal radiographic anatomy of an anteroposterior X-ray of the skull

Figure 8.72 shows the major features of an anteroposterior (AP) view of the skull.

Normal radiographic anatomy of a lateral X-ray of the skull

In Figure 8.73 shows the major features of a lateral X-ray of the skull.

CLINICAL NOTE

ENT

Sinusitis is inflammation of the sinuses, usually frontal or maxillary. A dull pain is felt over the affected sinus

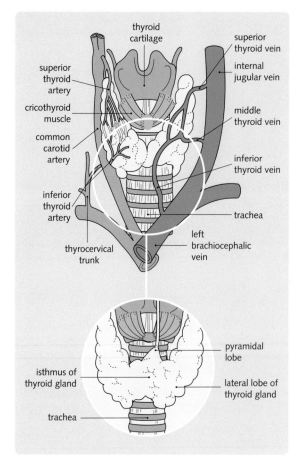

Fig. 8.71 Anterior view of the thyroid gland. The left side of the figure shows the arterial supply, and the right side shows the venous drainage. Inset shows thyroid gland anatomy.

with tenderness of the overlying skin (referred pain due to the same nerve supplying the skin and sinus mucosa) and nasal discharge (a runny nose). If the ethmoid or sphenoidal sinus is affected, a deep pain is usually felt at the root of the nose.

How to examine a skull X-ray

- Check that the name, date of birth, date and time of the X-ray, and the type of X-ray (including which side) are correct.
- Ensure that the area of concern is fully visible.
- Comment on any major abnormalities, then go on to examine the X-ray in a logical sequence.
- Examine the cortex of each bone. Look at the outline for any breaks in continuity and thickening, thinning or alterations in a normally smooth cortex.

- Check the sutures ensuring that no fracture line is crossing them.
- Check any natural curves of skull, e.g. the orbital rim, ensuring that no fracture line crosses it.
- Check sinuses for radiolucency (an opacity could indicate fluid).
- Finally, if you have found one abnormality, e.g. a fracture, keep looking because there may be more.

> **CLINICAL NOTE**
>
> **Radiology**
>
> As an individual ages the pineal gland within the brain undergoes calcification. This is sometimes seen on X-ray, giving a midline landmark but is of no clinical significance.

CT/MRI SCANNING OF THE BRAIN

CT and MRI scans of the brain are performed to look for various types of pathology within the brain and skull including strokes, haemorrhages and tumours. Figure 8.74 shows an MRI scan (transverse section) of the normal brain. 3D angiograms can be used to detect disease of vessels supplying the head and neck, e.g. aneurysms and areas of stenosis (Figs 8.75 and 8.76).

In suspected stroke, CT scanning does not always show abnormality in the first 24 hours after the onset of ischaemia. However, it is important in the exclusion of acute haemorrhage (essential if thrombolysis is being considered) or other diseases, which may present with symptoms similar to a stroke (e.g. brain tumour). Areas of infarction appear dark (areas of low attenuation) on CT scans (Fig. 8.77).

In contrast the presence of blood (haemorrhage) within the cranial cavity or the brain substance will be immediately apparent on a CT scan. Blood appears white on CT scans (an area of high attenuation). Figure 8.78 shows the typical lens-shaped (biconvex) appearance of an extradural haematoma. Extradural haematoma commonly occurs secondary to laceration of meningeal arteries, often the middle meningeal artery, as a consequence of skull fracture (the middle meningeal artery lies deep to the pterion).

In contrast to an extradural haematoma, a subdural haematoma appears crescent shaped. A large haematoma may result in increased intracranial pressure (the skull is a fixed compartment which cannot expand) resulting in midline shift (Fig. 8.79).

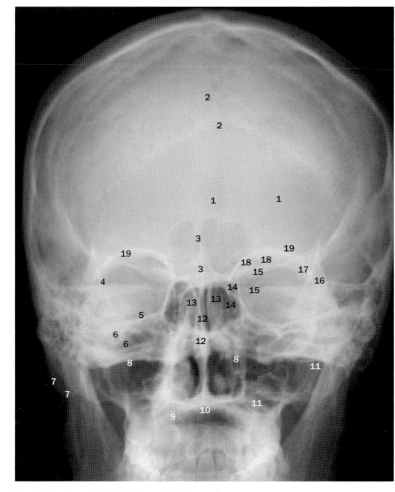

1. Frontal sinus
2. Sagittal suture
3. Crista galli
4. Lambdoid suture
5. Petrous part of temporal bone
6. Internal acoustic meatus
7. Mastoid process
8. Basi-occiput
9. Lateral mass of atlas
   (1st cervical vertebra)
10. Odontoid process (Dens) of axis
11. Floor of maxillary sinus (antrum)
12. Nasal septum
13. Sella turcica
14. Ethmoidal air cells
15. Superior orbital fissure
16. Zygomatic process of frontal bone
17. Temporal surface of greater
    wing of sphenoid
18. Lesser wing of sphenoid
19. Orbital rim

Fig. 8.72   Occipitofrontal view of skull.

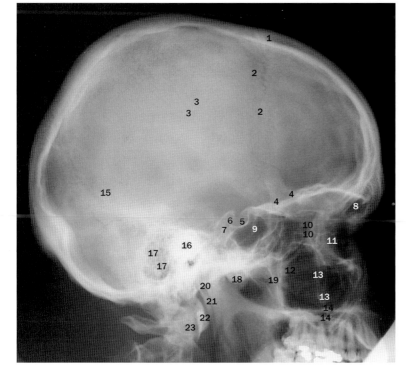

1. Diploë
2. Coronal suture
3. Grooves for middle meningeal
   vessels
4. Greater wing of sphenoid
5. Pituitary fossa (sella turcica)
6. Dorsum sellae
7. Clivus
8. Frontal sinus
9. Sphenoid sinus
10. Ethmoidal air cells
11. Frontal process of zygoma
12. Arch of zygoma
13. Maxillary process of maxilla
14. Palatine process
15. Lambdoid process
16. External acoustic meatus
17. Mastoid air cells
18. Articular tubercle for
    temporomandibular joint
19. Coronoid process of mandible
20. Condyle of mandible
21. Ramus of mandible
22. Anterior arch of atlas
23. Odontoid process (Dens) of axis

Fig. 8.73   Lateral view of skull.

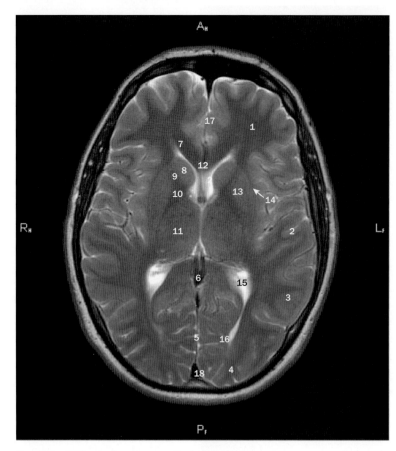

Fig. 8.74 MRI scan (transverse section) of the brain.

1. Frontal lobe
2. Temporal lobe
3. Parietal lobe
4. Occipital lobe
5. Falx cerebri
6. Inferior sagittal sinus
7. Frontal horn of lateral ventricle
8. Caudate nucleus
9. Globus pallidus
10. Posterior limb of internal capsule
11. Thalamus
12. Genu of corpus callosum
13. Putamen
14. External capsule
15. Choroid plexus
16. Occipital horn of lateral ventricle
17. Falx cerebri
18. Superior sagittal sinus

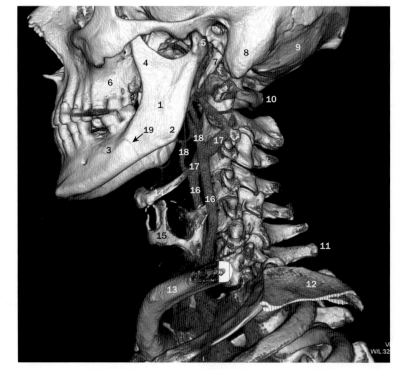

Fig. 8.75 3D CT angiogram of the carotid arteries.

1. Ramus of the mandible
2. Angle of the mandible
3. Body of the mandible
4. Coronoid process of the mandible
5. Condylar process of the mandible
6. Maxilla
7. Styloid process of sphenoid bone
8. Mastoid process of temporal bone
9. Occipital bone
10. Posterior arch of C1 vertebra
11. Vertebra prominens of C7 vertebra
12. Left scapula
13. Left clavicle
14. Hyoid bone
15. Thyroid cartilage of the larynx (partially ossified)
16. Left and right common carotid arteries
17. Left and right internal carotid arteries
18. Left and right external carotid arteries

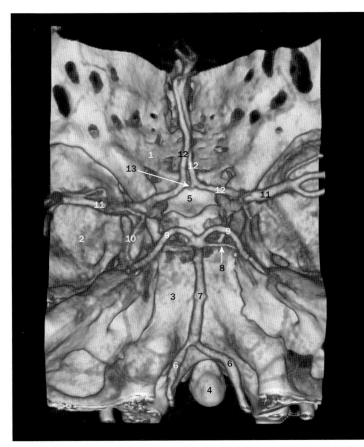

Fig. 8.76 3D CT angiogram of the circle of Willis.

1. Anterior cranial fossa
2. Middle cranial fossa
3. Posterior cranial fossa
4. Odontoid process within the foramen magnum
5. Pituitary fossa (sella turcica)
6. Left and right vertebral arteries
7. Basilar artery
8. Left superior cerebellar artery
9. Left and right posterior cerebral arteries
10. Right posterior communicating artery
11. Left and right middle cerebral arteries
12. Left and right anterior cerebral arteries
13. Position of the anterior communicating artery

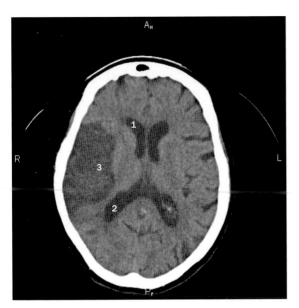

1. Anterior horn of lateral ventricle
2. Posterior horn of lateral ventricle
3. Area of infarction

Fig. 8.77 Infarct affecting the territory supplied by the right middle cerebral artery.

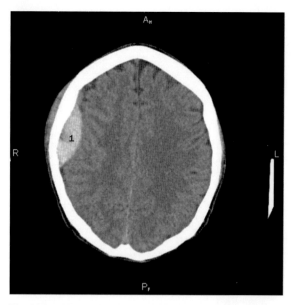

1. Infarct

Fig. 8.78 CT scan (transverse section) showing an extradural haematoma

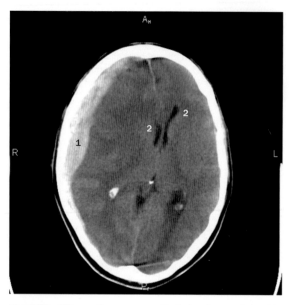

1. Infarct
2. Lateral ventricles

Fig. 8.79 CT scan (transverse section) showing a subdural haemorrhage with left midline shift.

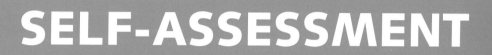

SELF-ASSESSMENT

Best-of-five questions (BOFs)

Chapter 1 Basic concepts of anatomy

1. A 50-year-old builder comes to your surgery. He has noticed an enlarging mole on his shoulder. You refer him to the dermatology department of his local hospital, where he is diagnosed with a malignant melanoma. He is required to undergo further tests to stage his disease (determine the extent of any spread). To which of the following regions of the body are metastases from melanoma likely to spread?
   a. Colon, liver, bones, brain
   b. Colon, liver, bones, kidney
   c. Kidneys, liver, bones, lung
   d. Liver, bones, lung, brain
   e. Liver, bones, lung, colon

2. A 70-year-old man presents to his GP with generalized weakness. The GP tests his muscle power as part of his examination. He decides that the patient is able to contract his muscles against resistance. According to the MRC scale what level of power does the patient have?
   a. Grade 1
   b. Grade 2
   c. Grade 3
   d. Grade 4
   e. Grade 5

3. A 75-year-old woman who is known to have breast cancer is admitted to hospital with back pain and urinary incontinence, which she has not experienced before. Her symptoms, along with her known history of cancer suggest that she may have spinal cord compression. After your initial examination, which of the following tests are likely to be most helpful in reaching a diagnosis?
   a. CT scan of the spine
   b. MRI of the spine
   c. Plain X-ray of the vertebral column
   d. Urinalysis
   e. White blood cell count

4. The anatomical position is the standard reference for describing the position of the body.
   What is the position of the hands in the anatomical position?
   a. The hands are adducted at the wrist
   b. The little fingers lie lateral to the thumbs
   c. The palms face anteriorly
   d. The palms lie in the sagittal plane
   e. The thumbs point medially

5. A 35-year-old man is diagnosed with leukaemia. He is found to have a pancytopenia (a deficiency of all types of blood cells) due to infiltration of his bone marrow with leukaemic cells. In the adult, which of the following sites contain red marrow?
   a. Fibula
   b. Phalanges
   c. Radius
   d. Sternum
   e. Tibia

6. A 25-year-old man comes to see you with pain in his left shoulder. You examine him and in doing so you ask him to abduct his shoulder at the glenohumeral joint. Which of the following best describes abduction?
   a. Movement away from the median sagittal plane
   b. Movement in the coronal plane where there is a reduction in the angle between two parts of the body
   c. Movement in the sagittal plane where there is an increase in the angle between two parts of the body
   d. Movement in the sagittal plane where there is a reduction in the angle between two parts of the body
   e. Movement towards the median sagittal plane

7. An 80-year-old lady presents to the A&E department after a fall. She describes having put out her hands to break her fall and is now complaining of pain in her right wrist. After an examination and X-ray she is diagnosed with a Colles' fracture of her right wrist. Her past medical history includes hypertension and osteoporosis. Which other bones is this lady at particular risk of fracturing?
   a. Clavicle and distal fibula
   b. Clavicle and neck of femur
   c. Vertebrae and clavicle
   d. Vertebrae and distal fibula
   e. Vertebrae and neck of femur

8. You are asked to examine a 77-year-old woman who has been admitted to hospital with a left-sided weakness. As part of your assessment, you perform a cranial nerve examination. In which part of the brain do the nuclei of the cranial nerves originate?
   a. Brainstem
   b. Cerebellar cortex
   c. Cerebral cortex
   d. Corpus callosum
   e. Diencephalon

Chapter 2 **The back**

1. A 70-year-old woman undergoes an X-ray of her vertebral column. The X-ray shows arthritic changes. Which region of the vertebral column is most mobile and therefore, most likely to undergo arthritic change?
   a. Cervical
   b. Coccygeal
   c. Lumbar
   d. Sacral
   e. Thoracic

2. A 21-year-old woman presents to the A&E department complaining of a severe headache and photophobia. She has been vomiting over the past few hours and is becoming increasingly drowsy. The doctors are concerned that she may have meningitis and so after a CT scan, decide to perform a lumbar puncture. Below which of the following vertebral levels is a lumbar puncture safe to perform in an adult?
   a. T10−T1
   b. T11−T12
   c. T12−L1
   d. L1−L2
   e. L2−3

3. The lumbar region is an ideal site of access to the subarachnoid space where a sample of CSF may be obtained without damage to the spinal cord. What feature is used as a landmark when preparing to undertake a lumbar puncture?
   a. Disc between L1 and L2
   b. Disc between L3 and L4
   c. Line between the iliac crests
   d. Lower border of L5 vertebra
   e. Lower border of S2 vertebra

4. Following a car accident a 21-year-old man is taken to hospital with a suspected neck injury. His ability to shrug (elevate) his shoulder against resistance is very weak. Innervation of which muscle has been affected by the trauma?
   a. Deltoid
   b. Latissimus dorsi
   c. Rhomboids
   d. Supraspinatus
   e. Trapezius

5. A 50-year-old man presents to his GP with lower back pain, which radiates into the back of his left thigh and extends along the lateral aspect of his leg. He is diagnosed with a herniated intervertebral disc. Intervertebral joints may undergo degenerative changes resulting in prolapse of the nucleus pulposus, which is part of an intervertebral disc. Through which layer does the nucleus pulposus prolapse in a 'slipped disc'?
   a. Anulus fibrosus
   b. Anterior longitudinal ligament
   c. Articular cartilage
   d. Fibrous capsule
   e. Ligamentum flavum

6. With regard to the patient above, in which direction does the nucleus pulposus most commonly herniate?
   a. Anteriorly
   b. Anterolaterally
   c. Anteromedially
   d. Posteriorly
   e. Posterolaterally

7. A man undergoes a laminectomy (removal of the lamina of a vertebra) in order to relieve pressure on a spinal nerve. Which ligament is attached to the lamina, and therefore would also be removed during this procedure?
   a. Anulus fibrosus
   b. Anterior longitudinal ligament
   c. Ligamentum flavum
   d. Posterior longitudinal ligament
   e. Supraspinous ligament

8. A 39-year-old man presents to his GP with neck pain. As part of the examination his GP asks him to move his head to the left and to the right. At which joint does this movement occur?
   a. Atlanto-axial joint
   b. Atlanto-occipital joint
   c. Intervertebral disc between vertebrae C1 and C2
   d. Intervertebral disc between vertebrae C2 and C3
   e. Zygapophyseal joints between vertebrae C2 and C3

9. A 23-year-old woman is admitted to hospital after a road traffic accident. She sustains whiplash. Whiplash injuries may occur as the result of hyperextension of the cervical region of the vertebral column. Which ligament is most likely to be damaged in a whiplash injury?

   a. Anterior longitudinal ligament
   b. Interspinous ligament
   c. Ligamentum flavum
   d. Ligamentum nuchae
   e. Posterior longitudinal ligament

Chapter 3 **The upper limb**

1. You are an FY1 doctor on the acute receiving ward of your local hospital. A 70-year-old lady presents to you with a left-sided weakness affecting her face, arm and leg. As part of your examination you must perform a neurological examination. You test her upper limb reflexes and find that her biceps reflex is absent on the left. Which nerve roots does this reflex test?
   a. C4/5
   b. C5/6
   c. C6
   d. C6/7
   e. C7

2. A 60-year-old man with known hypothyroidism comes into your surgery for a routine blood test in order to measure his thyroid stimulating hormone level and his

T4 level. Which of the following is the most common site of venepuncture?

a. Basilic vein
b. Brachial artery
c. Cephalic vein
d. Median cubital vein
e. Radial artery

3. A 30-year-old man presents to his GP complaining of pain in his right shoulder. He is eventually diagnosed with a rotator cuff muscle tear. The rotator cuff is composed of which of the following muscles?

a. Deltoid, infraspinatus, supraspinatus, teres major
b. Deltoid, infraspinatus, supraspinatus, teres minor
c. Deltoid, supraspinatus, teres major, teres minor
d. Infraspinatus, subscapularis, supraspinatus, teres minor
e. Infraspinatus, subscapularis, teres major, teres minor

4. A 3-year-old boy is walking in the park with his parents. He trips on a step and his father, who is holding his hand, pulls him upwards to prevent him from falling. Afterwards the child complains of pain in his elbow. In A&E he is diagnosed with a pulled elbow. Pulled elbow results in subluxation of the radial head. Through which structure does the radial head sublux?

a. Anular ligament
b. Radial collateral ligament
c. Tendon of biceps brachii
d. Tendon of triceps brachii
e. Ulnar collateral ligament

5. A 20-year-old man is involved in a motorcycle accident. He suffers a brachial plexus injury, leading to loss of motor and sensory function in his upper limb. The brachial plexus is formed from which nerves?

a. The anterior rami of the C4–C8 spinal nerves
b. The posterior rami of the C4–C8 spinal nerves
c. The anterior rami of the C5–T1 spinal nerves
d. The posterior rami of the C5–T1 spinal nerves
e. The posterior rami of the C6–T2 spinal nerves

6. With regard to the brachial plexus which is the correct order, from proximal to distal, of the divisions of the plexus?

a. Cords, divisions, roots, trunks, branches
b. Cords, roots, branches, divisions, trunks
c. Divisions, cords, roots, branches, trunks
d. Roots, branches, trunks, cords, divisions
e. Roots, trunks, divisions, cords, branches

7. A 60-year-old woman presents to A&E after a fall. She complains of pain in her left hand and upon examination of the hand you elicit tenderness over the anatomical snuffbox.
Which of the following bones has she fractured?

a. Hamate
b. Lunate

c. Pisiform
d. Scaphoid
e. Triquetrum

8. Which of the following comprise the borders of the anatomical snuffbox?

a. Abductor pollicis brevis, extensor pollicis brevis, extensor pollicis longus
b. Abductor pollicis brevis, extensor pollicis brevis, opponens pollicis
c. Abductor pollicis brevis, extensor pollicis longus, opponens pollicis.
d. Abductor pollicis brevis, abductor pollicis longus, extensor pollicis brevis
e. Abductor pollicis longus, extensor pollicis brevis, extensor pollicis longus

9. A 10-year-old boy presents to the accident and emergency department having fallen off a wall. An X-ray confirms a fracture of the clavicle. At which point along his clavicle is the fracture most likely to be?

a. Junction of the middle and lateral thirds
b. Junction of the outer and middle thirds
c. Lateral third
d. Middle third
e. Outer third

10. A 15-year-old girl fell off a horse while riding, landing on her shoulder. On examination she was unable to abduct her right arm to 90°, and had loss of sensation of the skin over the superolateral aspect of the right arm. Which structure is most likely to be damaged?

a. Right axillary nerve
b. Right median nerve
c. Right musculocutaneous nerve
d. Right radial nerve
e. Right ulnar nerve

11. One of your flatmates who went to a party the previous evening complains of weakness in his left fingers and wrist. You perform a neurological examination and find that he has weakness of wrist and finger extension, and loss of sensation over the dorsum of the left hand. He tells you that he fell asleep with his left arm over the back of a chair. Which nerve is he likely to have injured?

a. Left axillary nerve
b. Left median nerve
c. Left musculocutaneous nerve
d. Left radial nerve
e. Left ulnar nerve

12. A 45-year-old woman comes to see you in her surgery complaining of a pain and pins and needles in her left thumb, index and middle fingers, and lateral half of her ring finger. She says the symptoms are worse at night. On examination you notice that the thenar muscles of her left hand appear wasted compared to those on the right. Which structure is affected?

a. The left axillary nerve
b. The left median nerve

c. The left musculocutaneous nerve
d. The left radial nerve
e. The left ulnar nerve

13. A 45-year-old man who works in a factory injures his right hand with a saw. On examination in the A&E department you find lacerations across the anterior surfaces of his right index, middle and ring fingers. On examination he is able to flex the distal interphalangeal joints of these fingers, however, he is unable to flex the proximal interphalangeal joints of these fingers. Which structure has he damaged?
a. Flexor digitorum profundus muscle
b. Flexor digitorum superficialis muscle
c. Median nerve
d. Palmaris longus muscle
e. Ulnar nerve

14. A 50-year-old man presents with clumsiness affecting his hands. The doctor tests the function of the muscles in his hands. She asks him to spread his fingers against resistance. Which muscles are being tested?
a. Dorsal interossei
b. Hypothenar muscles
c. Lumbricals
d. Palmar interossei
e. Thenar muscles

15. A 16-year-old rugby player presents to A&E with a painful left shoulder. An examination and X-ray of the shoulder reveals dislocation of the left glenohumeral joint. In which direction is his shoulder most likely to have dislocated?
a. Anteriorly
b. Inferiorly
c. Posteriorly
d. Posterolaterally
e. Superiorly

16. What would you tell the patient in question 15 when he asks if his shoulder is likely to dislocate again?
a. That he has approximately a 10% chance of recurrence
b. That he has approximately a 20% chance of recurrence
c. That he has approximately a 40% chance of recurrence
d. That he has approximately a 60% chance of recurrence
e. That he has approximately an 80% chance of recurrence

17. A 39-year-old woman presents to you having noticed a lump in her right breast. On examination you feel a lump in the upper outer quadrant of the breast. As part of the examination you must also palpate nearby lymph nodes. To which nodes does the majority of the lymph from the breast drain?
a. Apical
b. Central
c. Lateral

d. Pectoral
e. Subscapular

18. A 42-year-old woman comes to see you complaining of weakness in her left hand. She has also noticed that her ring and little fingers feel numb. On examination you find reduction in power of the intrinsic muscles of the hand, and loss of sensation on the skin of her little finger and the medial half of her ring finger. Which nerve is affected?
a. Axillary nerve
b. Median nerve
c. Musculocutaneous nerve
d. Radial nerve
e. Ulnar nerve

Chapter 4 The thorax

1. Whilst on attachment to an orthopaedic ward you are asked to perform an ECG on a patient who is experiencing chest pain. What is the correct placement of the chest leads when performing an ECG?
a. V1 in the suprasternal notch. V2 and V3 in the 5th intercostal space on either side of the sternum. V4 in the 5th intercostal space in the midclavicular line. V3 between V2 and V4. V6 in the midaxillary line, with V5 between V4 and V6
b. V1 in the 2nd intercostal space on the left, V2 and V3 in the 5th intercostal space on either side of the sternum. V4 in the 5th intercostal space in the midclavicular line. V6 in the midaxillary line, with V5 between V4 and V6
c. V1 and V2 in the 4th intercostal space on either side of the sternum. V4 in the 5th intercostal space in the midclavicular line. V3 between V2 and V4. V6 in the midaxillary line, with V5 between V4 and V6
d. V1 and V2 in the 5th intercostal space on either side of the sternum. V4 in the 5th intercostal space in the midclavicular line. V3 between V2 and V4. V6 in the midaxillary line, with V5 between V4 and V6
e. V1 and V2 in the 5th intercostal space on either side of the sternum. V5 in the 5th intercostal space in the midclavicular line. V3 and V4 between V2 and V5. V6 in the midaxillary line

2. A 25-year-old woman presents with abdominal pain. She is to undergo an exploratory laparoscopy. She is informed by the surgeon that postoperatively, she may experience referred pain around her shoulder. He explains that this is because the carbon dioxide used to inflate the abdomen during laparoscopy accumulates under the diaphragm, causing irritation. Which nerve is responsible for this effect?
a. Accessory
b. Axillary
c. Phrenic

d. Sympathetic trunk
e. Vagus

3. A 68-year-old male smoker presents to you with a 3-month history of worsening cough, unintentional weight loss and that morning, an episode of haemoptysis. You notice that his left eyelid appears to be drooping. What is the likely diagnosis given this combination of symptoms and signs?
   a. A tumour at the apex of his left lung
   b. A tumour at the hilum of his left lung
   c. A tumour at the apex of his right lung
   d. A tumour at the lower lobe of his right lung
   e. A tumour at the lower lobe of his right lung

4. The presence of a partial ptosis makes you suspect this patient may have Horner's syndrome. What other signs would you look for to confirm your diagnosis?
   a. Dilated pupil and facial redness on the left
   b. Dilated pupil and facial sweating on the left
   c. Constricted pupil and facial redness on the left
   d. Constricted pupil and exophthalmos on the left
   e. Dilated pupil, and a dry eye on the right

5. In this man, paralysis of which muscle is responsible for his partial ptosis.
   a. Frontalis
   b. Orbicularis oculi (lacrimal part)
   c. Orbicularis oculi (palpebral part)
   d. Superior oblique
   e. Superior tarsal muscle (smooth muscle portion of levator palpebrae superioris)

6. Some months later the man develops a hoarse voice. He undergoes a CT scan which shows enlargement of the left hilar lymph nodes. Which structure is being affected by the enlarged nodes and thus causing his hoarse voice?
   a. Left main bronchus
   b. Left phrenic nerve
   c. Left recurrent laryngeal nerve
   d. Left sympathetic trunk
   e. Left vagus nerve

7. A 55-year-old woman undergoes a mammogram which reveals an abnormality in her right breast. She attends a breast clinic where she is examined for signs of breast cancer. With regard to the anatomy of the breast which of the following statements is true?
   a. The breasts lie in the deep fascia
   b. The breast lies deep to pectoralis major and serratus anterior muscles
   c. The breast is composed of 15–20 lobules
   d. The base of the breast lies between the 1st and 8th rib vertically
   e. The majority of lymph from the breast drains to the parasternal nodes

8. She is diagnosed with a malignant tumour for which she undergoes a right-sided radical mastectomy.

At a follow-up examination, you note that she has winging of her right scapula. This has occurred due to injury to:
   a. Right accessory nerve
   b. Right long thoracic nerve
   c. Right supraclavicular nerve
   d. Right suprascapular nerve
   e. Right thoracodorsal nerve

9. A 15-year-old boy chokes on a peanut. Where in the respiratory tract is the peanut most likely to lodge?
   a. Left lower lobar bronchus
   b. Left main bronchus
   c. Left superior segmental bronchus
   d. Right lower lobar bronchus
   e. Right main bronchus

10. A 30-year-old man presents with acute dyspnoea, tachycardia and tachypnoea. He is diagnosed with a left-sided pneumothorax and a chest drain is inserted. What is the correct order of the layers through which a chest drain must be passed?
    a. Skin, endothoracic fascia, superficial fascia, external intercostal, internal intercostal, innermost intercostal, parietal pleura
    b. Skin, external intercostal, internal intercostal, innermost intercostal, superficial fascia, endothoracic fascia, parietal pleura
    c. Skin, superficial fascia, endothoracic fascia, external intercostal, internal intercostal, innermost intercostal, parietal pleura
    d. Skin, superficial fascia, external intercostal, internal intercostal, innermost intercostal, endothoracic fascia, parietal pleura
    e. Skin, superficial fascia, external intercostal, internal intercostal, innermost intercostal, parietal pleura, endothoracic fascia

11. With reference to the patient above, which of the following describes the correct location for the insertion of a chest drain?
    a. At the apex of the left lung between the clavicle and the first rib
    b. Costodiaphragmatic recess on the left
    c. Left 2nd intercostal space in the midclavicular line
    d. Left 5th intercostal space in the midaxillary line
    e. Left 2nd intercostal space in the midaxillary line

12. An 18-year-old man presents to A&E after a fight. He complains of pain in his chest, and is tender to palpation. A chest X-ray confirms fractures of the 4th–6th ribs. The intercostal neurovascular bundles are vulnerable to damage from fractured ribs because of their position. What is the position of the intercostal neurovascular bundle?
    a. Between the external and internal intercostal muscles
    b. Deep to the endothoracic fascia
    c. Deep to the posterior intercostal membrane
    d. In the costal groove
    e. Superficial to the ribs

13. A 65-year-old man presents to A&E with chest pain. The pain is crushing, radiates to his left arm and jaw and is associated with nausea and sweating. An ECG shows he is having a myocardial infarction. He undergoes primary coronary intervention (PCI) and is found to have occlusions in several of his coronary arteries, secondary to atheroma. Which coronary artery is most likely to be affected by atheroma?
    a. Anterior interventricular artery
    b. Circumflex artery
    c. Left marginal artery
    d. Posterior interventricular artery
    e. Right marginal artery

14. Several months later the man is readmitted to hospital suffering from a further myocardial infarction. He is bradycardic with a heart rate of 36 beats per minute. It is thought that the infarction has affected his sinoatrial (SA) node. Which artery most commonly supplies the SA node?
    a. Anterior interventricular artery
    b. Circumflex artery
    c. Left coronary artery
    d. Posterior interventricular artery
    e. Right coronary artery

15. The patient continues to suffer from angina, and eventually undergoes a coronary artery bypass. During surgery, the anterior interventricular artery is located. Which vein lies adjacent to the anterior interventricular artery?
    a. Anterior cardiac vein
    b. Coronary sinus
    c. Great cardiac vein
    d. Middle cardiac vein
    e. Small cardiac vein

16. The veins of the heart drain into the coronary sinus. Into which structure does the coronary sinus drain?
    a. Inferior vena cava
    b. Left atrium
    c. Right atrium
    d. Right auricular appendage
    e. Superior vena cava

17. A 25-year-old man presents to A&E. He has been stabbed in the neck on the right side. He complains of shortness of breath and is tachypnoeic. A chest X-ray shows a pneumothorax and a raised right hemidiaphragm. Which of the following is true with regard to the diaphragm?
    a. The centre is muscular and the periphery is tendinous
    b. The diaphragm is pierced by the IVC at T12
    c. The diaphragm is pierced by the oesophagus at T8
    d. The left dome is higher than the right
    e. The motor supply arises from the phrenic nerve

18. Several important structures pass through the diaphragm. Which structure passes through at the level of T10?
    a. Aorta
    b. Azygos vein
    c. Branches of the left gastric artery
    d. Right phrenic nerve
    e. Thoracic duct

Chapter 5 The abdomen

1. A 45-year-old man presents to his local hospital complaining of pain in his back which radiates around his right side and extends into his groin. He is diagnosed with renal calculi. At which site are renal calculi most likely to lodge?
    a. Neck of the bladder
    b. Nephron of the kidney
    c. Pelvic brim
    d. Where the ureter is crossed by the colic vessels
    e. Where the ureter crosses the transverse processes of the lumbar vertebrae

2. An 18-year-old girl presents with pain in the right iliac fossa, pyrexia and vomiting. She is diagnosed with appendicitis and undergoes appendicectomy. The base of the appendix lies deep to McBurney's point. Which of the following best describes the location of McBurney's point?
    a. It lies one-third of the way between ASIS and the umbilicus
    b. It lies one-third of the way between the umbilicus and ASIS
    c. It lies two-thirds of the way between ASIS and the umbilicus
    d. It lies one-third of the way between PSIS and the umbilicus
    e. It lies two-thirds of the way between ASIS and the umbilicus

3. When the surgeon makes an incision in order to reach the appendix, what is the correct order of the layers of the abdominal wall, through which the scalpel must pass in order to reach the appendix?
    a. Internal oblique, external oblique, peritoneum, transversus abdominis
    b. External oblique, internal oblique, peritoneum, transversus abdominis
    c. External oblique, internal oblique, transversus abdominis, peritoneum
    d. Internal oblique, peritoneum, external oblique, transversus abdominis
    e. Rectus abdominis, external oblique, internal oblique, peritoneum

4. The appendicular artery supplies the appendix. It is a branch of which of the following arteries?
    a. Anterior caecal artery
    b. Ileal artery
    c. Ileocolic artery
    d. Inferior mesenteric artery
    e. Right colic artery

5. A 24-year-old male comes to see you complaining of a dragging sensation in his scrotum. On examination you find that he has a visible and palpable swelling in the right side of his scrotum, which feels like a sac of worms. When the patient lies down the area of swelling disappears. Which of the following conditions accounts for this patient's symptoms and signs?
   a. Haematocoele
   b. Hydrocoele
   c. Spermatocoele
   d. Testicular torsion
   e. Varicocoele

6. A 30-year-old man who presented with a lump in his left testicle is diagnosed with a malignant tumour. To which lymph nodes do testicular tumours most commonly metastasize?
   a. Deep inguinal
   b. Femoral nodes
   c. Lumbar nodes
   d. Para-aortic nodes
   e. Superficial inguinal

7. A 75-year-old man presents to his GP complaining of a swelling in his groin. On examination the GP observes a visible bulge in his right groin, which has a cough impulse and can be reduced by gentle pressure. He suspects it is a direct inguinal hernia. Which of the following is true with regard to direct inguinal hernias?
   a. They arise medial to the inferior epigastric artery
   b. They occur only in young men
   c. They occur secondary to a patent processus vaginalis
   d. They pass lateral to the inferior epigastric artery
   e. They pass through the deep inguinal ring

8. The next patient of the GP in the question above presents with a swelling in his scrotum. The patient is a 25-year-old builder who is otherwise fit and well. He says the swelling appeared after he had been lifting some heavy equipment at work. On examination the GP observes that his scrotum is enlarged on the left side. He suspects that this patient has an indirect inguinal hernia. Which of the following is true with regard to indirect inguinal hernias?
   a. They arise medial to the inferior epigastric artery
   b. They occur mostly in older men
   c. They occur secondary to a defect in the transversus abdominis muscle
   d. They pass lateral to the inferior epigastric artery
   e. They pass through Hesselbach's triangle

9. Inguinal hernias may exit the superficial inguinal ring. The spermatic cord also exits through the superficial inguinal ring. The external spermatic fascia is one of the coverings of the spermatic cord. From which of the following layers does it arise?
   a. Aponeurosis of external oblique
   b. Aponeurosis of internal oblique
   c. Extraperitoneal fascia

   d. Transversalis fascia
   e. Tunica vaginalis

10. Direct inguinal hernias pass through Hesselbach's triangle in the posterior wall of the inguinal canal. What are the boundaries of Hesselbach's triangle?
    a. Conjoint tendon, inferior epigastric vessels, inguinal ligament
    b. Conjoint tendon, inferior epigastric vessels, rectus sheath
    c. Conjoint tendon, superior epigastric vessels, inguinal ligament
    d. Rectus sheath, inferior epigastric vessels, inguinal ligament
    e. Rectus sheath, superior epigastric vessels, inguinal ligament

11. Inguinal hernias may extend into the scrotum. Which of the following lists the correct order of the layers within the wall of the scrotum?
    a. Skin, cremasteric fascia, superficial fascia, internal spermatic fascia, external spermatic fascia, parietal layer of the tunica vaginalis
    b. Skin, superficial fascia, cremasteric fascia, external spermatic fascia, internal spermatic fascia, parietal layer of the tunica vaginalis
    c. Skin, superficial fascia, external spermatic fascia, cremasteric fascia, internal spermatic fascia, parietal layer of the tunica vaginalis
    d. Skin, superficial fascia, external spermatic fascia, internal spermatic fascia, cremasteric fascia, parietal layer of the tunica vaginalis
    e. Skin, superficial fascia, internal spermatic fascia, cremasteric fascia, external spermatic fascia, visceral layer of the tunica vaginalis

12. A 17-year-old boy presents to A&E with a painful swollen right testicle. He appears to be in severe pain and has vomited twice since arrival in A&E. When you see him you suspect he may have testicular torsion. In testicular torsion the spermatic cord becomes twisted. Which of the following describes the contents of the spermatic cord?
    a. Ductus deferens, artery to the ductus deferens, cremasteric artery, testicular artery, genitofemoral branch of the genitofemoral nerve, sympathetic nerves, lymph vessels, pampiniform plexus of veins, processus vaginalis
    b. Ductus deferens, artery to the ductus deferens, inferior epigastric artery, testicular artery, femoral branch of the genitofemoral nerve, sympathetic nerves, lymph vessels, pampiniform plexus of veins, processus vaginalis
    c. Ductus deferens, artery to the ductus deferens, femoral artery, testicular artery, genitofemoral branch of the genitofemoral nerve, sympathetic nerves, lymph vessels, pampiniform plexus of veins, processus vaginalis
    d. Ductus deferens, artery to the ductus deferens, femoral artery, testicular artery, ilioinguinal nerve,

sympathetic nerves, lymph vessels, pampiniform plexus of veins, processus vaginalis

e. Ductus deferens, external pudendal artery, cremasteric artery, testicular artery, genitofemoral branch of the genitofemoral nerve, sympathetic nerves, lymph vessels, pampiniform plexus of veins, processus vaginalis

13. A 50-year-old woman who was admitted with worsening jaundice, dark urine, pale stools and pain in the right upper quadrant is diagnosed with gallstones. The common bile duct drains into which of the following?
   a. 1st part of the duodenum
   b. 2nd part of the duodenum
   c. 3rd part of the duodenum
   d. 4th part of the duodenum
   e. Junction of the 2nd and 3rd parts of the duodenum

14. The patient undergoes cholecystectomy. The fundus of the gallbladder lies posterior to which costal cartilage, at the intersection of the transpyloric plane with the costal margin?
   a. 6th costal cartilage
   b. 7th costal cartilage
   c. 8th costal cartilage
   d. 9th costal cartilage
   e. 10th costal cartilage

15. An 80-year-old man presents with severe abdominal pain. He undergoes a CT scan which shows ischaemic bowel. At laparotomy, he has a region of ischaemic gut extending from approximately two-thirds of the way along his transverse colon to the distal part of his sigmoid colon. Which blood vessel has become occluded, causing this pattern of ischaemia?
   a. Coeliac trunk
   b. Inferior mesenteric artery
   c. Rectal artery
   d. Sigmoid artery
   e. Superior mesenteric artery

16. An erect chest X-ray reveals air under the right hemi-diaphragm. What is the diagnosis?
   a. No pathology − this is a normal finding
   b. Perforated abdominal viscus
   c. Pneumonia
   d. Right-sided pneumothorax
   e. Small bowel obstruction

17. A 35-year-old man presents with haematemesis (vomiting blood). He undergoes an emergency endoscopy and is diagnosed with a gastric ulcer on the posterior wall of the stomach. Which blood vessel is most likely to have been eroded by the presence of the ulcer?
   a. Gastroduodenal artery
   b. Hepatic artery
   c. Left gastric artery
   d. Right gastric artery
   e. Splenic artery

18. A 15-year-old girl presents with abdominal pain. Her history reveals that her pain is around the umbilical region. Which part of the gastrointestinal tract is likely to be the cause of her pain?
   a. Ascending colon
   b. Duodenum
   c. Ileum
   d. Jejunum
   e. Stomach

19. A 38-year-old man, who is an alcoholic and is known to have cirrhosis of the liver, is admitted to A&E after having vomited a large amount of blood. He undergoes an upper gastrointestinal endoscopy which reveals the presence of oesophageal varices. The anastomosis of which vessels results in the formation of oesophageal varices?
   a. Hepatic portal vein and right gastric vein
   b. Left gastric vein and azygos vein
   c. Right gastric vein and azygos vein
   d. Splenic vein and azygos vein
   e. Splenic vein and hepatic portal vein

20. With regard to the liver, which of the following is true?
   a. It is completely covered by peritoneum except over its anterior surface
   b. Deoxygenated blood exits the liver via the porta hepatis
   c. The bare area of the liver lies in direct contact with the stomach
   d. The division into left, quadrate and caudate lobes is based on function
   e. The falciform ligament attaches the liver to the anterior abdominal wall

Chapter 6 The pelvis and perineum

1. A 36-year-old woman is a pedestrian in a road traffic accident. She sustains a fracture of her pelvis. Which of the following is true with regard to the pelvis?
   a. The greater or false pelvis lies below the pelvic brim
   b. The sacrum is attached to the hip bones via two synovial joints
   c. The pubic tubercle lies in the midline
   d. When standing upright, the anterior inferior iliac spines and pubic symphysis lie in the same vertical plane
   e. The male pubic arch is wider than the female pubic arch

2. Which of the following correctly describes the boundaries of the pelvic inlet?
   a. Inferior border of the pubic symphysis, posterior border of the pubic crest, pectineal line, arcuate line of the ilium, anterior borders of the ala of the sacrum, sacral promontory
   b. Inferior border of the pubic symphysis, superior border of the pubic crest, pectineal line, arcuate

line of the ilium, anterior borders of the ala of the sacrum, sacral promontory

c. Superior border of the pubic symphysis, posterior border of the pubic crest, pectineal line, arcuate line of the ilium, anterior borders of the ala of the sacrum, sacral promontory

d. Superior border of the pubic symphysis, posterior border of the pubic crest, pectineal line, arcuate line of the ilium, superior borders of the ala of the sacrum, sacral promontory

e. Superior border of the pubic symphysis, posterior border of the pubic crest, pectineal line, arcuate line of the ilium, posterior borders of the ala of the sacrum, sacral promontory

3. Following the birth of her second child, a 40-year-old woman presents to her GP with faecal incontinence. She attends the gynaecology department of her local hospital where investigation reveals that she sustained damage to the muscles of her pelvic floor during the delivery of her baby. Injury to which structure is responsible for her faecal incontinence?
   a. Deep transverse perineal muscle
   b. External anal sphincter
   c. Iliococcygeus
   d. Internal anal sphincter
   e. Puborectalis

4. Which nerve supplies the muscle responsible for this patient's incontinence?
   a. Inferior rectal nerve
   b. Nerve to obturator internus
   c. Obturator nerve
   d. Pudendal nerve
   e. Superior rectal nerve

5. Which of the following is true with regard to the rectum?
   a. It commences where the sigmoid mesocolon ends
   b. The rectum is supplied by branches of the superior mesenteric artery
   c. The rectum has taeniae coli
   d. The rectovesical pouch in females separates the rectum from the bladder
   e. The middle third of the rectum is covered laterally by peritoneum

6. A 47-year-old woman presents with pain and swelling in the perineal area. Her past medical history includes arthritis and Crohn's disease. She is diagnosed with an abscess in the ischioanal fossa. The ischioanal fossa lies in the perineum. Which of the following is true with regard to the perineum?
   a. It can be divided into an anterior (anal) triangle and a posterior (urogenital) triangle
   b. The line dividing anal and urogenital triangles runs between the two ischial tuberosities
   c. The structures of the perineum are supplied by the obturator artery and nerve
   d. The urogenital triangle contains the perineal membrane, which lies above the pelvic floor

e. The ischioanal fossa is filled with venous plexuses which enlarge to form haemorrhoids

7. A 75-year-old man presents to his GP with difficulty in passing urine. He describes frequency, urgency, nocturia and terminal dribbling. He is diagnosed with benign prostatic hyperplasia. Which region of the prostate is most likely to be affected by BPH?
   a. Anterior lobe
   b. Lateral lobes
   c. Middle lobe
   d. Peripheral zone
   e. Posterior lobe

8. An 80-year-old man who presented with weight loss, back pain, nocturia, frequency and urgency is diagnosed with prostate cancer. Which lobe of the prostate is most likely to be affected by prostate cancer?
   a. Anterior
   b. Posterior
   c. Left lateral
   d. Right lateral
   e. Middle

9. A 25-year-old woman presents to her GP with pelvic pain. She undergoes an examination including a bimanual vaginal examination. In which position is the GP most likely to find her uterus?
   a. Anteflexed and anteverted
   b. Anteflexed and inverted
   c. Anteflexed and retroverted
   d. Retroflexed and anterverted
   e. Retroflexed and retroverted

10. A 65-year-old woman presents to her GP having noticed blood in her urine. She has also, for the past few weeks experienced urinary frequency and urgency. She undergoes a cystoscopy and biopsy and is diagnosed with a malignant tumour of the bladder. What type of epithelium lines the internal surface of the bladder?
    a. Columnar epithelium
    b. Cuboidal epithelium
    c. Keratinized stratified squamous epithelium
    d. Stratified squamous epithelium
    e. Transitional epithelium

11. With reference to the patient above, to which lymph nodes is this tumour most likely to metastasize?
    a. Coeliac nodes
    b. Iliac nodes
    c. Inguinal nodes
    d. Para-aortic nodes
    e. Sacral nodes

12. Which of the following is true with regard to the bladder and the ureters?
    a. The ureters turn posteriorly towards the bladder at the level of the ischial spines
    b. The base of the bladder is related to internal sexual organs in both sexes

c. In the female the uterine artery passes inferior to the ureter
d. Detrusor muscle has a sympathetic nerve supply
e. The trigone is a ridged area of mucosa lying between urethral and ureteric orifices

13. A 59-year-old woman undergoes a hysterectomy after a diagnosis of endometrial cancer. When ligating the uterine arteries, the surgeon must be particularly careful to avoid damage to which structure?
a. Obturator artery
b. Pudendal nerve
c. Ureters
d. Uterine vein
e. Uterine tube

14. A 34-year-old woman attends her GP as she believes she is pregnant. Where in the uterine tube does fertilization normally occur?
a. Ampulla
b. Infundibululm
c. Isthmus
d. Ovary
e. Uterus

15. A 20-year-old woman is admitted to A&E with pain in the right iliac fossa. She is tachycardic and hypotensive, with a mild pyrexia. She is diagnosed with appendicitis. In this patient, what is the most important differential diagnosis which must be excluded?
a. Cholecystitis
b. Ectopic pregnancy
c. Gastroenteritis
d. Pancreatitis
e. Perforated peptic ulcer

Chapter 7 The lower limb

1. A 60-year-old man presents to you complaining of difficulty in walking. When you ask the patient to lift their right foot off the floor, Trendelenburg's sign is positive. Which muscles are the cause of the abnormal test result?
a. Gluteus maximus and gluteus medius on the left
b. Gluteus maximus and gluteus medius on the right
c. Gluteus maximus and gluteus minimus on the right
d. Gluteus medius and gluteus minimus on the left
e. Gluteus medius and gluteus minimus on the right

2. With reference to the patient above, which nerve supplies the affected muscles?
a. Femoral nerve
b. Inferior gluteal nerve
c. Pudendal nerve
d. Sciatic nerve
e. Superior gluteal nerve

3. Concerning the gluteal region:
a. Abduction of the hip is performed by all three gluteal muscles
b. All the structures that pass from the greater sciatic foramen to supply the gluteal region and lower limb lie inferior to the piriformis muscle
c. Cutaneous innervation is supplied by the gluteal branches of the anterior rami of lumbar and sacral nerves
d. The close fit of the femoral head in the acetabulum does not contribute to the stability of the hip joint
e. The pudendal nerve exits the pelvis through the greater sciatic foramen and re-enters through the lesser sciatic foramen

4. Through which foramen does the left superior gluteal nerve pass to reach the muscles it supplies?
a. Left greater sciatic foramen
b. Left lesser sciatic foramen
c. Left obturator foramen
d. Right greater sciatic foramen
e. Right lesser sciatic foramen

5. An 18-year-old man presents to A&E after a fall. He has injured his ankle and despite being able to weight-bear his ankle appears swollen and bruised. He is diagnosed with a sprained ankle. Which ligament is the most commonly injured in ankle sprains?
a. The anterior talofibular ligament on the lateral side
b. The calcaneofibular ligament on the lateral side
c. The deltoid ligament on the lateral side
d. The deltoid ligament on the medial side
e. The posterior talofibular ligament on the medial side

6. A 75-year-old woman presents with pain in her left hip. On examination you find that she has difficulty in all movements of the hip, although she appears to have the greatest difficulty with extension of the joint. Which of the following is true with regard to movements at the hip joint?
a. Flexion is limited by the pubofemoral and iliofemoral ligaments
b. The anteroposterior axis of abduction-adduction passes through the femoral neck
c. The axis of rotation passes through the femoral neck and femoral medial condyle
d. The gluteus medius and minimus muscles resist excessive adduction
e. The ischiofemoral ligament is stretched by lateral rotation

7. You are called to see a 35-year-old man who was admitted to hospital earlier that day. He was involved in a road traffic accident and sustained a fracture of his left tibia. He is now complaining of pain, and on examination his leg appears white and cold. You are unable to palpate his foot pulses. He is diagnosed with compartment syndrome affecting the extensor

compartment of his leg. Which nerve supplies the extensor compartment of the leg?
a. Deep peroneal nerve
b. Femoral nerve
c. Sciatic nerve
d. Superficial peroneal nerve
e. Sural nerve

8. As part of your examination you palpate his peripheral pulses in both lower limbs. Which of the following correctly describes the location of the peripheral pulses of the lower limbs?
a. Femoral pulse – one-third of the way between ASIS and the pubic symphysis
b. Femoral pulse – two-thirds of the way between ASIS and the pubic symphysis
c. Dorsalis pedis pulse – between the tendons of extensor hallucis brevis and extensor digitorum longus
d. Popliteal pulse – in the popliteal fossa
e. Posterior tibial pulse – posterior to the lateral malleolus

9. An 80-year-old woman undergoes an X-ray of her right knee after complaining of pain and stiffness, which is worse after exertion. The X-ray shows changes that indicate that she has osteoarthritis of her knee. What are the typical X-ray changes found in osteoarthritis?
a. Loss of joint space, subchondral sclerosis, osteophytes and joint erosion
b. Loss of joint space, subchondral sclerosis, osteophytes and subchondral cysts
c. Soft tissue swelling, loss of joint space, osteophytes and subchondral cysts
d. Soft tissue swelling, loss of joint space, subchondral sclerosis and marginal erosion
e. Soft tissue swelling, subchondral sclerosis, osteophytes and subchondral cysts

10. A 13-year-old boy falls from his skateboard and lacerates the lateral side of his left leg several centimetres below his knee. On examination in A&E, the wound appears to be superficial, the skin is sutured and the boy is sent home. The next day he notices that the toe of his shoe is scraping the ground whilst he is walking. He returns to A&E where examination reveals he has sustained damage to a nerve in his leg. Which nerve has been damaged?
a. Common peroneal nerve
b. Saphenous nerve
c. Sciatic nerve
d. Sural nerve
e. Tibial nerve

11. An 80-year-old man is brought into A&E having been found unconscious at home. You are asked to gain intravenous access in order to take blood samples and give intravenous fluids. However, the patient is clinically shocked and you are unable to do so. Your consultant decides to gain intravenous access via a saphenous cutdown (an incision is made allowing

access to the great saphenous vein). At which of the following points should the incision be made?
a. Anterior to the lateral malleolus
b. Anterior to the medial malleolus
c. Lateral to the extensor hallucis longus tendon
d. Posterior to the lateral malleolus
e. Posterior to the medial malleolus

12. A 50-year-old woman undergoes surgery for varicose veins, particularly affecting her great saphenous vein. Which of the following is true with regard to the great saphenous vein?
a. It passes posterior to the medial malleolus
b. It drains into the femoral vein
c. It lies in the deep fascia of the leg
d. It passes posterior to the lateral malleolus
e. It receives blood from the inferior epigastric vein

13. The femoral vein lies in the femoral triangle. Which of the following is true with regard to the femoral triangle?
a. The femoral vein, artery and nerve lie in the femoral sheath
b. The femoral nerve lies most laterally in the femoral triangle
c. The medial border of the femoral triangle is formed by the medial border of the adductor magnus muscle
d. The femoral canal is bounded proximally by the conjoint tendon, lacunar ligament, pectinate line (of pubis) and femoral vein
e. The floor of the femoral triangle is formed by the iliopsoas, pectineus, adductor longus and vastus medialis muscles

14. A 25-year-old man presents to his GP, having injured his knee the previous day, playing football. His knee is swollen and painful, and he is unable to extend it fully. After examining his knee his GP decides he has probably ruptured his anterior cruciate ligament (ACL). Which of the following is true with regard to the ACL?
a. It passes between the lateral femoral condyle and the anterior intercondylar area of the tibia
b. It passes between the lateral femoral condyle and the posterior intercondylar area of the tibia
c. It passes between the medial femoral condyle and the anterior intercondylar area of the tibia
d. It passes between the medial femoral epicondyle and the anterior intercondylar area of the tibia
e. It passes between the medial femoral epicondyle and the posterior intercondylar area of the tibia

15. Which of the following is true with regard to the knee joint?
a. The knee joint is an articulation between the femur, tibia and fibula
b. Only flexion and extension movements are possible at the knee joint
c. The cavity of the knee joint communicates with the suprapatellar bursa
d. The anterior cruciate ligament prevents anterior displacement of the femur when tibia is fixed

e. Inflammation of the prepatellar bursa is known as clergyman's knee

16. A 60-year-old man presents to his GP with a swelling in his popliteal fossa. He complains that his knee is stiff. After examining the man's knee the GP suspects the swelling is a Baker's cyst (a posterior herniation of the knee joint capsule, which allows synovial fluid to enter one of the posterior bursae of the knee). Many of the structures in the popliteal fossa are difficult to palpate upon examination. Which of the following is true?
   a. The popliteal vein is the deepest structure of the popliteal fossa
   b. The popliteal artery has no branches in the popliteal fossa
   c. The small saphenous vein joins the popliteal vein in the popliteal fossa
   d. The upper boundaries of the fossa are formed by the semimembranosus and biceps femoris muscles only
   e. The popliteus muscle locks the knee joint

Chapter 8 The head and neck

1. The mother of a 10-day-old baby girl tells her midwife she is concerned about her baby as she can feel a soft spot on the top of her head. The midwife reassures the woman that this is normal, explaining that the soft area she can feel is known as the anterior fontanelle. The anterior fontanelle lies at the junction between the frontal and parietal bones. What type of joint connects the bones of the skull?
   a. Fibrous joint − syndesmosis
   b. Fibrous joint − sutures
   c. Primary cartilaginous joint
   d. Secondary cartilaginous joint
   e. Synovial joint

2. A 20-year-old man presents to A&E with a reduced level of consciousness (Glasgow coma score − 13: E3, V4, M6) and confusion. His girlfriend tells you that he fell over earlier that day and hit the side of his head on some steps. He briefly lost consciousness, but recovered quickly and did not appear to have any injuries as a result of the fall. An X-ray and CT scan show that the patient has suffered a skull fracture and an extradural haemorrhage. In which region of the skull is the fracture most likely to have occurred?
   a. Bregma
   b. Lambda
   c. Occiput
   d. Orbit
   e. Pterion

3. Given the location of the patient's fracture, which vessel has been ruptured?
   a. Middle cerebral artery
   b. Middle meningeal artery

c. Occipital artery
d. Superficial temporal artery
e. Supraorbital artery

4. With reference to the previous question, through which of the following foramina does the middle meningeal artery pass?
   a. The foramen ovale
   b. The foramen lacerum
   c. The foramen magnum
   d. The foramen rotundum
   e. The foramen spinosum

5. A 45-year-old woman presents to you with loss of vision in her right eye which has come on over a few hours. She also complains of pain when she moves her eye and feels that colours are not as bright as they usually are when seen through her right eye. She is known to have multiple sclerosis. After testing her vision you suspect she has optic neuritis (inflammation of the optic nerve) secondary to multiple sclerosis. Which of the following is true regarding the optic nerve?
   a. It is the only structure to pass through the optic canal
   b. It passes through the optic canal with the ophthalmic vein
   c. It passes through the optic canal with the ophthalmic artery
   d. It reaches the eye by passing through the superior orbital fissure
   e. It reaches the eye by passing through the inferior orbital fissure

6. An 18-year-old man presents to A&E after a fight. His nose is bleeding and swollen and you suspect it might be broken. Which of the following is true with regard to the nasal cavity?
   a. The cribriform plate forms part of the roof
   b. The ethmoid bone forms the lateral wall
   c. The maxilla forms part of the roof
   d. The palatine bone forms part of the roof
   e. The vomer forms the lateral wall

7. A 50-year-old man presents to A&E with epistaxis (a nosebleed). He tells you that this is the second time this has happened in 24 hours, but on this occasion the bleeding is much heavier. Little's area is the region of the nose in which epistaxis is most likely to occur. In which part of the nose is Little's area located?
   a. Anteroinferior part of the nasal septum
   b. Floor of the nasal cavity
   c. Lateral wall of the nose
   d. Posterosuperior part of the nasal septum
   e. Roof of the nasal cavity

8. You are performing a cranial nerve examination on a 20-year-old woman. When you test her extraocular muscles you ask her to look to the right, and you find she is unable to adduct her left eye. Which muscle is affected?
   a. Inferior oblique

b. Lateral rectus
c. Medial rectus
d. Superior oblique
e. Trochlear

9. Which nerve supplies this muscle?
    a. Abducens nerve
    b. Facial nerve
    c. Nasociliary nerve
    d. Oculomotor nerve
    e. Trochlear nerve

10. You are asked to test the eye movements of a 10-year-old boy. How would you test the function of his left trochlear nerve? Ask him to move his left eye:
    a. Inward, toward the nose and downward
    b. Inward, toward the nose and upward
    c. Laterally, in a horizontal plan
    d. Medially, in a horizontal plane
    e. Outward, away from the nose and downward

11. A 25-year-old man presents to A&E with a temperature, headache, vomiting and photophobia. He undergoes a lumbar puncture for suspected meningitis. Cerebrospinal fluid (CSF) is removed and sent for microscopy and culture. CSF drains via arachnoid granulations, into which structure?
    a. Cavernous sinus
    b. Choroid plexus
    c. Jugular vein
    d. Petrosal sinus
    e. Superior sagittal sinus

12. A 38-year-old woman attends her optician as she has been experiencing problems with her vision. The results of her eye test concern her optician and so he refers her to the local hospital for further investigation. She undergoes a CT scan which reveals a pituitary adenoma, compressing the optic chiasma. This will result in which of the following?
    a. Complete blindness
    b. Loss of left and right inferior fields of vision
    c. Loss of left and right temporal (outer) fields of vision
    d. Loss of vision in the left eye
    e. Loss of vision in the right eye

13. A 69-year-old man presents with a right-sided facial weakness. He is unable to close the right eye. He also complains that noises seem particularly loud in his right ear (hyperacusis), and that he is unable to taste food properly. On examination there is loss of the corneal reflex in both eyes, and loss of taste over the anterior two-thirds of the tongue on the right. His inability to close the right eye is due to involvement of:
    a. Buccal branch of the trigeminal nerve
    b. Cervical branch of the facial nerve
    c. Glossopharyngeal nerve.
    d. Temporal branch of the facial nerve
    e. Zygomatic branch of the facial nerve

14. With reference to the patient above, hyperacusis is due to involvement of which of the following structures?
    a. Auditory nerve
    b. Chorda tympani nerve
    c. Lesser petrosal nerve
    d. Stapedius muscle
    e. Tensor tympani muscle

15. Which nerve conveys taste from the anterior two-thirds of the tongue?
    a. Buccal branch of the trigeminal nerve
    b. Chorda tympani
    c. Greater petrosal nerve
    d. Lesser petrosal nerve
    e. Mandibular branch of the facial nerve

16. Given this combination of symptoms and signs, where would a lesion of the facial nerve be located?
    a. Geniculate ganglion in the facial canal
    b. Internal auditory meatus
    c. Parotid gland
    d. Stylomastoid foramen
    e. Within the facial canal distal to the geniculate ganglion

17. An 18-year-old man presents to his GP with swollen lymph nodes in his neck. On examination the GP finds that the swollen nodes lie superficially in the posterior triangle of the neck. The man is referred to hospital for a biopsy of these nodes. Which nerve is at risk during this procedure?
    a. Accessory nerve
    b. Dorsal scapular nerve
    c. Long thoracic nerve
    d. Phrenic nerve
    e. Suprascapular nerve

18. A 45-year-old woman presents to her GP with a swelling in her neck. On examination the swelling is in the midline and moves upon swallowing and drinking a sip of water. The GP decides that the swelling is within the thyroid gland. Which of the following is true with regard to the thyroid gland?
    a. It lies posterior to the trachea and part of the larynx
    b. It is drained by two pairs of veins
    c. The superior and inferior thyroid arteries are both branches of the external carotid artery
    d. The inferior thyroid artery is closely associated with the recurrent laryngeal nerve
    e. Enlargement of the thyroid produces phrenic nerve palsy

19. A 20-year-old man sustains a fracture of the orbit after being involved in a fight. The area around his eye is swollen and there is loss of sensation over the ipsilateral cheek. Damage to which structure is responsible for this loss of sensation?
    a. Infraorbital nerve
    b. Lacrimal nerve
    c. Supraorbital nerve
    d. Supratrochlear nerve
    e. Zygomaticofacial nerve

20. The infraorbital nerve is a branch of which nerve?
   a. Facial nerve
   b. Mandibular division of the trigeminal nerve
   c. Maxillary division of the trigeminal nerve
   d. Oculomotor nerve
   e. Ophthalmic division of the trigeminal nerve

21. Fractures of the orbit can potentially damage structures within it. Which of the following is true with regard to the orbit?
   a. The long ciliary branch of the nasociliary nerve carries parasympathetic fibres
   b. The nasolacrimal duct empties into the middle meatus of the nasal cavity
   c. The parasympathetic fibres that supply the lacrimal gland synapse in the pterygopalatine ganglion
   d. The roof of the orbit is partially formed by the temporal bone
   e. The superior orbital fissure communicates with the pterygopalatine fossa

Extended matching questions (EMQs)

For each statement below, choose a single option from the list of answers.

1. The nervous system:

A. Central nervous system
B. Cranial nerves
C. Motor nerves
D. Parasympathetic nerves
E. Peripheral nervous system
F. Sacral nerves
G. Sensory nerves
H. Spinal nerves
I. Sympathetic nerves
J. Thoracic nerves

1. Nerves containing preganglionic fibres, which synapse in ganglia associated with organs
2. Nerves that innervate structures of the head and neck
3. Term that applies to the structures that comprise the brain and spinal cord
4. Nerves that have cell bodies in the anterior horn of the spinal cord
5. Nerves that arise from the thoracic and upper lumbar segments of the spinal cord only

2. The back:

A. Anterior longitudinal ligament
B. Atlas
C. Cervical vertebrae
D. Interspinous ligament
E. Ligamentum flavum
F. Lumbar vertebrae
G. Posterior longitudinal ligament
H. Sacrum
I. Supraspinous ligament
J. Thoracic vertebrae

1. Features foramina transversarii
2. Found between the lamina
3. Has fused vertebral bodies
4. Has circular vertebral foramina
5. Has kidney shaped vertebral bodies

3. Muscles of the upper limb:

A. Abductor pollicis brevis
B. Biceps brachii
C. Deltoid
D. Flexor carpi radialis
E. Flexor digitorum superficialis
F. Flexor pollicis longus
G. Opponens pollicis
H. Rhomboid major
I. Supraspinatus
J. Triceps

1. Abducts, flexes and medially rotates, extends, and laterally rotates arm
2. Extends the arm at the elbow
3. Flexes the arm at the elbow
4. Flexes the interphalangeal and metacarpophalangeal joints of the thumb
5. Flexes the proximal interphalangeal and metacarpophalangeal joints of the medial four digits

4. Osteology of the upper limbs:

A. Clavicle
B. Head of radius
C. Lunate
D. Medial epicondyle of humerus
E. Olecranon process of ulna
F. Scaphoid
G. Scapula
H. Spiral groove of humerus
I. Surgical neck of humerus
J. Ulna

1. A 70-year-old woman trips over her cat. On examination she is tender over the anatomical snuffbox region
2. A 20-year-old man falls down some steps. Subsequently he is unable to extend his wrist and fingers
3. Fracture of this structure can cause weakness in the interossei muscles, adductor pollicis, hypothenar eminence and anaesthesia (no sensation) in the medial one and a half digits

4. A 75-year-old woman suffering from osteoporosis falls while out walking. She complains of numbness over the lateral aspect of her arm and she is unable to abduct her arm at the glenohumeral joint

5. A small child almost trips on the edge of a pavement. His mother pulls him up sharply by the hand. Afterwards he complains of pain around the elbow and is holding his arm by his side

F. Gluteus medius
G. Peroneus tertius
H. Popliteus
I. Sartorius
J. Soleus

1. Inserts onto the head of the fibula
2. Unlocks the knee joint from full extension
3. Inserts into the iliotibial tract
4. Dorsiflexes the ankle
5. Plantarflexes the foot at the ankle

5. Nerve injuries affecting the upper limb:

A. Axillary nerve
B. Long thoracic nerve
C. Medial pectoral nerve
D. Median nerve
E. Musculocutaneous nerve
F. Radial nerve
G. Subscapular nerve
H. Suprascapular nerve
I. Thoracodorsal nerve

1. A 40-year-old man presents to A&E with a traumatic injury to his left arm. An X-ray reveals a midshaft fracture of the humerus. On examination, you find he cannot extend his wrist
2. A 45-year-old woman has a left sided mastectomy with removal of her left axillary lymph nodes. After the operation, she complains that she cannot wash or comb her hair with her left hand. Examination reveals winging of the left scapula
3. A 40-year-old woman presents with pain and loss of sensation in her lateral 3½ digits of her hand. She finds it difficult to perform fine movements requiring pinch grip
4. A 20-year-old man presents with a left shoulder dislocation after playing rugby. Afterwards he experiences a loss of sensation over the upper lateral aspect of his left arm.
5. A 25-year-old man is involved in a fight at a nightclub. He presents with a puncture wound to the anterior aspect of his right wrist. Examination reveals paraesthesia (numbness) in the lateral three and a half digits and weak abduction of the pollicis (thumb)

6. Muscles of the lower limb:

A. Biceps femoris
B. Flexor digitorum brevis
C. Flexor hallucis brevis
D. Gemellus inferior
E. Gluteus maximus

7. Nerve injuries affecting the lower limb:

A. Common peroneal nerve
B. Femoral nerve
C. Lateral cutaneous nerve of thigh
D. Lateral plantar nerve
E. Medial plantar nerve
F. Obturator nerve
G. Saphenous nerve
H. Sciatic nerve
I. Sural nerve
J. Tibial nerve

1. A 35-year-old woman is involved in a road traffic accident. Examination reveals that she is unable to dorsiflex her right foot (clinically known as foot drop). An X-ray demonstrates a fracture of the neck of the fibula
2. A 50-year-old man presents with back pain due to a herniated intervertebral disc. The pain radiates down the posterior aspect of the thigh and the lateral side of the leg
3. A 40-year-old woman undergoes surgery for varicose veins of the lower limb. Post operatively she complains of numbness over the medial aspect of the foot
4. A 75-year-old man sustains a pelvic fracture. Some weeks later he complains of numbness over his medial thigh
5. Following hip surgery involving an anterior approach, a 67-year-old man is aware of a reduction in sensation over his outer thigh

8. Osteology of the lower limbs:

A. Adductor tubercle
B. Greater trochanter of the femur
C. Head of fibula
D. Lateral condyle of femur

E. Linea aspera

F. Medial condyle of femur

G. Medial malleolus

H. Neck of femur

I. Patella

J. Shaft of femur

1. Its larger surface area allows rotation and locking of the knee joint during knee extension
2. A 90-year-old woman falls in her garden and fractures a bone in her lower limb. This results in shortening and lateral rotation of the affected limb
3. The insertion of the hamstring part of adductor magnus
4. A 15-year-old female gymnast falls dislocating her patella. Which structure normally contributes to the stability of the patella?
5. An 18-year-old man is kicked on the lateral aspect of his leg, inferior to the knee, whilst playing football. Subsequently he suffers from foot drop

9. Surface markings of the thorax:

A. Angle of Louis

B. Azygos vein

C. Brachiocephalic trunk

D. Brachiocephalic vein

E. Common carotid artery

F. Right atrium

G. Subclavian artery

H. Superior vena cava

I. Trachea (carina)

J. Ventricular apex

1. A structure that begins at the level of right first costal cartilage
2. The surface landmark used to determine the level of the second costal cartilage
3. A structure that joins the superior vena cava at the level of the right second costal cartilage
4. A structure found in the left fifth intercostal space
5. A structure that bifurcates at the level of the sternoclavicular joint

10. Anatomy of the heart:

A. Atrioventricular (coronary) groove

B. Atrioventricular node

C. Bundle of His

D. Chordae tendineae

E. Interventricular groove

F. Left atrium

G. Left atrioventricular bundle branch

H. Moderator band

I. Right atrium

J. Sinoatrial node

1. On an anteroposterior chest X-ray, this heart structure is adjacent to the middle lobe of the right lung
2. The location of the right coronary artery, part of the left coronary and its circumflex branch
3. The term that is used for the area of the heart that controls its inherent rhythmicity
4. The structure which conducts electrical activity in the interventricular septum and has three branches
5. The structure which attaches the papillary muscles to the cusps of the atrioventricular valve

11. The thorax:

A. Aorta

B. Azygos vein

C. Brachiocephalic trunk

D. Intercostal nerves

E. Oesophagus

F. Phrenic nerve

G. Recurrent laryngeal nerve

H. Thoracic duct

I. Trachea

J. Vagus nerve

1. Accompanies the inferior vena cava through the diaphragm
2. Accompanies the vagus nerves through the diaphragm
3. May be affected by tumours around the hilum of the lung
4. Provides sensory innervation to the periphery of the diaphragm
5. Lies on the surface of scalenus anterior muscle

12. Inguinal hernia:

A. Abdominal wall

B. Deep inguinal ring

C. Direct inguinal hernia

D. Indirect inguinal hernia

E. Inferior epigastric artery

F. Inguinal ligament

G. Inguinal triangle

H. Processus vaginalis

I. Spermatic cord

J. Superficial inguinal ring

1. An 80-year-old man presents to his GP with a swelling in his left groin which is reducible and has a cough impulse. The GP diagnoses an inguinal hernia. Given the patient's age, which type of inguinal hernia is this likely to be?
2. The structure which lies medial to the neck of an indirect inguinal hernia
3. The structure which an indirect inguinal hernia may pass through before entering the scrotum
4. The structure through which a direct inguinal hernia enters the inguinal canal
5. An indirect inguinal hernia always lies inside this structure

13. The gastrointestinal tract:

A. Azygos vein and brachiocephalic vein
B. Azygos vein and left gastric vein
C. Coeliac trunk
D. Cystic artery
E. Hepatic artery
F. Inferior mesenteric artery
G. Inferior thyroid artery
H. L1
I. Superior mesenteric artery
J. T12

1. Arterial supply to the upper third of the oesophagus
2. Arterial supply to the gallbladder
3. Level of origin of the coeliac trunk
4. Vessel giving rise to the pancreaticoduodenal artery
5. Vessels forming the portosystemic anastomosis at the lower end of the oesophagus

14. Anatomy of the pelvis:

A. 5th sacral nerve
B. Anteroposterior diameter
C. Bulbiospongiosus muscle
D. Motor nerves
E. Obturator internus muscle
F. Parasympathetic nerves
G. Piriformis muscle
H. Pudendal nerve
I. Sympathetic nerves
J. Transverse diameter

1. Forms part of the lateral wall of the pelvis
2. Nerves contracting the detrusor muscle of the bladder
3. Nerves responsible for ejaculation in males
4. Part of the innervation to levator ani muscle
5. The largest diameter of the pelvic inlet

15. Autonomic supply of abdomen and pelvis:

A. Coeliac plexus
B. Ganglion impar
C. Inferior hypogastric plexus
D. Parasympathetic
E. Pelvic splanchnic nerves
F. Superior hypogastric plexus
G. Sympathetic
H. Sympathetic trunks
I. Thoracic and lumbar splanchnic nerves
J. Vagal trunks

1. Type of innervation provided by greater splanchnic nerves
2. Autonomic plexus supplying the stomach with sympathetic innervation
3. Origin of parasympathetic innervation for the bladder
4. Origin of parasympathetic innervation for foregut structures
5. The structure formed in the pelvis by the hypogastric nerves

16. Foramina of the skull:

A. Foramen lacerum
B. Foramen magnum
C. Foramen ovale
D. Foramen rotundum
E. Foramen spinosum
F. Internal acoustic meatus
G. Jugular foramen
H. Optic canal
I. Optic nerve
J. Superior orbital fissure

1. The facial nerve exits the cranium through this foramen
2. The internal carotid artery passes through this foramen
3. The maxillary division of the trigeminal nerve passes through this foramen
4. The nasociliary nerve passes through this foramen
5. The middle meningeal artery passes through this foramen.

17. Nerve palsy and the eye:

A. Abducent nerve CNVI
B. Constricted pupil
C. Convergent squint

D. Dilated pupil

E. Divergent squint

F. Horner's syndrome

G. Oculomotor nerve CN III

H. Ptosis

I. Trigeminal nerve CN V

J. Trochlear nerve CN IV

1. The cranial nerve most vulnerable to damage due to its long intracranial course
2. A 65-year-old man presents with a ptosis and a dilated pupil. Which nerve is affected?
3. The sign other than ptosis that is observed in Horner's syndrome
4. A 20-year-old man with an infection of his left cavernous sinus presents with a convergent squint of his left eye. Which nerve is damaged?
5. As part of a cranial nerve examination you gently touch the surface of your patient's eyeball with a piece of cotton wool. This makes her blink. Which nerve provides general sensory innervation to the conjunctiva?

---

18. Intracranial haemorrhage:

A. Arachnoid

B. Cavernous sinus

C. Circle of Willis

D. Dural venous sinuses

E. Endocranium

F. Extradural haemorrhage

G. Subaponeurotic haematoma

H. Subarachnoid haemorrhage

I. Subarachnoid space

J. Subdural haemorrhage

1. A 30-year-old man is involved in a fight. He suffers rib fractures and a fracture of the pterion. A fracture of the pterion may lead to which injury?
2. Term used to describe bleeding into the CSF
3. A 50-year-old man who is a known alcoholic presents to A&E having fallen over and bumped his head. He undergoes a CT scan which shows he has sustained a subdural haemorrhage. This type of haemorrhage occurs between the dura and what layer?
4. Structure into which CSF drains
5. An 18-year-old man presents with pain around the eye and loss of vision. He has recently been treated for cellulitis (an infection of the skin) of his face. To which site has the infection spread (via the ophthalmic veins)?

19. Spinal meninges and lumbar puncture:

A. Arachnoid mater

B. Cauda equina

C. Conus medullaris

D. Dura mater

E. Extradural space

F. L2

G. L3

H. L4

I. Pia mater

J. Subarachnoid space

1. The lumbar cistern typically commences at the level of this vertebra in adults
2. A lumbar puncture needle is inserted directly above or below this vertebra
3. The lumbar cistern contains CSF and what structure?
4. Separates the dura from the vertebral periosteum and is a site for injection of anaesthesia?
5. Which is the last layer of the meninges to be penetrated when sampling CSF?

---

20. Cranial nerves:

A. Cranial nerve I

B. Cranial nerve II

C. Cranial nerve III

D. Cranial nerve IV

E. Cranial nerve V

F. Cranial nerve VI

G. Cranial nerve VII

H. Cranial nerve VIII

I. Cranial nerve IX

J. Cranial nerve X

1. Sensory supply to the conjunctiva
2. Motor supply to stylopharyngeus
3. Sensation of the skin of the forehead
4. Supplies inferior oblique muscle
5. Taste to anterior two-thirds of tongue

BOF answers

Chapter 1 Basic concepts of anatomy

1. d.
2. d.
3. b. Since the patient's history and symptoms are suggestive of spinal cord compression, MRI is the imaging modality of choice. It provides the best resolution of the spinal cord and spinal canal.
4. c.
5. d.
6. a.
7. e. Vertebrae and neck of femur – patients with osteoporosis are at increased risk of fractures in general. However, they are particularly at risk of radial, vertebral and neck of femur fractures.
8. a.

Chapter 2 The back

1. a.
2. e. The spinal cord ends at the L2 vertebra in adults.
3. c.
4. e.
5. a.
6. e.
7. c.
8. a.
9. a.

Chapter 3 The upper limb

1. b. Biceps brachii is innervated by C5/C6 nerve roots. After a stroke, reflexes are often hypoactive (reduced), becoming brisk (increased) at a later stage.
2. d. The median cubital vein in the cubital fossa is the most common site for venipuncture.
3. d.
4. a.
5. c.
6. e. Remember the mnemonic – Robert Taylor Drinks Cold Beer (roots, trunks, divisions, cords, branches).
7. d. The scaphoid lies within the anatomical snuffbox.
8. e.

9. b. This is the thinnest part of the clavicle, therefore is the region most likely to fracture.
10. a. The axillary nerve supplies deltoid and teres minor. Loss of innervation to these muscles can occur due to damage to the axillary nerve – resulting in failure of abduction of the arm to 90° and loss of sensation of the skin over deltoid.
11. d. The radial nerve lies in the spiral groove of the humerus. Radial nerve palsy can occur due to compression of the nerve in the spiral groove. This is often due to hanging the arm over the back of a chair (often when drunk – hence its alternative name – 'Saturday night palsy') resulting in loss of wrist and finger extension, with paraesthesia over the dorsum of the hand.
12. c. The median nerve is responsible. It is the only nerve which passes through the carpal tunnel at the wrist. Compression of the nerve in the carpal tunnel leads to pain and paraesthesia over the area supplied by the median nerve, i.e. the lateral 3½ digits of the hand.
13. b. Since he can flex his distal interphalangeal joints, the innervation of flexor digitorum profundus (via the ulnar and anterior interosseous nerves) is intact. Flexion of the proximal interphalangeal joints is brought about by the flexor superficialis muscle the tendons of which lie superficially on the fingers.
14. a.
15. a.
16. e. In people under the age of 20, recurrence of shoulder dislocation is greater than 80%.
17. d.
18. e.

Chapter 4 The thorax

1. c.
2. c.
3. a.
4. c. Horners syndrome results in partial ptosis, miosis and anyhydrosis, often accompanied by facial redness. This is due to loss of sympathetic innervation of the eyelid, pupil, and blood vessels of the face on the affected side.
5. e. Levator palpebrae superioris (LPS) along with the superior tarsal muscle (which is attached to LPS) both elevate the eyelid. LPS is innervated by the oculomotor nerve. The superior tarsal muscle is

innervated by sympathetic fibres from the superior cervical ganglion. A tumour at the apex of the lung may affect the cervical sympathetic chain, resulting in a partial ptosis (LPS is unaffected).

6. c.

7. c.

8. b. The long thoracic nerve innervates serratus anterior which apposes the scapula to the thoracic wall. Injury to the long thoracic nerve, therefore, leads to winging of the scapula.

9. d.

10. d.

11. d. Emergency decompression of a pneumothorax involves insertion of a needle into the 2nd intercostal space in the midclavicular line, on the affected side. A chest drain is inserted into the 5th intercostal space in the midaxillary line, on the affected side.

12. d.

13. a.

14. e.

15. c.

16. c.

17. e.

18. c.

Chapter 5 The abdomen

1. c. There are three points of narrowing, at which renal calculi are most likely to become lodged – the pelvi-ureteric junction, the point at which the ureter crosses the pelvic brim and the point at which the ureter enters the bladder.

2. a.

3. c.

4. c.

5. e.

6. d. The testes originate on the posterior abdominal wall, close to the kidney and descend into the scrotum during fetal development. Lymphatic drainage is, therefore, to the para aortic nodes in the abdomen and not to the inguinal nodes

7. a.

8. d.

9. a.

10. d.

11. c.

12. a.

13. d.

14. d.

15. b.

16. b. Rupture of an intra abdominal viscus will produce air under the diaphragm on an erect chest X-ray. This is because free air rises. The presence of a gastric air bubble below the diaphragm is a normal finding on the LEFT side of a chest X-ray.

17. e. The splenic artery passes posterior to the stomach. A gastric ulcer eroding the posterior stomach wall may erode into the splenic artery causing massive haemorrhage.

18. a. The ascending colon is formed from the fetal midgut. Pain from structures formed from the fetal midgut is felt around the umbilical region. b, c, d and e are part of the fetal foregut (therefore pain is felt in the epigastric region).

19. c.

20. e.

Chapter 6 The pelvis and perineum

1. b.

2. c.

3. e.

4. d.

5. a.

6. b.

7. b.

8. b.

9. a.

10. e.

11. b.

12. b.

13. c.

14. a.

15. b.

Chapter 7 The lower limb

1. d.

2. e.

3. e.

4. a.

5. a.

6. d.

7. a.

8. d.

9. b. Typical changes of osteoarthritis are loss of joint space, subchondral sclerosis, osteophytes and subchondral cysts. Rheumatoid arthritis is characterized by soft tissue swelling, initial joint space widening followed by joint space narrowing and erosion around the joint margins.

10. a. Damage to the common peroneal nerve may result in foot drop. The common peroneal nerve originates from the sciatic nerve in the thigh. It supplies the muscles of the lateral compartment of the leg and the dorsum of the foot, peroneus longus and brevis muscles. The deep peroneal nerve supplies tibialis anterior and extensor hallucis longus muscles, as well as extensor digitorum longus and peroneus tertius muscles. The nerve may be injured as a result of many causes including trauma, a tight plaster cast, injury during knee surgery and habitually crossing the legs. Individuals who spend long hours in a squatting position can also present with clinical evidence of peroneal nerve compression (strawberry picker's palsy). This is likely the result of compression of the common peroneal nerve as it penetrates the fibro-osseous opening in the peroneus longus muscle in persons with a fibrous or tight peroneal tunnel.

11. b.

12. b.

13. b.

14. a.

15. c.

16. c.

Chapter 8 The head and neck

1. b.

2. e. The pterion (the point at which the parietal, frontal, temporal and sphenoid bones meet) is the weakest part of the skull.

3. b. The pterion overlies the middle meningeal artery. The middle meningeal artery lies in the extradural space and so injury to this vessel leads to bleeding into space between the dura and the skull (the extradural space). An extradural haematoma has a crescentic appearance on CT scan.

4. e. The foramen spinosum transmits the middle meningeal artery (page 178).

5. c.

6. a.

7. a. Little's area is located on the anteroinferior part of the nasal septum. It is an area of anastomosis between the anterior ethmoidal artery, posterior ethmoidal artery, sphenopalatine artery, greater palatine artery, superior labial artery.

8. c.

9. d.

10. a. The superior oblique muscle is innervated by the trochlear nerve.

11. e.

12. c.

13. e.

14. d.

15. b.

16. e.

17. a.

18. d.

19. a.

20. c.

21. c

1. The nervous system:

1. D   Parasympathetic nerves. Arise from the cranial and sacral portions of the central nervous system.
2. B   Cranial nerves. There are 12 pairs of these nerves that supply the sense organs, muscles and skin of the head and neck.
3. A   Central nervous system. Consists of aggregated nerve cell bodies (nuclei) and fibres that run together in tracts.
4. C   Motor nerves. These innervate muscle cells via a synapse, which forms a motor end plate.
5. I   Sympathetic nerves. These fibres synapse in a sympathetic ganglion and then enter a spinal nerve or innervate an organ.

2. The back:

1. C   Cervical vertebrae contain foramina transversarii for passage of the vertebral arteries.
2. E   The ligamentum flavum unites adjacent laminae; plays a role in flexion and extension and preserves the curvatures of the vertebral column.
3. H   The sacrum consists of five fused vertebrae. It has anterior and posterior foramina for passage of the anterior and posterior rami of sacral spinal nerves. The median sacral crest represents the fused spinous processes of the sacral vertebrae.
4. J   The thoracic vertebral bodies have circular vertebral foramina. The cervical bodies above and the lumbar below have triangular vertebral bodies.
5. F   The lumbar vertebrae have kidney shaped vertebral bodies whilst the cervical vertebrae have small vertebral bodies and the thoracic vertebrae have heart shaped bodies.

3. Muscles of the upper limb:

1. C   Deltoid originates from the clavicle, acromion and spine of scapula. It inserts onto the deltoid tubercle of the humerus. It abducts, flexes and medially rotates, extends and laterally rotates the arm.
2. J   Triceps has three heads which originate from the infraglenoid tubercle of the scapula and the posterior surface of the humerus. All three heads insert onto the olecranon process of the ulna. It extends the elbow joint.
3. B   Biceps brachii flexes the elbow joint. It also supinates the flexed forarm and assists in flexion of the shoulder joint.
4. F   Flexor pollicis longis originates from the radius and the interosseus membrane. It inserts onto the distal phalynx of the thumb. It flexes the interphalangeal and MCP joints.
5. E   Flexor digitorum superficialis has two heads. It originates from the common flexor origin and the coronoid process of the ulna, and the anterior oblique line of the radius. It inserts onto the middle phalanges of the medial four digits.

4. Osteology of the upper limbs:

1. F   A scaphoid fracture commonly occurs due to a fall onto an outstretched hand. This causes hyper-extension of the wrist which places pressure on the scaphoid, resulting in fracture. The scaphoid lies within the anatomical snuffbox.
2. H   The radial nerve lies in the spiral groove of the humerus. Fractures may result in damage to the radial nerve which innervates the extensors of the wrist and fingers.
3. D   The ulnar nerve runs in a groove on the posterior aspect of the medial epicondyle of the humerus.
4. I   The axillary nerve lies in close contact with the surgical neck of the humerus. Fractures of the surgical neck may lead to damage to the nerve, which innervates deltoid (abduction of the arm) and a patch of skin over the lateral aspect of the arm.
5. B   In young children (under approximately 6 years of age) the head of the radius can sublux from the annular ligament due to the fact that at this age the radial head is spherical and is largely composed of cartilage.

5. Nerve injuries affecting the upper limb:

1. F   Radial nerve. It runs in the spiral (radial) groove of the humerus. Damage at this level causes loss of function in the forearm extensors. The triceps brachii muscle is unaffected as its branches arise more proximally.

2. B   Long thoracic nerve. Arises from the brachial plexus roots C5–C7. It crosses the lateral chest wall and supplies the serratus anterior muscle. This muscle rotates the scapula, allowing the arm to be raised above the head.

3. D   The symptoms described in this scenario represent the classic symptoms of carpal tunnel syndrome, where the median nerve is compressed in the carpal tunnel.

4. A   Axillary nerve. It has a branch (upper lateral cutaneous branch) that supplies the skin of the lateral aspect of arm over the deltoid.

5. D   Median nerve. This supplies the skin over the thenar eminence and the palmar surface of the lateral three and a half digits. Damage causes loss of sensation in this area as well as loss of abduction and opposition of thumb due to thenar eminence paralysis. Flexor pollicis longus still allows flexion.

6. Muscles of the lower limb:

1. A   Biceps femoris originates from the ischial tuberosity and inserts onto the head of fibula. It flexes the leg at knee joint and extends the thigh at the hip joint.

2. H   With the knee in full extension, the femur is medially rotated upon the fixed tibia. Popliteus laterally rotates the femur on the tibia, unlocking the knee joint.

3. E   Gluteus maximus originates from the ilium, sacrum, coccyx and sacrotuberous ligament. It inserts onto the iliotibial tract and gluteal tuberosity of femur. It extends and laterally rotates the thigh at the hip joint and extends the knee joint.

4. G   Peroneus tertius originates from the fibula and the interosseous membrane in the leg. It inserts onto the base of the 5th metatarsal bone. It dorsiflexes the ankle and everts the foot.

5. J   Soleus muscle originates from the tibia and fibula. It inserts onto the calcaneus. It plantarflexes the foot at the ankle along with plantaris and gastrocnemius muscles.

7. Nerve injuries affecting the lower limb:

1. A   Common peroneal nerve. It winds around the neck of the fibula and passes beneath the peroneus longus muscle to divide into superficial and deep branches supplying the lateral and anterior leg compartments respectively. Damage causes loss of foot dorsiflexors. To compensate, the patient develops a high-stepping gait to prevent the foot hitting the floor while the foot swings forward during walking.

2. H   The herniated intervertebral disc is compressing the nerve roots of L4 and L5. These are components of the sciatic nerve.

3. G   The saphenous nerve accompanies the great saphenous vein on the medial side of the leg. This may be damaged during surgery for varicose veins.

4. F   The obturator nerve supplies the skin of the medial thigh; it is closely related to the pelvic brim.

5. C   The lateral cutaneous of thigh is vulnerable to damage during hip surgery of this type. It supplies the skin over the lateral aspect of the thigh.

8. Osteology of the lower limbs:

1. F   During knee extension the anterior cruciate ligament (ACL) becomes taut, preventing the lateral condyle of the femur from extending further. The medial condyle has a larger surface area which allows extension to continue medially around the ACL.

2. H   Shortening and lateral rotation occurs in neck of femur fractures due to the pull of the muscles of the hip (abductors, flexors and external rotators) on the proximal fragment and the pull of the adductors on the distal fragment.

3. A   The adductor part of adductor magnus inserts onto the posterior surface of femur, while the hamstring part inserts onto the adductor tubercle of the femur.

4. D   The anterior prominence of the lateral condyle of the femur prevents dislocation of the patella.

5. C   The common peroneal nerve winds around the neck of the fibula. Trauma to this region may affect the innervation to the extensor muscles of the foot.

9. Surface markings of the thorax:

1. H   Superior vena cava – see Chapter 4.
2. A   Angle of Louis – see Chapter 4.
3. B   Azygos vein – see Chapter 4.
4. J   Ventricular apex (apex of heart) – see Chapter 4.
5. C   Brachiocephalic trunk – see Chapter 4.

10. Anatomy of the heart:

1. I   Blurring or loss of the right atrium border on X-ray suggests middle lobe pathology in the right lung, e.g. pneumonia.

2. A   Atrioventricular (coronary) groove. It is a superficial feature demarcating atria from ventricles.

3. J   Sinoatrial node. Its inherent rhythmicity causes the heart to beat 70 times a minute.

4. C Bundle of His. It conducts electrical impulses to the left side of the heart via an anterior and a posterior branch and to the right side of the heart via a single branch.

5. D Chordae tendineae. They are composed of collagen and hold the atrioventricular valves closed during ventricular contraction.

11. The thorax:

1. F the IVC and the right phrenic nerve pass through the diaphragm at the level of T8.

2. E The right and left vagus nerves pass through the diaphragm with the oesophagus at the level of T12.

3. G The recurrent laryngeal nerve may be compressed by tumours of the hilum of the lung producing hoarseness and a bovine cough.

4. D The intercostal nerves provide sensory innervation to the periphery of the diaphragm. The phrenic nerve provides sensory innervation to the central tendon as well as providing a motor supply.

5. F The phrenic nerves pass over the anterior surface of scalenus anterior as it passes through the neck.

12. Inguinal hernia:

1. C Indirect hernias are common in younger people, often due to a persistent processus vaginalis. Direct hernias tend to occur in older people due to weakening of the muscles of the abdominal wall.

2. E Or inside the inguinal triangle.

3. J Sometimes within a persistent processus vaginalis.

4. A An indirect inguinal hernia enters via the deep inguinal ring.

5. H It may lie within a persistent processus vaginalis.

13. The gastrointestinal tract:

1. G Arterial supply to the upper third of the oesophagus arises from the inferior thyroid artery, the middle third from the oesophageal branches of the aorta, the lower third from oesophageal branches of the left gastric artery.

2. D The cystic artery is a branch of the right hepatic artery.

3. J The coeliac trunk arises from the abdominal aorta at the level of T12. The SMA arises at the level of L1 (transpyloric plane). The IMA arises opposite the L3 vertebra.

4. I The SMA gives rise to the inferior pancreaticoduodenal, jejunal, ileal, ileocolic, right colic and middle colic arteries.

5. B There are several areas of portosystemic anastomoses. The anastomosis at the lower end of the oesophagus is formed by the oesophageal tributary of the left gastric vein, and the oesophageal tributaries of the azygos vein.

14. Anatomy of the pelvis:

1. E The side walls of the pelvis are formed by the hip bone and obturator internus muscle.

2. F Parasympathetic nerves contract the detrusor muscle and relax urethral sphincters. Sympathetic nerves relax the detrusor muscle and contract urethral sphincters.

3. I Sacral sympathetic trunk gives branches to the inferior hypogastric plexus. Its branches micturition, defaecation, erection, ejaculation and orgasm.

4. H Levator ani is supplied by the pudendal nerve and the 4th sacral nerve.

5. J The largest diameter of the pelvic inlet is the transverse diameter. The largest diameter of the pelvic outlet is the anteroposterior diameter.

15. Autonomic supply of abdomen and pelvis:

1. G They pierce the diaphragm to synapse in the coeliac ganglion.

2. A The sympathetic trunks do not give branches to abdominal viscera.

3. E If these nerves are impaired, continence problems and impotence can result.

4. J Distally the hindgut is supplied by pelvic splanchnic nerves.

5. C This then gives origin to several subsidiary plexuses, innervating pelvic viscera.

16. Foramina of the skull:

1. F Internal acoustic meatus – see page 178.
2. A Foramen lacerum – see page 178.
3. D Foramen rotundum – see page 178.
4. J Superior orbital fissure – see page 189.
5. E Foramen spinosum – see page 182.

17. Nerve palsy and the eye:

1. J The trochlear nerve originates from the dorsal aspect of the brainstem.

2. G The oculomotor nerve innervates levator palpabrae superioris (elevates the eyelid). It also carries

parasympathetic fibres, which constrict the pupil. Damage results in ptosis and a dilated pupil (loss of parasympathetic action).

3. B   Horners syndrome produces a ptosis, miosis and anhydrosis.
4. A   The abducens nerve passes through the cavernous sinus. Damage to this nerve affects the action of lateral rectus, and so medial rectus acts unopposed resulting in a convergent squint.
5. I   The trigeminal nerve has three divisions – it divides into ophthalmic, maxillary and manibular divisions. It provides sensory innervation to the cornea via the ophtalmic division of the 5th cranial nerve.

18. Intracranial haemorrhage:

1. F   The middle meningeal artery lies just behind this region of the skull and may be damaged in a fracture.
2. H   As the name implies, via bleeding into the subarachnoid space.
3. A   Blood fills the potential space between the two.
4. D   CSF drains into the dural venous sinuses.
5. B   This gives rise to a 'danger area of the face' centred on the nose.

19. Spinal meninges and lumbar puncture:

1. F   It commences at the level of L4 in children.
2. H   Level with the highest points of the iliac crests.
3. B   Composed of lumbar and sacral nerve roots.
4. E   It contains fat, connective tissue and the internal vertebral venous plexus.
5. A   CSF is taken from the subarachnoid space.

20. Cranial nerves:

1. E   – see Chapter 8.
2. I   – see Chapter 8.
3. E   – see Chapter 8.
4. C   – see Chapter 8.
5. E   – see Chapter 8.

A- Absence of; lacking, e.g. avascular – absence of a blood supply.

Abscess A localized collection of pus.

Afferent Carrying towards a given point. Afferent nerve impulses (i.e. sensory) are carried towards the brain and spinal cord.

Agonist A muscle that, when it contracts, causes a specific movement (prime mover), e.g. biceps brachii causes flexion of the elbow. Contraction of the agonist usually requires the relaxation of the antagonist. See antagonist.

Anaesthesia Loss of feeling due to nerve damage, resulting from disease or trauma.

Anastomosis Network of communicating arteries, veins or nerves (plural - anastomoses).

Aneurysm A dilatation of an arterial wall.

ANS The autonomic nervous system regulates bodily functions not under conscious control. It is divided into sympathetic and parasympathetic divisions.

Antagonist A muscle which has the opposite action of the agonist muscle. It returns limbs to their original position.

Antigen-presenting cell A cell which displays foreign material (antigen), to immune cells (lymphocytes). Antigen presenting cells may be macrophages, dendritic cells, or B-cells.

Apex Pointed end of a cone-shaped structure, e.g. apex of the axilla.

Aponeurosis Strong, flattened tendon with a wide area of attachment, e.g. external oblique aponeurosis.

Appendicular Relating to the appendages (the limbs) e.g. appendicular skeleton.

Arteriogram Digital image or film produced as a result of arteriography.

Arteriography The use of contrast medium and X-rays, to visualize the lumina of arteries, or of the chambers of the heart.

Arthro- Relates to joints, e.g. arthrodesis, arthritis, arthroscope.

Atherosclerosis Disease involving the endothelium, tunica intima and tunica media of arteries. It is characterized by build-up of lipids and cholesterol within the walls of arteries, resulting in obstruction of the lumen with decreased blood flow and hence oxygen, to organs.

Atrophy Wasting of a tissue or organ due to cell loss e.g muscle atrophy after prolonged bedrest.

Axial Relating to the axis of the body, as in axial skeleton, which consists of the skull, vertebral column and thoracic cage.

Axilla Region where the upper limb joins the trunk (commonly known as the armpit).

Axon A neuron consists of a nerve cell body, and an axon which conducts impulses away from the cell body.

Barium sulfate An insoluble compound which is used as a contrast medium in imaging of the gastrointestinal tract.

Bifurcation The point at which an anatomical structure, e.g. trachea, divides into two parts, i.e. primary bronchi.

Bipennate Usually a term which describes the structure of a muscle. A bipennate muscle is one in which the tendon lies in the centre of the muscle and the muscle fibres pass to it from either side (e.g. rectus femoris). See unipennate and multipennate.

Brachial Relates to the arm (between the shoulder and elbow) – hence brachial artery.

Branchial At the cranial end of the embryonic digestive system there are a series of branchial arches (primitive gill arches) which give rise to specific structures of the head and neck.

Bronchiole A microscopic branch of the bronchi.

Bronchus First branches of the trachea (plural – bronchi, adjective – bronchial).

Buccal Relating to the mouth.

Bursa Small sac lined by synovial membrane which ensures free movement of tendons close to joints, e.g. infrapatellar bursa.

Bursitis Inflammation of a bursa.

Canal A tubular passage, e.g. adductor canal of the thigh.

Cancer A malignant tumour, arising as a result of abnormal and uncontrolled cell division which may spread to other tissues.

Carcinoma Cancer of epithelial origin.

Cardia Heart (adjective — cardiac).

Cerebellum Part of the brain which controls co-ordinated movement, balance and muscle tone (adjective – cerebellar).

Cerebrum Largest part of the brain composed of the two cerebral hemispheres (adjective – cerebral).

Cerebrospinal fluid Fluid surrounding the central nervous system and filling the ventricles of the brain.

Cerebrovascular accident (CVA) – see stroke.

Cervix Literally means 'the neck'. Also used to refer to the narrow part or 'neck' of an organ. In anatomy 'cervix' usually refers to the neck of the uterus (adjective – cervical).

Chondro- Relates to cartilage, e.g. chondrocytes – cartilage cells.

Coeliac disease An autoimmune disease which occurs due to sensitivity to gliadin protein, resulting in production of antigliadin antibodies. It is characterized by crypt cell hyperplasia and loss of intestinal villi.

Collateral Accessory or secondary, e.g. collateral circulation is an accessory route of blood flow to an organ.

Condyle Literally means 'knuckle'. A rounded articular surface, e.g. femoral condyles.

Connective tissue A tissue composed of cells, fibres and extracellular matrix which supports and separates more specialized tissues and organs.

Contrast studies A procedure involving the use of contrast medium, allowing improved visualization of structures on plain X-rays, CT or MRI scans.

Coronary Encircling like a crown, e.g. coronary arteries, arteries which encircle and supply the heart.

Cortex Outer part of a structure, e.g. cortex of the kidney (adjective – cortical); see also medulla.

Costa Literally means 'rib' (adjective - costal), e.g. intercostal muscles lie between the ribs.

Cranial nerves 12 pairs of nerves which emerge from the brain (the majority from the brainstem) – unlike spinal nerves which emerge from the spinal cord.

Cranium The section of the skull containing the brain.

Crohn's disease An autoimmune disease of the gastrointestinal tract characterized by inflammation and ulceration, usually affecting the bowel wall (but it may affect any part of the gastrointestinal tract from mouth to anus). It is one of the inflammatory bowel diseases (IBD) – the other major IBD is ulcerative colitis.

Cruciate Structures arranged like a cross, e.g. the cruciate ligaments.

Cusp Leaflet of a heart valve. Hence bicuspid valve means a valve comprising two leaflets.

Cutaneous Relating to the skin.

Cystic fibrosis An inherited disease (autosomal recessive) which is characterized by production of thick mucus mainly in the lungs, pancreas and gastrointestinal tract.

Deep vein thrombosis (DVT) The formation of a venous blood clot usually in the lower limbs, most commonly in the calf.

Dendrite A short branch of the neuron cell body which forms synapses with other neurons.

Dental Related to teeth (the dens is a tooth-shaped structure).

Depolarization A change in the membrane potential of a cell usually resulting in an action potential.

Dermatome An area of skin supplied by a single spinal segment.

Diastole Relaxation phase of the cardiac cycle (adjective – diastolic).

Discharge The release of fluid or pus from its site of production, e.g. an infected wound.

Dislocate Joint displacement where the contact between the articular surface of bones is lost.

Dural venous sinuses Venous spaces lying between the endosteal and meningeal layers of the dura, within the cranium, e.g. superior sagittal sinus.

Dyspnoea Difficulty in breathing.

Electrocardiogram (ECG) Records the electrical activity of the heart.

Efferent Carrying away from. Efferent (i.e. motor) nerve impulses are carried away from the central nervous system.

Endo- Within or inner part of a structure, e.g. endocardium – the innermost layer of the heart.

Epi- Above or on the surface of a structure, e.g. epidermis – outermost layer of the skin.

Epithelium One of the four basic tissue types. It forms glands, covers all surfaces and lines the body cavities (adjective – epithelial).

Erythema Reddening of the skin due to dilatation of dermal capillaries.

Eversion Turning the sole of the foot outwards (laterally).

ex- extra- Out, e.g. expiration – to breathe out, extracapsular – outside a joint capsule.

Facet A flat articular surface of a bone, e.g. facet joints of the vertebra.

Fissure A groove or cleft, e.g. the oblique fissure of the left lung separates upper and lower lobes.

Foramen Opening or passage through a bone, e.g. foramen magnum through which the spinal cord passes (plural – foramina).

Fossa Literally means 'a ditch', therefore a depression, hollow or pit (antecubital fossa of the elbow).

Fracture A break in the continuity of a bone.

Fundus Base of a hollow organ, or the part furthest from the opening (stomach, uterus).

Ganglion A swelling. In the nervous system, it is a collection of nerve cell bodies outside the CNS, e.g. a sensory ganglion (without synapses), or an autonomic ganglion (with synapses). See nucleus.

Gastro- Relates to the stomach, e.g. gastric artery, gastrointestinal (GI) tract, gastroscopy.

Genicular Relates to the knee joint, e.g. genicular arteries which supply the knee.

Glosso- Relates to the tongue. The hypoglossal nerve lies below the tongue.

Glottis Gap between the vocal folds (adjective – glottal).

Gonads Sex organs – ovaries and testes (adjective – gonadal).

Greater sac General peritoneal cavity.

Gyrus Raised area of the cerebral cortex (pleural – gyri). See sulcus.

Haemo- Relates to blood, e.g. haematology is the study of blood, haematoma (bruising) is the swelling caused by bleeding into the tissues.

Haemoptysis Coughing up blood, commonly a sign of infection or malignancy.

Hemi- Denotes one half of the body or a structure, e.g. hemi-diaphragm, hemiplegia.

Hepato- Relates to the liver, e.g. hepatic artery, hepatitis – inflammation of the liver.

Hernia Protrusion of an organ or tissue through the wall of a cavity which normally encloses it, e.g. femoral and inguinal hernias.

Hiatus An opening, e.g. adductor hiatus of adductor canal.

Hilum Place where vessels and nerves enter or leave an organ, e.g. hilum of the lung (plural – hila, adjective - hilar).

Hyper- Literally 'above', or 'excessive', e.g. hyperextension – forced extension of a joint beyond normal limits, hypertrophy – increase in size.

Hypo- Literally 'below' or 'depressed', e.g. hypochondrium – below the costal cartilages, hypoglossal – below the tongue.

Ilium Part of the hip bone, along with the pubis and ischium (adjective – iliac).

Infra- Below or lower, e.g. infraorbital, below the orbit of the skull, infrahyoid below the hyoid bone.

Infundibulum A funnel-shaped passage.

Inguinal Relates to the groin where the lower limb meets the trunk, e.g. inguinal hernia, inguinal ligament.

Insertion Relates to the more distal attachment of a muscle, which moves on contraction of the muscle.

Inter- Between, e.g. interosseous membrane lies between the bones, intercostal between the ribs.

Intra- Inside, e.g. an intracapsular tendon lies inside the capsule of the joint (see extra-).

Intraperitoneal A viscus suspended from the posterior abdominal wall by a mesentery, e.g. the ileum and jejunum.

Intervertebral discs Secondary cartilaginous joints between the vertebrae.

Ischaemia Reduction of blood flow to a tissue or organ, often resulting in damage to the tissue or organ.

Isthmus Narrow region connecting two parts, e.g. isthmus of the thyroid gland.

-itis Inflammation, e.g. gastritis – inflammation of the stomach, arthritis – inflammation of joints.

Labium Lip (pleural – labia, adjective – labial).

Labrum Lip or a lip-like structure, e.g. glenoid labrum of the glenoid fossa of the shoulder joint.

Larynx The part of the airway, between the pharynx and trachea containing the vocal cords (adjective – laryngeal).

Lesser sac Diverticulum of peritoneum posterior to the stomach.

Ligament Tough connective tissue bands which conenct two or more structures, most commonly bones (adjective – ligamentous).

Lingula Tongue (adjective – lingual).

Loculus A small, enclosed cavity or space (plural – loculi, adjective – loculated).

Lumen Central cavity of a tube, e.g. artery, vein, intestine, etc. (adjective – luminal).

Macro- Indicates the large size of a structure (macroscopic – visible with the naked eye).

Mast- Relating to the breast, e.g. mastectomy – removal of the breast, mastitis – inflammation of the breast.

Mediastinum The space within the thorax, between the two pleural cavities.

Medulla Inner part of a solid organ (adjective – medullary), e.g. medulla of the kidney. See cortex.

Mesentery Double layer of peritoneum attaching viscera to the posterior abdominal wall (adjective – mesenteric).

Metastasis The spread of a malignant tumour to distant sites, e.g. breast carcinoma to axillary lymph nodes.

Mitral Describes the valve between the left atrium and left ventricle (also known as the atrioventricular valve).

Motor Relates to structures or activities involving transmission of nerve impulses away from the CNS. See efferent.

Motor endplate The enlarged end of a motor neuron which forms a synapse with part of the muscle membrane.

MRC Medical Research Council.

Mucus A thick glycoprotein secretion produced by glands (adjective – mucous).

Multipennate A term which describes the structure of a muscle. A multipennate muscle may be arranged as a series of bipennate muscles lying alongside one another (e.g. the acromial fibres of the deltoid) or may have the tendon lying within its centre and the muscle fibres passing to it from all sides, converging as they go (e.g. tibialis anterior).

Myo- Relating to muscle, e.g. myocardium – muscle of the heart, myometrium – uterine muscle, myalgia – muscle pain.

Necrosis Death of a tissue, e.g. cardiac muscle, resulting from a myocardial infarction.

Nerve A term that may be used rather loosely. Strictly it should refer to a large collection of nerve fibres that can be seen with the naked eye, e.g. the ulnar nerve. However, it may be used when referring to a single neuron, or its axon.

Neuro- Relates to nerves, e.g. neurology – study of the nervous system.

NMJ Neuromuscular junction is the synapse between a neuron and the muscle cell membrane.

Noxious Harmful, e.g. a substance that causes damage to cells.

Nucleus In terms of the CNS, a nucleus describes a collection of nerve cell bodies which share a similar function. See ganglion.

-oma Denotes a tumour, e.g. lymphoma (of the lymph nodes), carcinoma (of an epithelium), melanoma (of the skin).

Omental bursa See lesser sac.

Omentum Folds of peritoneum linking the stomach to other viscera, e.g. lesser omentum connects the stomach to the liver.

Orifice An opening to a cavity.

Oss-, Osteo- Relates to bones, e.g. ossification – process of bone formation, osteoporosis – abnormal loss of bone density.

-ostomy Making a permanent opening, e.g. colostomy – opening of the colon onto the surface of the abdomen, ileostomy – opening of the ileum onto the surface of the abdomen.

-otomy Making a small, temporary opening, e.g. laparotomy, emergency opening of the abdomen.

Palpebral Relates to the eyelids (palpebrae), e.g. the muscle which lifts the eyelids is levator palpebrae superioris.

Papilloedema Swelling of the optic disc, seen on fundoscopy. Often a sign of raised intracranial pressure.

Para- By the side of, e.g. paravertebral muscles, alongside the vertebral column, para-aortic, beside the aorta, paranasal air sinuses.

Paraesthesia Abnormal sensation in the distribution of a peripheral nerve, e.g. pins and needles along the medial border of the forearm and medial one-and-a-half digits in ulnar nerve damage.

Paralysis Loss of muscle function.

Parietal Relates to the surface of the inner walls of a body cavity, e.g. parietal pleura. Also relates to the parietal bone of the skull.

Pectoral (adj) Relating to the chest.

Perforation The formation of a hole in an organ or tissue, usually through a disease process.

Peri- Around or near, e.g. periosteum - membrane covering the surface of bone, pericardium – sac surrounding the heart.

Perineum The region between the anus and external genitalia, inferior to the pelvic diaphragm and bounded by the pelvic outlet.

Peristalsis Motion by which intestinal contents are moved through the alimentary tract.

Peritoneum Membrane lining the abdominal cavity.

Phrenic Relating to the diaphragm.

Pia Innermost, vascular layer of the meninges.

Pleura The epithelial covering of the lungs.

Plexus Network, e.g. brachial plexus is the network of nerves that supply the upper limb.

Pneumothorax A condition in which there is air within the pleural cavity around the lungs.

Portal system Venous system carrying blood through a second capillary bed before returning blood to the heart, e.g. hepatic portal vein delivers blood from the GI tract to the capillaries of the liver before it is returned to the right atrium via the hepatic vein and the inferior vena cava.

Post- After or following, e.g. postganglionic describes a neuron that leaves a ganglion and terminates in an effector (muscle or gland).

Pre- Preceding or before, e.g. preganglionic describes a neuron that leaves the spinal cord and terminates in a ganglion.

Process A thin prominence or protuberance, e.g. spinous process of vertebrae.

Prominence A projection of bone.

Prone Lying face down.

Proprioception Ability to sense the position of the body in space. Proprioceptors are present in muscles and tendons and register mechanical changes in position.

Protuberance A rounded projection of bone.

Ptosis Drooping of the eyelid. Complete ptosis is due to damage to levator palpebrae superioris muscle or its nerve supply (oculomotor nerve). Partial ptosis is due to damage to the superior tarsal muscle or nerve supply (sympathetic fibres).

Pulmonary circulation Vessels which carry blood from the right side of the heart to the alveolar capillaries of the lungs and back to the left side of the heart. In the process, gaseous exchange occurs with oxygen entering the blood and carbon dioxide leaving it.

Radiolucent A structure that does not absorb X-rays and appears dark on an X-ray film.

Radiopaque A structure which absorbs X-rays and appears white on an X-ray film.

Raphe Literally 'a seam'. A line of union between two muscles such as is found in the pharyngeal constrictors.

Recess A depression or hollow cavity of an organ.

Reflex An unconscious, autonomic and involuntary action, e.g. muscle contraction through a neuronal circuit.

Regurgitation The backflow of a liquid against its normal direction, e.g. blood flows from the left ventricle to left atrium through a defective mitral valve.

Renal Relating to the kidneys, e.g. renal artery.

Retinaculum A thickened connective tissue band holding other tissues in position, e.g. extensor tendons held by the extensor retinaculum in the forearm.

Retro- At the back or behind a structure, e.g. retroperitoneal.

Retroperitoneal A viscus lying against the posterior abdominal wall and covered by peritoneum on its anterior surface only, e.g. pancreas, kidneys, etc.

Sarcoma Cancer of connective tissue origin.

Sclerosis Hardening of a tissue.

Sensory Relates to structures or activities which involve transmitting nerve impulses towards the CNS from the periphery. See afferent.

Septum A partition which divides an anatomical structure, e.g. interventricular septum – between the ventricles.

Serous Thin, watery secretions, secreted by a serous membrane like the pleura. See mucus.

Sesamoid An oval or round shaped bone within a tendon that slides over another bone, e.g. the patella within the patellar tendon which slides over the patellar surface of the femur.

Sheath A connective tissue envelope that surrounding anatomical structures, e.g. nerve, muscle or tendon.

Sinus Cavity or channel; has many meanings, e.g. paranasal sinus, hepatic sinus, dural venous sinus.

Somatic Relating to the structures which make up the body wall, or its primitive divisions, known as somites.

Sphincter Muscular valve which controls the diameter of a tube, e.g. the pyloric sphincter lies between the stomach and duodenum.

Sphygmomanometer The instrument used to measure arterial blood pressure.

Splanchnic Equivalent to visceral – splanchnic is derived from Greek, visceral from Latin.

Squamous Flattened, scale-like cells, e.g. squamous epithelium consists of very flattened cells.

Stroke Sudden onset of weakness due to interruption of blood flow to the brain.

Sub- Below or underlying, e.g. subcostal - below the ribs.

Sulcus Gutter or depression, particularly used in relation to the surface of the cerebrum where sulci lie between the gyri, e.g. central sulcus of the cerebral cortex (plural – sulci).

Supine Lying on the back, face up.

Supra- Above, e.g. supraorbital nerve, suprarenal gland.

Synapse Junction between two neurons or between a nerve and an effector e.g. a muscle.

Synovial Synovial means 'like an egg'. Describes joints which are freely movable. Synovial fluid secreted by synovial membrane has the consistency of egg white and lubricates and nourishes the joint surfaces.

Systemic circulation Vessels carrying blood from the left side of the heart, to the capillary beds of the entire body (except the lungs), and returning blood to the right side of the heart. In the process gaseous exchange occurs with oxygen leaving the blood to enter the tissues, and carbon dioxide exiting the tissues and entering the blood.

Systole Contraction phase of the cardiac cycle (adjective – systolic). See diastole.

Tachycardia An increased heart rate.

Tachypnoea An increased respiratory rate.

Tamponade An abnormal pressure on a part of the body, e.g. the presence of fluid within the pericardial cavity, compressing the heart.

Tendon The tough extension of the connective tissue associated with muscles, which forms the attachment of muscle to bone.

Thermoregulation Regulation of body temperature through shivering or peripheral capillary dilatation and sweating.

Thoraco- Relating to the thorax.

Thrombus A blood clot.

Tissue A collection of similar cells which perform specialized functions. There are four basic tissue types: epithelia, muscle, nerve and connective tissues.

Transverse A plane dividing a structure into superior and inferior parts.

Tubercle A small rounded bony protuberance, e.g. lesser tubercle of the humerus.

Tuberosity A large rounded bony protuberance, e.g. the greater tuberosity of the femur.

Tunica A layer of an anatomical structure, e.g. tunica media – the smooth muscle layer of an artery.

Umbilicus Abdominal site of attachment of the umbilical cord.

Unipennate Relates usually to muscle. Describes a muscle in which the tendon lies along one side of the muscle, and the muscle fibres pass obliquely to it. See bipennate and multipennate.

Ureter Muscular tube which carries urine between the kidney and bladder.

Urethra Muscular tube which carries urine from the bladder to the exterior.

Varicose Enlarged and twisted superficial veins, especially in the lower limb.

Vaso- Relating to vessels, e.g. vasoconstriction - physiological narrowing of blood vessels (plural - vasa).

Venae comitantes Veins which closely accompany arteries, e.g. the deep veins of the limbs.

Venepuncture The puncture of a vein to obtain a sample of blood or administer medication, e.g. antibiotics.

Ventricle Chamber, e.g. chambers of the heart. There are also four ventricles in the brain.

Vinculae A band of synovial tissue, connecting the flexor tendons to the phalanges.

Visceral Relates to internal organs. Visceral nerves tend to be under involuntary control, and sensation tends to be vague, imprecisely perceptible or even imperceptible. See somatic.

Viscus Internal organ, e.g. heart, spleen, etc. (plural – viscera).

Index